New Insights into DNA Damage and Repair

New Insights into DNA Damage and Repair

Editor: Albert Douglas

MURPHY & MOORE
www.murphy-moorepublishing.com

www.murphy-moorepublishing.com

MURPHY & MOORE

Cataloging-in-Publication Data

New insights into DNA damage and repair / edited by Albert Douglas.
p. cm.
Includes bibliographical references and index.
ISBN 978-1-63987-392-0
1. DNA damage. 2. DNA repair. 3. Mutation (Biology). 4. Biochemical genetics. I. Douglas, Albert.
QH465.A1 N49 2022
616.042--dc23

Murphy & Moore Publishing,
1 Rockefeller Plaza,
New York City, NY 10020, USA

ISBN 978-1-63987-392-0 (Hardback)

Contents

Preface VII

Chapter 1 **Application of Host Cell Reactivation in Evaluating the Effects of Anticancer Drugs and Environmental Toxicants on Cellular DNA Repair Activity in Head and Neck Cancer** 1
Yi-Shan Tsai, Jau-Ling Huang and Chang-Shen Lin

Chapter 2 **The Nuclear Compartmentation of Glutathione: Effect on Cell Cycle Progression** 19
Jelena Markovic, Nancy Mora, Amparo Gimeno, Consuelo Burguete, José Luis García-Gimenez and Federico V. Pallardó

Chapter 3 **DNA Repair in Pathogenic Eukaryotic Cells: Insights from Comparative Genomics of Parasitic Protozoan** 41
Laurence A. Marchat, Mavil López-Casamichana, Esther Orozco and César López-Camarillo

Chapter 4 **Role for PKCδ on Apoptosis in the DNA Damage Response** 61
Kiyotsugu Yoshida

Chapter 5 **The Influence of Individual Genome Sensitivity in DNA Damage Repair Assessment in Chronic Professional Exposure to Low Doses of Ionizing Radiation** 73
Mirta Milić, Ružica Rozgaj, Vilena Kašuba, Ana Marija Jazbec, Patrizia Hrelia and Sabrina Angelini

Chapter 6 **New Players in Recognition of Intact and Cleaved AP Sites: Implication in DNA Repair in Mammalian Cells** 101
Svetlana Khodyreva and Olga Lavrik

Chapter 7 **DNA Radiosensitization: The Search for Repair Refractive Lesions Including Double Strand Breaks and Interstrand Crosslinks** 127
Tsvetan G. Gantchev, Marie-Eve Dextraze and Darel J. Hunting

Chapter 8 **DNA Damage Protection and Induction of Repair by Dietary Phytochemicals and Cancer Prevention** 147
Alice A. Ramos, Cristóvão F. Lima and Cristina Pereira-Wilson

Chapter 9 **SiDNA and Other Tools for the Indirect Induction of DNA Damage Responses** 181
Maria Quanz, Amélie Croset and Marie Dutreix

Chapter 10 **Mechanisms of Mutagenic DNA Nucleobase Damages and their Chemical and Enzymatic Repairs Investigated by Quantum Chemical Methods** 217
Eric A. C. Bushnell, Jorge Llano, Leif A. Eriksson and James W. Gauld

Permissions

List of Contributors

Index

Preface

In my initial years as a student, I used to run to the library at every possible instance to grab a book and learn something new. Books were my primary source of knowledge and I would not have come such a long way without all that I learnt from them. Thus, when I was approached to edit this book; I became understandably nostalgic. It was an absolute honor to be considered worthy of guiding the current generation as well as those to come. I put all my knowledge and hard work into making this book most beneficial for its readers.

DNA damage refers to an abnormal chemical structure in DNA. It hinders the proper working of the replication mechanism and causes alterations in the structure of the genetic material. The group of processes through which the identification and correction of damage to the DNA takes place within a cell is called DNA repair. DNA damage can be caused due to various factors, both environmental and metabolic. This leads to a large number of molecular lesions in the cells. These lesions may trigger structural damage to the DNA. The pace at which the DNA is repaired depends on various factors such as the type and age of the cell, and the extracellular environment. This book discusses the fundamentals as well as modern approaches of DNA damage and repair. It will also provide interesting topics for research which interested readers can take up. Those in search of information to further their knowledge will be greatly assisted by this book.

I wish to thank my publisher for supporting me at every step. I would also like to thank all the authors who have contributed their researches in this book. I hope this book will be a valuable contribution to the progress of the field.

Editor

1

Application of Host Cell Reactivation in Evaluating the Effects of Anticancer Drugs and Environmental Toxicants on Cellular DNA Repair Activity in Head and Neck Cancer

Yi-Shan Tsai[1], Jau-Ling Huang[2] and Chang-Shen Lin[3]

[1]*Center of Excellence for Environmental Medicine, Kaohsiung Medical University, Kaohsiung*

[2]*Department of Bioscience Technology, Chang Jung Christian University, Tainan*

[3]*Graduate Institute of Medicine, Kaohsiung Medical University, Kaohsiung Taiwan*

1. Introduction

DNA repair pathways are targets of numerous anticancer drugs including natural and chemical compounds, which direct cancer cells toward apoptosis. However, different types of cancer cells consist of various alterations in DNA repair genes that make cancer cells become drug-resistant and lead to treatment failure and disease recurrence. On the contrary, cancer cells may also possess defects in certain DNA repair pathway that make them are susceptible to certain compounds, which inhibit another DNA repair pathway inside the cancer cells. As a result, these compounds selectively kill the cancer cells and are less harmful to the normal ones. Understanding the effects of anticancer drugs on DNA repair as well as the DNA repair activity of cancer cells themselves are important for improvement of anticancer treatment. Similarly, this information is helpful for elucidation of the carcinogenicity of environmental toxicants. This chapter introduces the crosstalk between anticancer drugs, environmental toxicants and DNA repair pathways in head and neck cancer. In addition, the application of an easy, fast and measurable *in vivo* functional assay for nucleotide excision repair (NER) and DNA repair via homologous recombination (HR) and non-homologous end-joining (NHEJ) pathways is shown to examine the cellular DNA repair activity responding to anticancer drugs or environmental toxicants. By which the functional roles of DNA repair genes in response to anticancer treatments and genotoxic substances could be evolved in head and neck cancer cells.

2. Roles of DNA repair genes/pathways in cancer development and treatment

DNA repair genes play a pivotal role in the maintenance of genome integrity. Defects or dysregulation of DNA repair genes can result in genomic instability (GIN), which is a common feature of cancer cells (Hanahan & Weinberg, 2000). To prevent this, human cells evolve several

DNA repair pathways that may interplay each other to repair various types of DNA damages. These DNA repair mechanisms include pathways of base excision repair (BER), nucleotide excision repair (NER), mismatch repair (MMR), double strand break (DSB) repair through homologous recombination (HR) or non-homologous end-joining (NHEJ) and direct repair of DNA lesions such as O^6-methylguanine by O^6-methylguanine-DNA methyltransferase (Sancar et al., 2004). Collectively, there are hundreds of DNA repair genes involved in various DNA repair pathways that include processes of sense and recognition of DNA lesions, amplification and transmission of the damage signal, recruitment of repair proteins to the damage sites, and execution of DNA repair (Sancar et al., 2004; Wood et al., 2005).

2.1 DNA repair genes/signaling in HR and NER pathways

Upon DNA damaged, histone H2AX, a histone H2A variant, is quickly phosphorylated (denoted as γ-H2AX) in an ataxia telangiectasia mutated (*ATM*)-dependent manner (Uziel et al., 2003). The phosphorylated H2AX serves as an important marker for DNA damages. Some genes are also involved in the recognition of DNA damages. They are members of MRN complex (*Mre11A, RAD50, NBN*) for DSB and damage-specific DNA binding protein 1 and 2 (*DDB1* and *DDB2*), Xeroderma pigmentosum (XP) complementation group C (*XPC*) for UV-induced damages and bulky DNA adducts, which are produced by DNA-damaging chemotherapeutic drugs and can be repaired through NER pathway. In addition to H2AX, ATM also phosphorylates p53, BRCA1, CHEK1/2 and results in activation of various DNA repair pathways as well as induction of cell cycle arrest (Sancar et al., 2004). Generally, the genes involved in HR repair include *BRCA1, BRCA2*, members of *RAD51* and Fanconi anemia (FA) families, as well as the Bloom syndrome, RecQ helicase-like (*BLM*) and Werner syndrome, RecQ helicase-like (*WRN*). The genes in NER pathway consists of XP complementation group A to G (*XPA* to *XPG*), XP complementation group variant (*XPV*), excision repair cross-complementing rodent repair deficiency, complementation group 1 (*ERCC1*), replication protein A (*RPA*), and so on (Sancar et al., 2004; Wood et al., 2005).

ATM is the key gene for initiating DNA repair signaling. Its downstream targets, both *TP53* and *BRCA1* are capable of regulating multiple DNA repair pathways (Deng, 2006; Helton & Chen, 2007). *BRCA1* encodes a multifunctional protein that maintains genome integrity through regulating gene transcription, cell cycle checkpoints, DNA repair (Deng, 2006; Yoshida & Miki, 2004), and centrosome duplication (Deng, 2002; Xu et al., 1999). In addition to the role in HR, BRCA1 is involved in NER through transactivating the expression of *DDB2* and *XPC* (Hartman & Ford, 2002; Takimoto et al., 2002), both of them can also be transactivated by p53 (Adimoolam & Ford, 2002; Hwang et al., 1999). Thus, both *BRCA1* and *TP53* can regulate NER pathway. RAD51 is the human homolog of bacteria *recA* and forms a complex with BRCA1 and BRCA2. This interaction is important for proper regulation of RAD51 activity inside a cell. Loss of the binding between RAD51 and BRCA complex may be a key event leading to GIN and tumorigenesis (Martin et al., 2007). RAD51 contributes the key step of HR by mediating homologous pairing and strand exchange between two homologous DNA (Richardson, 2005). It has been shown that *RAD51* overexpression is correlated with GIN and that p53 can transcriptionally inhibits *RAD51* expression (Arias-Lopez et al., 2006; Richardson et al., 2004).

2.2 DNA repair activity is important for preventing cancer development

Activation of DNA repair genes has been shown as a critical anticancer barrier in early human tumorigenesis. By examining various stages from precancerous lesions to late-stage tumor tissues, DNA repair genes, including *ATM, CHEK1/2,* and *TP53,* are found predominantly to be highly activated in the precancerous stage of bladder, colon and lung epithelia when DNA damages are emerging inside these cells (Bartkova et al., 2005; Gorgoulis et al., 2005; Venkitaraman, 2005). Further, DNA repair genes also play a key role in the oncogene-induced senescence and prevent cell transformation (Bartkova et al., 2006; Braig et al., 2005; Di Micco et al., 2006). In other word, cells that are unable to activate DNA repair genes in the early-stage of tumorigenesis are susceptible for malignant transformation. These data demonstrated in somatic cancers strongly indicate that defects or inactivations of DNA repair genes/pathways are prerequisite for tumor development. Besides, several cancer predisposition syndromes are linked to hereditary mutations or deletions of DNA repair genes, such as *ATM* in ataxia telangiectasia, *BRCA1* and *BRCA2* in familial breast and ovarian cancers, *XPC* and *DDB2* in Xeroderma pigmentosum. Hence, people with, either inherited or sporadic, inactivated DNA repair genes/pathways are prone to cancer development. In this chapter, we will use head and neck cancer as an example to illustrate the important role of DNA repair genes/pathways in the development and treatment of this malignancy, and demonstrate the application of a functional DNA repair assay, host cell reactivation (HCR), in cancer research.

2.3 DNA repair activity is a critical determinant for efficacy of anticancer treatment using chemotherapy or radiotherapy

The cell-killing mechanisms of radiotherapy and most regimens of chemotherapy are dependent on the induction of severe DNA damages, which result in apoptosis of cancer cells. Therefore, the DNA repair activity of cancer cells can play an important role in modulating patient's response to these anticancer treatments. For example, the platinum-based anticancer chemical, cisplatin is one of the most popular DNA-damaging chemotherapeutic drugs used in clinical management. It causes DNA adducts by interstrand crosslinking, which is repaired by a combination of NER and HR (Helleday et al., 2008; Miyagawa, 2008). Mutations of NER genes, such as *XPF* or *ERCC1,* may increase the sensitivity of cells toward cisplatin (Martin et al., 2008; Saldivar et al., 2007). In contrast, elevated expression of NER genes usually confers resistance to chemotherapy using DNA-damaging regimens. The expression level of *BRCA1,* which plays a primary role in HR and may has a regulatory role in NER (Hartman & Ford, 2002; Takimoto et al., 2002), is also correlated with chemotherapy efficacy. It has been shown that cells with reduced or inactivated *BRCA1* are more sensitive to cisplatin but, in contrast, are resistant to taxanes, the microtubule-interfering drugs (Husain et al., 1998; Lafarge et al., 2001; Mullan et al., 2001). Overexpression of *RAD51,* a member of BRCA/FA complex involved in HR, is also correlated with cisplatin resistance (Bhattacharyya et al., 2000). For *ATM,* an *in vitro* study showed that partial loss of distal 11q (*ATM* locus) was associated with decreased IR sensitivity in head and neck cancer cell lines (Parikh et al., 2007). Therefore, understanding the status of DNA repair genes/activity is thought to be important for the selection of appropriate chemotherapeutic regimens and may have a great impact on the clinical treatment as well as the patient's outcome.

3. Head and neck cancer

Head and neck squamous cell carcinoma (HNSCC) is the most popular head and neck cancer and is the sixth most common cancer in the world. They include malignancies originated from the epithelia of larynx, pharynx, oral and nasal cavities.

3.1 Some HNSCC risk factors are able to inhibit DNA repair

Epidemiological evidences have demonstrated that alcohol drinking, betel quid (BQ) chewing (especially in South Asia and South-West Pacific area including Taiwan), cigarette smoking, and infection of human papillomavirus are risk factors for HNSCC development (Haddad & Shin, 2008; IARC, 2004). The carcinogenicity of betel nut has been approved by the International Agency for Research on Cancer (IARC), a WHO organization, in 2004 (IARC, 2004), although the molecular mechanism underlying its carcinogenicity is not fully elucidated. In this regard, we have explored the possible effect of arecoline, a major alkaloid in betel nut, on DNA repair activity using HCR. We found that arecoline could inhibit the repair of UV-induced DNA damages, at least partly, through inactivating p53's expression and transactivation activity (Tsai et al., 2008). Besides, we also showed that arecoline could affect mitotic spindles and deregulated mitotic checkpoint, another key guardian of genome integrity (Wang et al., 2010). These results provide molecular explanation for BQ-associated carcinogenicity that has been shown previously by an increase of mitosis errors and micronucleus (MN) in mammalian cells (Lin, 2010). Micronucleus is a typical sign of GIN and is derived from either DNA strand breaks (clastogenic effect) or whole chromosome lagging during mitosis (aneugenic effect) (Norppa & Falck, 2003).

Epidemiological studies also show that the probability of HNSCC development is synergistically increased by simultaneous exposure of BQ, cigarette, and alcohols (Ko et al., 1995; Lee et al., 2005). Regarding the carcinogenic role of cigarette on the aspect of DNA repair, we also found that benzo(a)pyrene (BaP), an important carcinogen in cigarette (IARC, 2010), exhibited negative effects on DNA repair (Lin et al., 2011 manuscript in preparation). The mechanistic study regarding the synergistic effect of arecoline and BaP on regulating DNA repair, especially via p53- and aryl hydrocarbon receptor-dependent pathway, is worthy to be investigated further.

3.2 Alterations of DNA repair genes/activity in HNSCC and the relationship with HNSCC development, treatment, as well as patient's outcome

GIN is a hallmark of most human malignancies including HNSCC that elevated microsatellite instability, aneuploidy and various genomic alterations have been found by genome-wide analyses (Bockmuhl et al., 1996; Brieger et al., 2003; Friedlander, 2001; Partridge et al., 1999; Sparano et al., 2006), suggesting that GIN may be involved in the development of HNSCC. Some studies also show that DNA repair activity is reduced in the peripheral blood cells of HNSCC patients when compared with normal individuals (Cheng et al., 1998; Paz-Elizur et al., 2006), implying that altered DNA repair genes and/or activity may play a critical role in the development of HNSCC.

Studies using comparative genomic hybridization (CGH) have shown that gene copy numbers at chromosome 11q22-23 (*ATM* locus) are frequently lost in HNSCC (Bockmuhl et al., 1996; Brieger et al., 2003; van den Broek et al., 2007). Lazar et al. also showed loss of heterozygosity (LOH) at 11q23 in 25% (13/52) of primary HNSCC (Lazar et al., 1998). In addition, we have reported that *ATM* mRNA is down-regulated in 81.3% (65/80) of laryngeal and pharyngeal cancers, and further show that lower *ATM* expression (tumor/normal < 0.3) was an independent risk factor for patient's survival (Lee et al., 2011). This is the first study showing that *ATM* expression is a valuable prognostic marker for HNSCC. One study also shows an absent or reduced ATM protein expression in 31.25% (10/32) of oral cancer (He et al., 2008). These results suggest that alteration of *ATM*, either in gene sequence or in expression level may be associated with HNSCC.

Previous investigations showed that LOH of chromosome 17q (*BRCA1* locus) were found in 35% to 56% of laryngeal cancer (Kiaris et al., 1995; Rizos et al., 1998). In contrast, studies using CGH found an overrepresentation of 17q in 9% to 47% of HNSCC (Bockmuhl et al., 1996; Brieger et al., 2003), and one array-CGH reported the gain of 17q21 in 33% (7/21) of oral cancer (Sparano et al., 2006). These controversial results by genome-wide analyses may be due to the physically close localization of *ERBB2* (HER-2/neu) oncogene and the results need to be clarified by specifically looking at the *BRCA1* gene locus. Regarding the expression of *BRCA1* in HNSCC, one study showed that BRCA1 immunostaining positivity was lost in 34% (26/77) of tongue cancers, which might be correlated with early-stage tumor progression (Vora et al., 2003).

The results of genome-wide studies also suggest that genetic alterations at *RAD51* (15q15.1) and *XPC* (3p25) loci may be present in HNSCC (Bockmuhl et al., 1996; Brieger et al., 2003; Partridge et al., 1999; Sparano et al., 2006; van den Broek et al., 2007). Altered RAD51 protein expression has been reported by one pilot study with twelve head and neck cancer patients (Connell et al., 2006). The patients with high RAD51 protein levels in their pre-treatment tumor biopsies demonstrate poorer cancer-specific survival rates than those with lower RAD51 levels (33.3% vs. 88.9% at 2 years; $P = 0.025$). These results suggest that RAD51 expression may influence the outcome of with head and neck cancer patients who receive chemotherapy and radiotherapy (Connell et al., 2006). Other reports regarding altered expression of DNA repair genes in HNSCC include Ku80 (Chang et al., 2006), NBN and ERCC1 (Hsu et al., 2010; Yang et al., 2006). It has been shown that ERCC1 expression is associated with cisplatin resistance (Handra-Luca et al., 2007; Hsu et al., 2010) and NBN is correlated with outcome of advanced HNSCC patients (Yang et al., 2006). Inactivation of the BRCA/FA pathway via promoter methylation has also been described in HNSCC, and may be related to tobacco and alcohol exposure and survival of these patients (Marsit et al., 2004).

3.3 Treatment of HNSCC

Since HNSCC and its treatment can affect important physiological functions, such as speaking, breathing, and swallowing, it is important for choosing the appropriate treatment that not only cures but also benefits to the preservation of organs, physiological functions, and quality of life. The standard treatment for resectable HNSCC is surgical resection with or without postoperative concurrent chemotherapy (cisplatin plus 5-fluorouracil) and radiotherapy (CCRT). Around two-thirds of HNSCC are in advanced stage at time of diagnosis (Specenier & Vermorken, 2009). The majority of these patients with advanced stage tumors finally relapse locoregionally or at distant sites. These patients are usually qualified for palliative treatment only. Recent advances in using cetuximab (anti-EGFR) to prolong patient's survival time in locally advanced HNSCC is a big, but still not a fully satisfied progress (Vermorken et al., 2008). The use of docetaxel (a spindle poison and mitotic catastrophe inducer) can enhance the efficacy of chemotherapy using cisplatin/fluorouracil and improve slightly the overall survival rates of HNSCC patients (Hitt et al., 2005; Posner et al., 2007; Vermorken et al., 2007). These results suggest that a combination regimen exploiting different cell-killing mechanisms may be superior to monotherapy. However, an ideal combination regimen with lower adverse and side effects for efficient treatment of HNSCC is still under looking for.

3.4 Understanding the status of DNA repair genes in HNSCC is important for design of an effective therapeutic strategy for this malignancy

Since DNA repair genes/activity play a key role in cancer development and treatment, understanding their expression and genomic/functional alterations may facilitate the identification of new predictive or prognostic markers and new therapeutic targets for treatment of HNSCC. For example, recent studies using the strategy of synthetic lethal interaction (SLI) to improve efficacy of cancer treatment have become an attractive strategy (Helleday et al., 2008). Cancer cells that can survive from innumerable genetic alterations are largely dependent on the activities of multiple DNA repair pathways. However, cancer cells may also be defective in certain DNA repair pathway that is inherent or arises during tumorigenesis. Therefore, inhibition of one DNA repair pathway may increase selectively killing of cancer cells that already have another defective DNA repair pathway. For examples, some clinical trials have shown the efficient killing of *BRCA1*- or *BRCA2*-defective cancer cells (with defective HR repair) by using *PARP1* inhibitors, which block BER pathway (Annunziata & O'Shaughnessy, 2010; Bryant et al., 2005; Farmer et al., 2005; Underhill et al., 2010). Notably, such kind of treatment is less toxic than conventional radiotherapy and chemotherapy. This may benefit to organ preservation of HNSCC patients if one can identify SLI targets (DNA repair genes are good candidates) and develop corresponding regimens for treatment. For this reason, some clinical trials are ongoing to examine the efficacy of anticancer treatments by modulating DNA repair activities that are involved in different DNA repair pathways (Bolderson et al., 2009; Helleday, 2010; Helleday et al., 2008).

4. Host cell reactivation (HCR) assay

As mentioned above, DNA repair activity plays a critical role in maintaining genome integrity. Regardless the alterations of DNA repair genes at the levels of gene expression or DNA sequence, measurement of DNA repair activity can reflect the overall biological effects that are as consequences of these molecular changes and/or anticancer drug responses. Here we describe an easy and fast functional assay (HCR) to evaluate cellular DNA repair activity *in vivo*. This method uses a plasmid that can produce luciferase in mammalian cells as a reporter. We choose luciferase as a reporter since its characteristics of high sensitivity and wide dynamic linear range for quantification. Of course, other commonly used reporters, such as chloramphenicol acetyltransferase (CAT), secreted alkaline phosphatase (SEAP) or green fluorescent protein (GFP) can also be used.

The reporter is damaged *in vitro* first and is transfected into host cells. If the damaged reporter plasmid can be repaired in the host cells, the luciferase will be re-expressed. Otherwise, the luciferase activity will be much lower than that transfected with undamaged control plasmid. By this way, one can determine the DNA repair capacity by simply measuring luciferase activity. The reporter plasmid can be damaged using various methods such as UV, chemicals or restriction enzymes and serve as substrates for different DNA repair pathways. In this chapter, we will demonstrate the use of HCR in evaluating DNA repair capacities via NER, HR and NHEJ pathways.

4.1 HCR for NER

NER is responsible for the repair of bulky DNA lesions induced by UV and a lot of anticancer drugs. Here we use UV as a method to damage a luciferase reporter plasmid. Other chemicals (such as cisplatin) that cause bulky DNA adducts can also be used.

4.1.1 Materials

1. The reporter plasmid: pCMV-Luc (Liu et al., 2004). The firefly luciferase is driven by the cytomegalovirus (CMV) immediate early (IE) gene promoter.

2. The internal control plasmid used for calibrating transfection efficiency: pRL-CMV (Promega, Cat. No. E2261). The *Renilla* luciferase is driven by the CMV IE promoter.
3. Transfection reagents: Lipofectamine™ 2000 (Invitrogen, Cat. No. 11668) and Opti-MEM® I reduced serum medium (Invitrogen, Cat. No. 31985).
4. The Dual-Glo™ Luciferase assay system (Promega, Cat. No. E2940) for analyzing firefly and *Renilla* luciferase activities.

4.1.2 Substrate preparation for NER

1. Amplify the pCMV-Luc and pRL-CMV plasmids in *E. coli* (Fig. 1A).
2. Harvest bacteria by centrifugation at 13,000 rpm for 15 minutes, discard the supernatant completely and purify plasmids using the Plasmid Midi Kit (Geneaid, Cat. No. PI025).
3. Determine plasmid DNA concentration and purity by measuring the absorbance at 260 nm and 280 nm with a UV spectrophotometer.
4. Prepare UV-damaged luciferase reporter plasmid (pCMV-Luc) with a UV-crosslinker (CL-1000, UVP). The plasmids are placed within inner side of an opened eppendorf lid (Fig. 1B) or 35 mm petri dish without lid. The UV dose for irradiation is dependent on cell types because of differential intrinsic DNA repair capacities of various cells. We use 1000 J/m^2 for 293 (human embryonic kidney), Beas-2B (human bronchial epithelium), H1299 (human lung cancer), HEp-2 (human laryngeal cancer), SAS, Ca9-22, (human oral cancer) and 500 J/m^2 for KB (human oral cancer) cells. It is important to keep above parameters (the same plasmid amount in a fixed volume for UV irradiation) consistently in each experiment, or prepare an enough quantity of UV-dameged plasmids that can be stored in aliquots at -80°C once for all experiments.

4.1.3 Transfection

1. The HEp-2 cells (6×10^4) are seeded in 24-well plates 24 h prior to transfection (the appropriate cell numbers for seeding are dependent on cell types).
2. Prepare DNA-Lipofectamine™ 2000 (Invitrogen) complexes for each sample as follows:
   a. Add 0.5 μg of UV-damaged or undamaged (serve as a control) pCMV-Luc together with 0.05 μg of internal control plasmid (pRL-CMV, Promega) in 50 μl of Opti-MEM (Invitrogen) medium, mix gently.
   b. Mix 1 μl Lipofectamine™ 2000 gently in 50 μl of Opti-MEM medium and incubate for 5 minutes at room temperature.
   c. Combine the diluted DNA with the diluted Lipofectamine™ 2000 (total volume is 100 μl). Mix gently and incubate for 20 min at room temperature to allow the formation of DNA-Lipofectamine™ 2000 complexes.
3. Add the 100 μl of DNA-Lipofectamine™ 2000 complexes to each well and incubate at 37°C in a CO_2 incubator for 6 h. Then the cells can be treated with toxicants (such as arecoline) or anticancer drugs for another 24 h. Note: cells can be treated with toxicants or anticancer drugs prior to transfection that is dependent on experimental design.

4.1.4 Dual-luciferase assay

1. After 24 h post-transfection, cells are harvested in 100 μl (adjustable) lysis buffer (0.1 M HEPES, pH 7.8, 1% Triton X-100, 1 mM $CaCl_2$ and 1 mM $MgCl_2$) with cell scrapers.
2. The cell lysates are transferred to eppendorf tubes and centrifuged at 13,000 rpm at 20°C for one minute.

3. The supernatants (50 μl, adjustable) are transferred into a 96-well plate and 20 μl of Dual-Glo™ Luciferase Reagent (Promega) are added to each well.
4. Ten minutes later, the firefly luminescence is measured by a microplate luminometer (Centro LB 960, Berthold, Bad Wildbad, Germany).
5. Add 20 μl of Dual-Glo™ Stop & Glo® Reagent (Promega) to each well and wait for 10 minutes, then the *Renilla* luminescence is read.
6. The transfection efficiency-adjusted firefly luciferase activity is obtained by dividing the *Renilla* luciferase activity.

4.1.5 Representation of NER activity by HCR assay

Since the pCMV-Luc is damaged by UV, the DNA repair activity (responsible to UV) can be represented as the *Renilla*-calibrated firefly luciferase activity derived from UV-damaged pCMV-Luc verse to those from undamaged pCMV-Luc. By this way, one can compare the effects of various environmental toxicants on cellular DNA repair capacity. For example, an inhibitory effect of arecoline on the repair of UV-damaged pCMV-Luc can be found by using HCR assay (Fig. 1C).

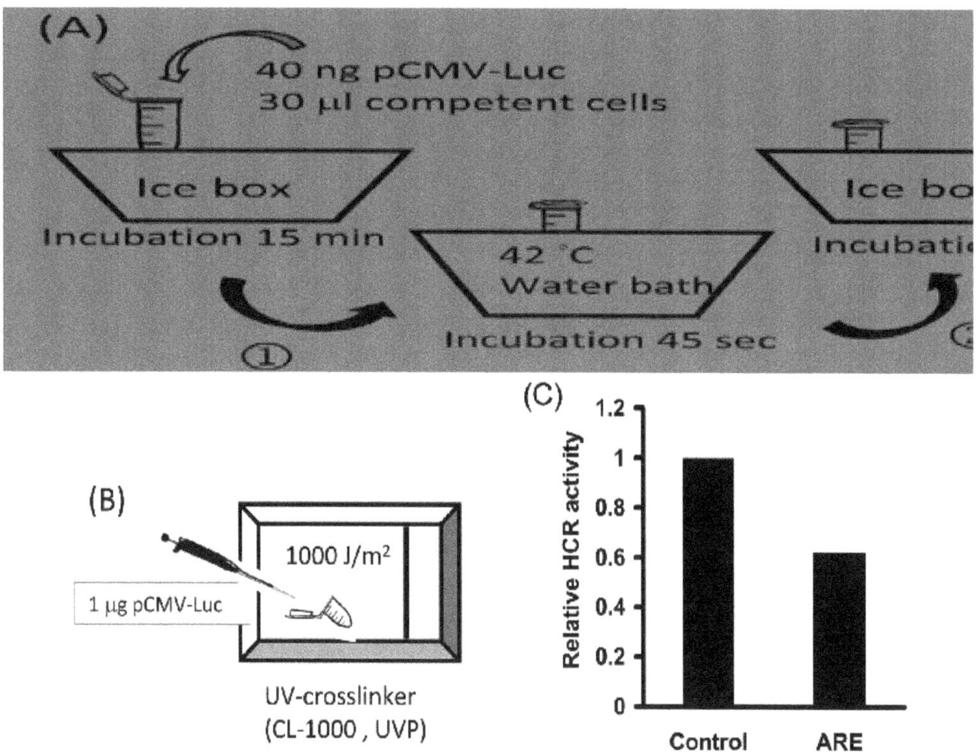

Fig. 1. Schematic illustration of host cell reactivation (HCR) assay for examination of nucleotide excision repair.
(A) The reporter plasmid pCMV-Luc is prepared in *E. coli*.
(B) The pCMV-Luc is damaged by 1000 J/m² of UV light.
(C) Comparison of the effects of arecoline (ARE, 0.3 mM) and its vehicle (distilled water) on the repair of UV-damaged pCMV-Luc in HEp-2 cells.

4.2 HCR for HR repair

HR is a reliable mechanism to accurately repair DNA double strand breaks. Here we use PCR to generate two overlapping DNA fragments that contain i) CMV IE promoter and 5′-part of *Renilla* luciferase gene, ii) 3′-part of *Renilla* luciferase gene and poly-A tail sequence from pRL-CMV (Fig. 2A) and serve as substrates for HR (Fig. 2B). The two overlapping DNA fragments can also be produced by restriction enzyme digestion and gel elution.

4.2.1 Materials

1. Plasmids: pRL-CMV (Promega, Cat. No. E2261) and pCMV-Luc (Liu et al., 2004).
2. PCR primers: RL_1: 5′-AGA TCT TCA ATA TTG GCC ATT AGC; RL_2: 5′-TTC TTA TTT ATG GCG ACA TGT TGT; RL_3: 5′-ACG AGG CCA TGA TAA TGT TGG ACG; RL_4: 5′-CTT ATC GAT TTT ACC ACA TTT GTA.
3. DNA Polymerase: *Ex Taq*™ Polymerase (Takara, Cat No. RR001A).
4. Gel-M™ Gel Extraction System (Viogene, Cat No. EG1002).

4.2.2 Substrate preparation for HR repair

1. Set up PCR reaction as below:

Reaction mixtures	HR_13 (µl)	HR_24 (µl)
10×PCR buffer	5	5
dNTP (2.5 mM)	4	4
RL_1 primer (10 µM)	2	-
RL_3 primer (10 µM)	2	-
RL_2 primer (10 µM)	-	2
RL_4 primer (10 µM)	-	2
ExTaq polymerase (5u/µl)	0.25	0.25
Template (40 ng/µl)	1	1
DNA/RNAase free- H_2O	35.75	35.75
Total volume (µl)	50	50

2. Incubate the PCR reaction mixtures at 94°C for 2 min, then run for 30 cycles of amplification (94°C, 45 sec; 55°C, 1 min; 72°C, 1 min) and additional extension step at 72°C for 5 min.
3. Purify the PCR products of HR13 fragments (1730 bp, containing CMV IE promoter and 5′-part of *Renilla* luciferase gene) and HR24 fregments (1023 bp, containing 3′-part of *Renilla* luciferase gene and poly-A tail) from 0.8% agarose gels (Fig. 2C) using the Gel-M™ Gel Extraction System kit (Viogene).
4. Determine DNA concentration and purity by measuring the absorbance at 260 nm and 280 nm with a UV spectrophotometer. Dilute the HR13-PCR products to 17 ng/µl and HR24-PCR products to 10 ng/µl with distilled H_2O to make the molar ratio of HR13:HR24 = 1:1, by which the same volume of the two DNA fragments can be used for transfection. Store the purified DNA in aliquots at -20°C.

Alternative: the two DNA fragments used for HR can also be generated by using a combination of restriction endonucleases *Bgl*II/*Nhe*I and *Pst*I/*Bam*HI for pRL-CMV (Progema). The use of former restriction enzymes will produce a DNA fragment containing

CMV IE promoter and 5′-part of *Renilla* luciferase gene, the later ones result in 3′-part of *Renilla* luciferase gene and the poly-A signal. These two DNA fragments contain a 222-bp overlapping region for recombination (Fig. 2D).

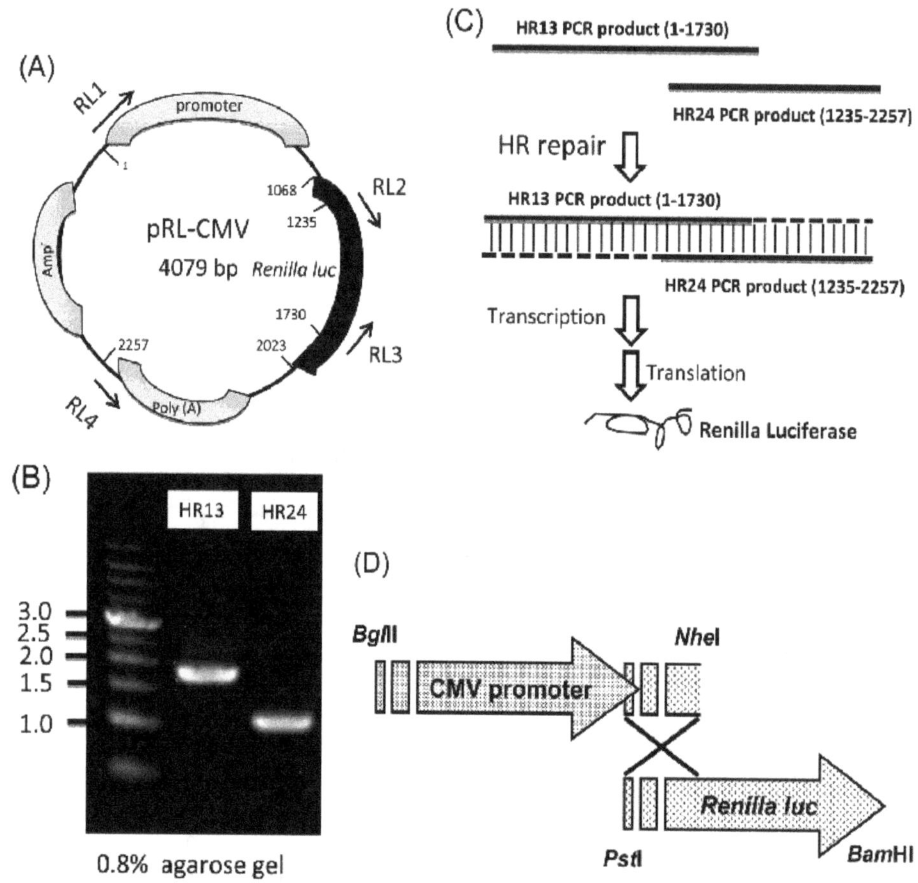

Fig. 2. Schematic representation of substrate preparation for HCR assay of homologous recombination (HR) repair.
(A) Location of PCR primers on the pRL-CMV reporter plasmid.
(B) Agarose gel electrophoresis of the PCR products, which serve as HR substrates.
(C) Homologous recombination of the two PCR fragments results in expression of luciferase.
(D) An alternative way to produce DNA fragments for HR by using restriction enzymes.

4.2.3 Transfection, dual-luciferase assay and representation of HR repair activity

1. The HEp-2 cells (6×10^4) are seeded in 24-well plates 24 h prior to transfection (the appropriate cell numbers for seeding are dependent on cell types).
2. Prepare DNA-Lipofectamine™ 2000 (Invitrogen) complexes for each sample as follows:
   a. Add 4 μl each of HR13 and HR24 DNA fragments together with 0.25 μg of internal control plasmid (pCMV-Luc) in 50 μl of Opti-MEM (Invitrogen) medium, mix gently.
   b. Mix 1 μl Lipofectamine™ 2000 gently in 50 μl of Opti-MEM medium and incubate for 5 minutes at room temperature.

   c. Combine the diluted DNA with the diluted Lipofectamine™ 2000 (total volume is 100 µl). Mix gently and incubate for 20 min at room temperature to allow the formation of DNA-Lipofectamine™ 2000 complexes.

3. Add the 100 µl of DNA-Lipofectamine™ 2000 complexes to each well and incubate at 37°C in a CO_2 incubator for 6 h. Then the cells can be treated with toxicants (such as areca nut extracts, ANE) or anticancer drugs for another 24 h. Note: cells can be treated with toxicants or anticancer drugs prior to transfection that is dependent on experimental design.
4. Perform dual-luciferase assay as section 4.1.4.
5. Determine the HR activity by comparing the firefly luciferase-calibrated *Renilla* luciferase activities between the environmental toxicants- or anticancer drugs-treated cells and vehicle-treated control cells. For examples, the treatment of anticancer drug camptothecin (CPT, a topoisomerase I inhibitor) can potentiate HR repair activity but the areca nut extracts (ANE) repress HR repair in HEp-2 cells (Fig. 3).

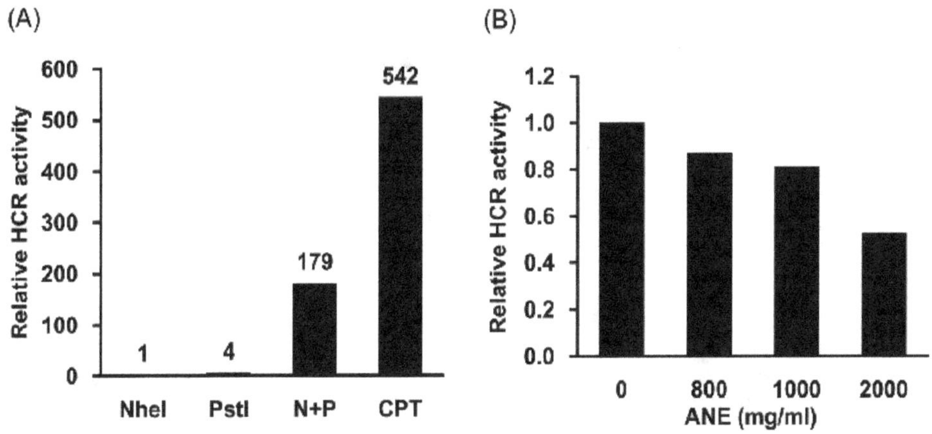

Fig. 3. The use of HCR assays in evaluating the effects of camptothecin and areca nut extracts on homologous recombination repair.
(A) Using the method illustrated in Fig. 2D, the *Renilla* luciferase activity (reflecting the HCR activity in Y-axis) can only be detected in the presence of both two DNA fragments (N+P, lane 3) but not in cells transfected with only one fragment (NheI or PstI, lanes 1 and 2). Treatment of camptothecin (CPT) stimulates HR repair efficiency in the cells (lane 4).
(B) Dose-dependent repression of HR repair activity by areca nut extracts (ANE).

4.3 HCR for NHEJ repair

NHEJ is another DNA repair mechanism responsible to DSB. Unlike HR repair using sister-chromatids as templates, NHEJ directly joins the broken DNA ends by trimming a few nucleotides on the ends. Therefore, it is thought as an error-prone repair system. In this regard, we prepare two kinds of reporter DNA substrates that are suitable for analyzing the precise and overall NHEJ repair activities, respectively.

For overall NHEJ repair, pRL-CMV is linearized with *Hin*dIII that cuts the flanking sequence between CMV promoter and the Renilla luciferase coding sequence. The luciferase will express after re-ligation regardless the loss of some nucleotides. For examining precise

NHEJ, *Afl* III that digests the coding region of *Renilla* luciferase gene is used and the luciferase can only be expressed after exact repair (Fig. 4A). The linearized reporter DNA fragments are purified, transfected into host cells and examined for luciferase activity as described above. Below is an example of evaluating the effect of areca nut extracts on precise and overall NHEJ repair (Fig. 4B).

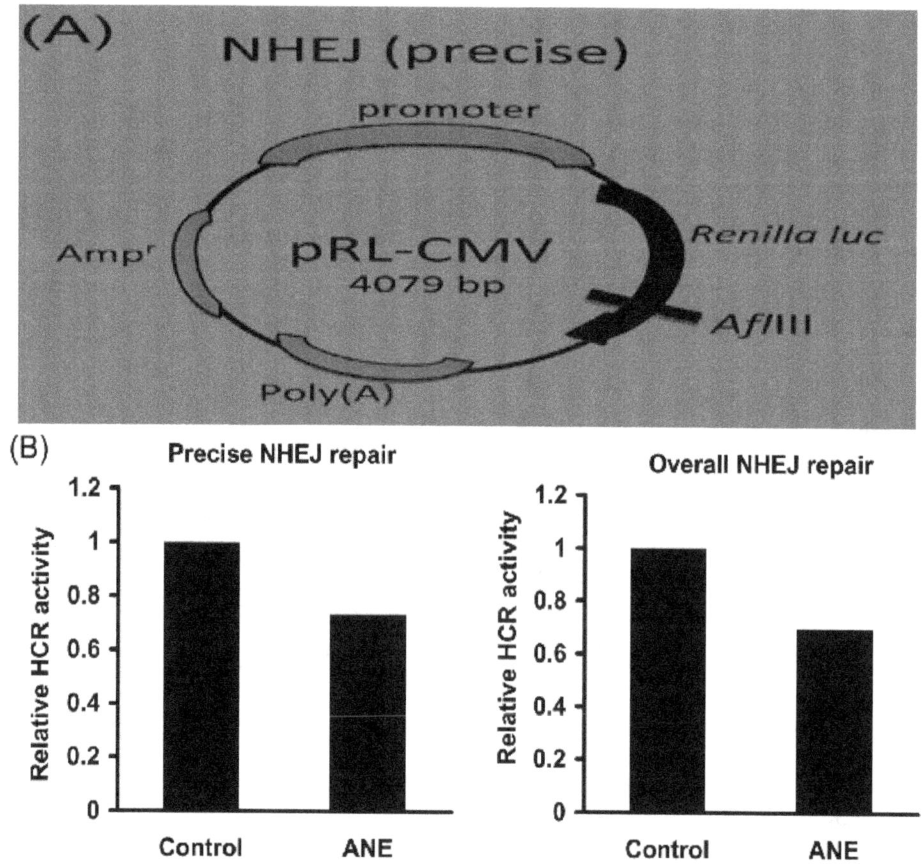

Fig. 4. HCR assay for non-homologous end-joining (NHEJ) repair.
(A) The *Afl* III-digested pRL-CMV is used as a substrate for analyzing precise NHEJ repair activity because of the need of exact joining of the *Renilla* luciferase coding sequence. For overall NHEJ, *Hind* III that cuts the flanking sequence between CMV promoter and the *Renilla* luciferase gene is used. The expression of luciferase is not affected by loss of a few nucleotides in this region during the end-joining process.
(B) The effect of areca nut extracts (ANE, 800 mg/ml for 24 h) on precise (left panel) and overall (right panel) NHEJ repair.

5. Conclusion

DNA repair genes play a pivotal role in the maintenance of genome integrity. Alterations of various DNA repair genes, either in gene sequence/structure or in gene expression, are frequently found in most of human malignancies. Since DNA repair activity is able to modulate cellular response to DNA-damaging anticancer drugs, alterations of DNA repair genes may be involved in the development of resistance to chemotherapy and radiotherapy. In addition, DNA repair activity plays an important role in preventing the mutagenicity and cytotoxicity induced by numerous environmental carcinogens and toxicants. Cells with reduced DNA repair activity may thus be prone to pathological transformation. Therefore, examining the DNA repair activity of a cell can help us to understand the probability of cellular tumorigenicity associated with exposure of environmental carcinogens and is able to assess the responses of various regimens of anticancer treatment. HCR assay is an easy and fast functional assay that can be applied to investigate several DNA repair pathways and is one of the most useful methods for evaluating cellular DNA repair activity *in vivo*.

6. Acknowledgment

The authors thank the financial support (grant No. NSC97-2311-B-037-002-MY3 to C.S.L. and NSC99-2314-B-309-004-MY2 to J.L.H.) from the National Science Council, Taiwan.

7. References

Adimoolam, S. & Ford, J.M. (2002) p53 and DNA damage-inducible expression of the xeroderma pigmentosum group C gene. *Proc Natl Acad Sci U S A*, Vol. 99, No.20, pp. 12985-12990.

Annunziata, C.M. & O'Shaughnessy, J. (2010) Poly (adp-ribose) polymerase as a novel therapeutic target in cancer. *Clin Cancer Res*, Vol. 16, No.18, pp. 4517-4526.

Arias-Lopez, C., Lazaro-Trueba, I., Kerr, P., Lord, C.J., Dexter, T., Iravani, M., Ashworth, A. & Silva, A. (2006) p53 modulates homologous recombination by transcriptional regulation of the RAD51 gene. *EMBO Rep*, Vol. 7, No.2, pp. 219-224.

Bartkova, J., Horejsi, Z., Koed, K., Kramer, A., Tort, F., Zieger, K., Guldberg, P., Sehested, M., Nesland, J.M., Lukas, C., Orntoft, T., Lukas, J. & Bartek, J. (2005) DNA damage response as a candidate anti-cancer barrier in early human tumorigenesis. *Nature*, Vol. 434, No.7035, pp. 864-870.

Bartkova, J., Rezaei, N., Liontos, M., Karakaidos, P., Kletsas, D., Issaeva, N., Vassiliou, L.V., Kolettas, E., Niforou, K., Zoumpourlis, V.C., Takaoka, M., Nakagawa, H., Tort, F., Fugger, K., Johansson, F., Sehested, M., Andersen, C.L., Dyrskjot, L., Orntoft, T., Lukas, J., Kittas, C., Helleday, T., Halazonetis, T.D., Bartek, J. & Gorgoulis, V.G. (2006) Oncogene-induced senescence is part of the tumorigenesis barrier imposed by DNA damage checkpoints. *Nature*, Vol. 444, No.7119, pp. 633-637.

Bhattacharyya, A., Ear, U.S., Koller, B.H., Weichselbaum, R.R. & Bishop, D.K. (2000) The breast cancer susceptibility gene BRCA1 is required for subnuclear assembly of Rad51 and survival following treatment with the DNA cross-linking agent cisplatin. *J Biol Chem*, Vol. 275, No.31, pp. 23899-23903.

Bockmuhl, U., Schwendel, A., Dietel, M. & Petersen, I. (1996) Distinct patterns of chromosomal alterations in high- and low-grade head and neck squamous cell carcinomas. *Cancer Res*, Vol. 56, No.23, pp. 5325-5329.

Bolderson, E., Richard, D.J., Zhou, B.B. & Khanna, K.K. (2009) Recent advances in cancer therapy targeting proteins involved in DNA double-strand break repair. *Clin Cancer Res*, Vol. 15, No.20, pp. 6314-6320.

Braig, M., Lee, S., Loddenkemper, C., Rudolph, C., Peters, A.H., Schlegelberger, B., Stein, H., Dorken, B., Jenuwein, T. & Schmitt, C.A. (2005) Oncogene-induced senescence as an initial barrier in lymphoma development. *Nature*, Vol. 436, No.7051, pp. 660-665.

Brieger, J., Jacob, R., Riazimand, H.S., Essig, E., Heinrich, U.R., Bittinger, F. & Mann, W.J. (2003) Chromosomal aberrations in premalignant and malignant squamous epithelium. *Cancer Genet Cytogenet*, Vol. 144, No.2, pp. 148-155.

Bryant, H.E., Schultz, N., Thomas, H.D., Parker, K.M., Flower, D., Lopez, E., Kyle, S., Meuth, M., Curtin, N.J. & Helleday, T. (2005) Specific killing of BRCA2-deficient tumours with inhibitors of poly(ADP-ribose) polymerase. *Nature*, Vol. 434, No.7035, pp. 913-917.

Chang, H.W., Kim, S.Y., Yi, S.L., Son, S.H., Song do, Y., Moon, S.Y., Kim, J.H., Choi, E.K., Ahn, S.D., Shin, S.S., Lee, K.K. & Lee, S.W. (2006) Expression of Ku80 correlates with sensitivities to radiation in cancer cell lines of the head and neck. *Oral Oncol*, Vol. 42, No.10, pp. 979-986.

Cheng, L., Eicher, S.A., Guo, Z., Hong, W.K., Spitz, M.R. & Wei, Q. (1998) Reduced DNA repair capacity in head and neck cancer patients. *Cancer Epidemiol Biomarkers Prev*, Vol. 7, No.6, pp. 465-468.

Connell, P.P., Jayathilaka, K., Haraf, D.J., Weichselbaum, R.R., Vokes, E.E. & Lingen, M.W. (2006) Pilot study examining tumor expression of RAD51 and clinical outcomes in human head cancers. *Int J Oncol*, Vol. 28, No.5, pp. 1113-1119.

Deng, C.X. (2002) Roles of BRCA1 in centrosome duplication. *Oncogene*, Vol. 21, No.40, pp. 6222-6227.

Deng, C.X. (2006) BRCA1: cell cycle checkpoint, genetic instability, DNA damage response and cancer evolution. *Nucleic Acids Res*, Vol. 34, No.5, pp. 1416-1426.

Di Micco, R., Fumagalli, M., Cicalese, A., Piccinin, S., Gasparini, P., Luise, C., Schurra, C., Garre, M., Nuciforo, P.G., Bensimon, A., Maestro, R., Pelicci, P.G. & d'Adda di Fagagna, F. (2006) Oncogene-induced senescence is a DNA damage response triggered by DNA hyper-replication. *Nature*, Vol. 444, No.7119, pp. 638-642.

Farmer, H., McCabe, N., Lord, C.J., Tutt, A.N., Johnson, D.A., Richardson, T.B., Santarosa, M., Dillon, K.J., Hickson, I., Knights, C., Martin, N.M., Jackson, S.P., Smith, G.C. & Ashworth, A. (2005) Targeting the DNA repair defect in BRCA mutant cells as a therapeutic strategy. *Nature*, Vol. 434, No.7035, pp. 917-921.

Friedlander, P.L. (2001) Genomic instability in head and neck cancer patients. *Head Neck*, Vol. 23, No.8, pp. 683-691.

Gorgoulis, V.G., Vassiliou, L.V., Karakaidos, P., Zacharatos, P., Kotsinas, A., Liloglou, T., Venere, M., Ditullio, R.A., Jr., Kastrinakis, N.G., Levy, B., Kletsas, D., Yoneta, A., Herlyn, M., Kittas, C. & Halazonetis, T.D. (2005) Activation of the DNA damage checkpoint and genomic instability in human precancerous lesions. *Nature*, Vol. 434, No.7035, pp. 907-913.

Haddad, R.I. & Shin, D.M. (2008) Recent advances in head and neck cancer. *N Engl J Med*, Vol. 359, No.11, pp. 1143-1154.

Hanahan, D. & Weinberg, R.A. (2000) The hallmarks of cancer. *Cell*, Vol. 100, No.1, pp. 57-70.

Handra-Luca, A., Hernandez, J., Mountzios, G., Taranchon, E., Lacau-St-Guily, J., Soria, J.C. & Fouret, P. (2007) Excision repair cross complementation group 1 immunohistochemical expression predicts objective response and cancer-specific survival in patients treated by Cisplatin-based induction chemotherapy for locally advanced head and neck squamous cell carcinoma. *Clin Cancer Res*, Vol. 13, No.13, pp. 3855-3859.

Hartman, A.R. & Ford, J.M. (2002) BRCA1 induces DNA damage recognition factors and enhances nucleotide excision repair. *Nat Genet*, Vol. 32, No.1, pp. 180-184.

He, Y., Chen, Q. & Li, B. (2008) ATM in oral carcinogenesis: association with clinicopathological features. *J Cancer Res Clin Oncol*, Vol. 134, No.9, pp. 1013-1020.

Helleday, T. (2010) Homologous recombination in cancer development, treatment and development of drug resistance. *Carcinogenesis*, Vol. 31, No.6, pp. 955-960.

Helleday, T., Petermann, E., Lundin, C., Hodgson, B. & Sharma, R.A. (2008) DNA repair pathways as targets for cancer therapy. *Nat Rev Cancer*, Vol. 8, No.3, pp. 193-204.

Helton, E.S. & Chen, X. (2007) p53 modulation of the DNA damage response. *J Cell Biochem*, Vol. 100, No.4, pp. 883-896.

Hitt, R., Lopez-Pousa, A., Martinez-Trufero, J., Escrig, V., Carles, J., Rizo, A., Isla, D., Vega, M.E., Marti, J.L., Lobo, F., Pastor, P., Valenti, V., Belon, J., Sanchez, M.A., Chaib, C., Pallares, C., Anton, A., Cervantes, A., Paz-Ares, L. & Cortes-Funes, H. (2005) Phase III study comparing cisplatin plus fluorouracil to paclitaxel, cisplatin, and fluorouracil induction chemotherapy followed by chemoradiotherapy in locally advanced head and neck cancer. *J Clin Oncol*, Vol. 23, No.34, pp. 8636-8645.

Hsu, D.S., Lan, H.Y., Huang, C.H., Tai, S.K., Chang, S.Y., Tsai, T.L., Chang, C.C., Tzeng, C.H., Wu, K.J., Kao, J.Y. & Yang, M.H. (2010) Regulation of excision repair cross-complementation group 1 by Snail contributes to cisplatin resistance in head and neck cancer. *Clin Cancer Res*, Vol. 16, No.18, pp. 4561-4571.

Husain, A., He, G., Venkatraman, E.S. & Spriggs, D.R. (1998) BRCA1 up-regulation is associated with repair-mediated resistance to cis-diamminedichloroplatinum(II). *Cancer Res*, Vol. 58, No.6, pp. 1120-1123.

Hwang, B.J., Ford, J.M., Hanawalt, P.C. & Chu, G. (1999) Expression of the p48 xeroderma pigmentosum gene is p53-dependent and is involved in global genomic repair. *Proc Natl Acad Sci U S A*, Vol. 96, No.2, pp. 424-428.

IARC. (2004) Betel-quid and areca-nut chewing and some areca-nut-derived nitrosamines. *IARC Monographs on the Evaluation of Carcinogenic Risks to Humans*, Vol. 85, The International Agency for Research on cancer, World Health Organization, Lyon, France.

IARC. (2010) Some non-heterocyclic polycyclic aromatic hydrocarbons and some related exposures. *IARC Monographs on the Evaluation of Carcinogenic Risks to Humans*, Vol. 92, The International Agency for Research on cancer, World Health Organization, Lyon, France.

Kiaris, H., Spanakis, N., Ergazaki, M., Sourvinos, G. & Spandidos, D.A. (1995) Loss of heterozygosity at 9p and 17q in human laryngeal tumors. *Cancer Lett*, Vol. 97, No.1, pp. 129-134.

Ko, Y.C., Huang, Y.L., Lee, C.H., Chen, M.J., Lin, L.M. & Tsai, C.C. (1995) Betel quid chewing, cigarette smoking and alcohol consumption related to oral cancer in Taiwan. *J Oral Pathol Med*, Vol. 24, No.10, pp. 450-453.

Lafarge, S., Sylvain, V., Ferrara, M. & Bignon, Y.J. (2001) Inhibition of BRCA1 leads to increased chemoresistance to microtubule-interfering agents, an effect that involves the JNK pathway. *Oncogene*, Vol. 20, No.45, pp. 6597-6606.

Lazar, A.D., Winter, M.R., Nogueira, C.P., Larson, P.S., Finnemore, E.M., Dolan, R.W., Fuleihan, N., Chakravarti, A., Zietman, A. & Rosenberg, C.L. (1998) Loss of heterozygosity at 11q23 in squamous cell carcinoma of the head and neck is associated with recurrent disease. *Clin Cancer Res*, Vol. 4, No.11, pp. 2787-2793.

Lee, K.W., Kuo, W.R., Tsai, S.M., Wu, D.C., Wang, W.M., Fang, F.M., Chiang, F.Y., Ho, K.Y., Wang, L.F., Tai, C.F., Kao, E.L., Chou, S.H., Lee, C.H., Chai, C.Y. & Ko, Y.C. (2005) Different impact from betel quid, alcohol and cigarette: risk factors for pharyngeal and laryngeal cancer. *Int J Cancer*, Vol. 117, No.5, pp. 831-836.

Lee, K.W., Tsai, Y.S., Chiang, F.Y., Huang, J.L., Ho, K.Y., Yang, Y.H., Kuo, W.R., Chen, M.K. & Lin, C.S. (2011) Lower ataxia telangiectasia mutated (ATM) mRNA expression is correlated with poor outcome of laryngeal and pharyngeal cancer patients. *Ann Oncol*, Vol. 22, No.5, pp. 1088-1093.

Lin, C.S. (2010) Carcinogenicity of arecoline, an alkaloid of betel nut. In: *SciTopics* , Date of access: 20 August 2010, Available from: http://www.scitopics.com/Carcinogenicity_of_arecoline_an_alkaloid_of_betel_nut.html

Liu, M.T., Chen, Y.R., Chen, S.C., Hu, C.Y., Lin, C.S., Chang, Y.T., Wang, W.B. & Chen, J.Y. (2004) Epstein-Barr virus latent membrane protein 1 induces micronucleus formation, represses DNA repair and enhances sensitivity to DNA-damaging agents in human epithelial cells. *Oncogene*, Vol. 23, No.14, pp. 2531-2539.

Marsit, C.J., Liu, M., Nelson, H.H., Posner, M., Suzuki, M. & Kelsey, K.T. (2004) Inactivation of the Fanconi anemia/BRCA pathway in lung and oral cancers: implications for treatment and survival. *Oncogene*, Vol. 23, No.4, pp. 1000-1004.

Martin, L.P., Hamilton, T.C. & Schilder, R.J. (2008) Platinum resistance: the role of DNA repair pathways. *Clin Cancer Res*, Vol. 14, No.5, pp. 1291-1295.

Martin, R.W., Orelli, B.J., Yamazoe, M., Minn, A.J., Takeda, S. & Bishop, D.K. (2007) RAD51 up-regulation bypasses BRCA1 function and is a common feature of BRCA1-deficient breast tumors. *Cancer Res*, Vol. 67, No.20, pp. 9658-9665.

Miyagawa, K. (2008) Clinical relevance of the homologous recombination machinery in cancer therapy. *Cancer Sci*, Vol. 99, No.2, pp. 187-194.

Mullan, P.B., Quinn, J.E., Gilmore, P.M., McWilliams, S., Andrews, H., Gervin, C., McCabe, N., McKenna, S., White, P., Song, Y.H., Maheswaran, S., Liu, E., Haber, D.A., Johnston, P.G. & Harkin, D.P. (2001) BRCA1 and GADD45 mediated G2/M cell cycle arrest in response to antimicrotubule agents. *Oncogene*, Vol. 20, No.43, pp. 6123-6131.

Norppa, H. & Falck, G.C. (2003) What do human micronuclei contain? *Mutagenesis*, Vol. 18, No.3, pp. 221-233.

Parikh, R.A., White, J.S., Huang, X., Schoppy, D.W., Baysal, B.E., Baskaran, R., Bakkenist, C.J., Saunders, W.S., Hsu, L.C., Romkes, M. & Gollin, S.M. (2007) Loss of distal 11q is associated with DNA repair deficiency and reduced sensitivity to ionizing radiation in head and neck squamous cell carcinoma. *Genes Chromosomes Cancer*, Vol. 46, No.8, pp. 761-775.

Partridge, M., Emilion, G., Pateromichelakis, S., A'Hern, R., Lee, G., Phillips, E. & Langdon, J. (1999) The prognostic significance of allelic imbalance at key chromosomal loci in oral cancer. *Br J Cancer*, Vol. 79, No.11-12, pp. 1821-1827.

Paz-Elizur, T., Ben-Yosef, R., Elinger, D., Vexler, A., Krupsky, M., Berrebi, A., Shani, A., Schechtman, E., Freedman, L. & Livneh, Z. (2006) Reduced repair of the oxidative 8-oxoguanine DNA damage and risk of head and neck cancer. *Cancer Res*, Vol. 66, No.24, pp. 11683-11689.

Posner, M.R., Hershock, D.M., Blajman, C.R., Mickiewicz, E., Winquist, E., Gorbounova, V., Tjulandin, S., Shin, D.M., Cullen, K., Ervin, T.J., Murphy, B.A., Raez, L.E., Cohen, R.B., Spaulding, M., Tishler, R.B., Roth, B., Viroglio Rdel, C., Venkatesan, V., Romanov, I., Agarwala, S., Harter, K.W., Dugan, M., Cmelak, A., Markoe, A.M., Read, P.W., Steinbrenner, L., Colevas, A.D., Norris, C.M., Jr. & Haddad, R.I. (2007) Cisplatin and fluorouracil alone or with docetaxel in head and neck cancer. *N Engl J Med*, Vol. 357, No.17, pp. 1705-1715.

Richardson, C. (2005) RAD51, genomic stability, and tumorigenesis. *Cancer Lett*, Vol. 218, No.2, pp. 127-139.

Richardson, C., Stark, J.M., Ommundsen, M. & Jasin, M. (2004) Rad51 overexpression promotes alternative double-strand break repair pathways and genome instability. *Oncogene*, Vol. 23, No.2, pp. 546-553.

Rizos, E., Sourvinos, G. & Spandidos, D.A. (1998) Loss of heterozygosity at 8p, 9p and 17q in laryngeal cytological specimens. *Oral Oncol*, Vol. 34, No.6, pp. 519-523.

Saldivar, J.S., Wu, X., Follen, M. & Gershenson, D. (2007) Nucleotide excision repair pathway review I: implications in ovarian cancer and platinum sensitivity. *Gynecol Oncol*, Vol. 107, No.1 Suppl 1, pp. S56-71.

Sancar, A., Lindsey-Boltz, L.A., Unsal-Kacmaz, K. & Linn, S. (2004) Molecular mechanisms of mammalian DNA repair and the DNA damage checkpoints. *Annu Rev Biochem*, Vol. 73, No., pp. 39-85.

Sparano, A., Quesnelle, K.M., Kumar, M.S., Wang, Y., Sylvester, A.J., Feldman, M., Sewell, D.A., Weinstein, G.S. & Brose, M.S. (2006) Genome-wide profiling of oral squamous cell carcinoma by array-based comparative genomic hybridization. *Laryngoscope*, Vol. 116, No.5, pp. 735-741.

Specenier, P.M. & Vermorken, J.B. (2009) Current concepts for the management of head and neck cancer: chemotherapy. *Oral Oncol*, Vol. 45, No.4-5, pp. 409-415.

Takimoto, R., MacLachlan, T.K., Dicker, D.T., Niitsu, Y., Mori, T. & el-Deiry, W.S. (2002) BRCA1 transcriptionally regulates damaged DNA binding protein (DDB2) in the DNA repair response following UV-irradiation. *Cancer Biol Ther*, Vol. 1, No.2, pp. 177-186.

Tsai, Y.S., Lee, K.W., Huang, J.L., Liu, Y.S., Juo, S.H., Kuo, W.R., Chang, J.G., Lin, C.S. & Jong, Y.J. (2008) Arecoline, a major alkaloid of areca nut, inhibits p53, represses DNA repair, and triggers DNA damage response in human epithelial cells. *Toxicology*, Vol. 249, No.2-3, pp. 230-237.

Underhill, C., Toulmonde, M. & Bonnefoi, H. (2011) A review of PARP inhibitors: from bench to bedside. *Ann Oncol*, Vol. 22, No. 2, pp. 268-279.

Uziel, T., Lerenthal, Y., Moyal, L., Andegeko, Y., Mittelman, L. & Shiloh, Y. (2003) Requirement of the MRN complex for ATM activation by DNA damage. *Embo J*, Vol. 22, No.20, pp. 5612-5621.

van den Broek, G.B., Wreesmann, V.B., van den Brekel, M.W., Rasch, C.R., Balm, A.J. & Rao, P.H. (2007) Genetic abnormalities associated with chemoradiation resistance of head and neck squamous cell carcinoma. *Clin Cancer Res*, Vol. 13, No.15 Pt 1, pp. 4386-4391.

Venkitaraman, A.R. (2005) Medicine: aborting the birth of cancer. *Nature*, Vol. 434, No.7035, pp. 829-830.

Vermorken, J.B., Mesia, R., Rivera, F., Remenar, E., Kawecki, A., Rottey, S., Erfan, J., Zabolotnyy, D., Kienzer, H.R., Cupissol, D., Peyrade, F., Benasso, M., Vynnychenko, I., De Raucourt, D., Bokemeyer, C., Schueler, A., Amellal, N. & Hitt, R. (2008) Platinum-based chemotherapy plus cetuximab in head and neck cancer. *N Engl J Med*, Vol. 359, No.11, pp. 1116-1127.

Vermorken, J.B., Remenar, E., van Herpen, C., Gorlia, T., Mesia, R., Degardin, M., Stewart, J.S., Jelic, S., Betka, J., Preiss, J.H., van den Weyngaert, D., Awada, A., Cupissol, D., Kienzer, H.R., Rey, A., Desaunois, I., Bernier, J. & Lefebvre, J.L. (2007) Cisplatin, fluorouracil, and docetaxel in unresectable head and neck cancer. *N Engl J Med*, Vol. 357, No.17, pp. 1695-1704.

Vora, H.H., Shah, N.G., Patel, D.D., Trivedi, T.I. & Choksi, T.J. (2003) BRCA1 expression in leukoplakia and carcinoma of the tongue. *J Surg Oncol*, Vol. 83, No.4, pp. 232-240.

Wang, Y.C., Tsai, Y.S., Huang, J.L., Lee, K.W., Kuo, C.C., Wang, C.S., Huang, A.M., Chang, J.Y., Jong, Y.J. & Lin, C.S. (2010) Arecoline arrests cells at prometaphase by deregulating mitotic spindle assembly and spindle assembly checkpoint: implication for carcinogenesis. *Oral Oncol*, Vol. 46, No.4, pp. 255-262.

Wood, R.D., Mitchell, M. & Lindahl, T. (2005) Human DNA repair genes, 2005. *Mutat Res*, Vol. 577, No.1-2, pp. 275-283.

Xu, X., Weaver, Z., Linke, S.P., Li, C., Gotay, J., Wang, X.W., Harris, C.C., Ried, T. & Deng, C.X. (1999) Centrosome amplification and a defective G2-M cell cycle checkpoint induce genetic instability in BRCA1 exon 11 isoform-deficient cells. *Mol Cell*, Vol. 3, No.3, pp. 389-395.

Yang, M.H., Chiang, W.C., Chou, T.Y., Chang, S.Y., Chen, P.M., Teng, S.C. & Wu, K.J. (2006) Increased NBS1 expression is a marker of aggressive head and neck cancer and overexpression of NBS1 contributes to transformation. *Clin Cancer Res*, Vol. 12, No.2, pp. 507-515.

Yoshida, K. & Miki, Y. (2004) Role of BRCA1 and BRCA2 as regulators of DNA repair, transcription, and cell cycle in response to DNA damage. *Cancer Sci*, Vol. 95, No.11, pp. 866-871.

2

The Nuclear Compartmentation of Glutathione: Effect on Cell Cycle Progression

Jelena Markovic, Nancy Mora, Amparo Gimeno, Consuelo Burguete, José Luis García-Gimenez and Federico V. Pallardó
University of Valencia School of Medicine, Spain

1. Introduction

The oxidizing environment, shared by all aerobic organisms and crucial for their survival, poses a continuous threat to cellular structures all the living beings are made of. Structural proteins and lipids, and cellular membranes they compose, nucleic acids and enzymes that govern vital cellular processes are all susceptible to oxidative damage. Dealing with this inevitable and constant danger is one of the greatest challenges the living being with aerobic metabolism has to meet.

2. The implication of cellular redox balance in cell proliferation

2.1 Reactive oxidative species in cell proliferation

Classical work of Kelvin Davies (Davies, 1999), more than ten years ago, showed that the cells show a whole range of responses to oxidative stress that depends on the intensity of the stress. Low level of hydrogen peroxide induced mitogenic responses and stimulation of proliferation; this observation was firstly reported by Oberly (Oberly et al., 1981) who have described that oxidative stimuli, such as superoxide and hydrogen peroxide, could activate signalling pathways that lead to proliferation. Davies et al. further assert that considerable increase in the oxidant concentrations caused temporary growth arrest which became permanent with a progressive increase. When high H_2O_2 concentrations were used, apoptosis took place and at very high oxidant levels the cells were killed by necrosis. A year later, (Pani et al., 2000) demonstrate a causal link between redox changes and growth control by cell density: they show that low level of oxygen species in the environment of proliferating cells was not only stimulating but necessary for the correct mitogenic signaling. This study was immediately followed by the work of Menon et al., 2003 who suggested that an oxidation event early in G1 phase may be a critical regulatory step in the progression of the cells into S phase. This lead to the development of the model of the "redox cycle within a cell cycle" proposed by the same group several years later (Menon & Goswami 2007).

According to this model, the transient change in ROS could modify the redox state of cell cycle regulatory proteins, at their critical cysteine residues, and thus determine progression or arrest in the proliferation. Antioxidant mechanism could scavenge ROS and reverse the process. In accordance to these reports, Barry Halliwell (Halliwell, 2007) draw a complete view of the present knowledge of the role of oxidative stress in promoting cancer, its damaging effects to DNA, and its action on cell proliferation and apoptosis. Malignant cells produce more radical species and, although antioxidant defence could also be induced in these cells, they display a pro-oxidant state. However, apparently the oxidative stress generated in these high proliferative cells does not exceed the level where oxidative damage becomes so severe that cell function is impaired. This finding is in line with previously cited reports and many others that support the role of reactive oxidative species mediated signalling in the promotion of cell growth.

2.2 The bridge between the oxidative stress and cell proliferation - Glutathione

Glutathione (GSH) is the most abundant non-protein thiol in mammalian cells (Meister & Anderson, 1983). It is considered essential for survival in mammalian cells (Viña, 1990) and yeast Meister & Anderson, 1983; Viña et al., 1978), but not in prokaryotic cells. The exact nature of this important difference has not been elucidated. Glutathione was discovered in 1888 by Rey Pailhade as "organic hydrogenate of sulphur" (Rey Paihade, 1988) and "rediscovered" and fully described by Sir Frederic Gowland Hopkins in the 1920s (Hopkins, 1929) and quoted by Sies several years later (Sies, 1999).

Glutathione has attracted the scientific interest with variable intensity along the century since its discovery and many important cellular functions of this tripeptide were revealed along the years. Glutathione shows a widespread localization within cells and considerably high concentration in cells and tissues (up to 10 mM) (Tateishi et al., 1974). Examples of normal physiological functions of glutathione known for a long time include regulation of the transport of certain amino acids (Viña & Viña, 1983) control of cytoskeleton assembly (Burchil et al. 1978) and regulation of enzymatic activity (Ernst et al., 1978; Ziegler, 1985). During 1960s, GSH was demonstrated to be a co-substrate for a number of important enzymatic reactions: GSH-S-transferase was described (Booth, 1961) and its role in a first-line defence against electrophilic insult, obviously dependent on glutathione, was suggested (Boyland, 1969). These pioneer works became the bases for many studies that lead to the development of concepts such as drug and foreign compound detoxification, and multidrug resistance (Smith, 1977) of crucial importance in the modern cancer therapy. Glutathione, as it lacks toxicity linked to cysteine (Viña et al., 1983), is considered perfect as a cellular thiol "redox buffer" with a purpose to maintain a given thiol/disulfide redox potential (Sies, 1999). Therefore, the redox properties and abundance that characterize this molecule grant it a major role in protecting the cell against oxidants and electrophiles, and during 1980s this particular role of glutathione is central in many research efforts.

Association of redox regulation with toxicity events lead to the introduction of the concept of "oxidative stress" at biochemical and cellular level (Sies & Cadenas, 1985). Oxidative stress is generally defined as an imbalance between prooxidants and antioxidants with a considerable effect on other cellular components, including redox sensitive functional groups of proteins. Nowadays, with the increasing awareness of the importance of ROS and glutathione in cellular signalling, and the cellular redox environment in fundamental physiological processes, a new definition of oxidative stress is proposed. According to Jones, 2006, oxidative stress may be better defined as a disruption of redox signaling and control. Interestingly, more than 10 years ago, searching for a molecular link between oxidative stress and cell proliferation, Cotgrave IA and Gerdes RG recommended similar term: "oxidant mediated regulation" (Cortgreave and Gerdes, 1998).

2.3 Glutathione in cell proliferation

Several studies from more than 20 years ago have suggested that changes in low molecular weight thiols (LMWT) are associated with regulation of cell growth. Harris and Patt published (Harris & Pat, 1969) that nonproliferating mouse tumour cells contained LMWT than proliferating cells and in early eighties various authors report similar results: human lung and ovarian tumour cells during the exponential growth demonstrate higher GSH levels than during nondividing state (Harris & Pat, 1969; Post, 1983). In accordance to these findings, Kosower and Kosower (Kosower & Kosower, 1978) have demonstrated that decrease of GSH biosynthesis in vivo inhibits tumour growth rate. Moreover, it was suggested that cellular GSH may have to reach certain critical levels before proliferation can be initiated and that variations in the protein sulphydryl redox status may directly relate to regulation of cell growth (Atzori et al. 1990).

Defining the intrinsic cellular redox environment by estimation of glutathione (GSH)/glutathione disulfide (GSSG) redox state, the group of Dean P. Jones (Nkabyo et al. 2002) concluded that each phase in the life of the cell is characterized by the certain redox state. Proliferating cells are in the most reduced state, with the values of Eh between -260mV and -230mV (Schafer & Buettner, 2001). Upon a growth arrest caused by differentiation (Nkabyo et al. 2002) or contact inhibition (Schafer & Buettner, 2001) cells are 40 mV more oxidised (-220mV to -190mV) while the apoptotic process is accompanied by further oxidation up to -165mV (Sun & Oberley, 1996).

Therefore, while the cell progresses from proliferation, through contact inhibition, differentiation, and finally apoptosis, there is an intrinsic and natural progression from more reduced to more oxidised cellular redox environment. The universality of this model which applies to various cells from different organisms (reviewed in Schafer & Buettner, 2001) inspired a daring hypothesis of Schafer and Buettner on the implication and function of thiols and disulfides as nano-switches. The GSSG/2GSH couple is imagined as a switchboard that move the cell from proliferation through differentiation towards programmed cell death, if the redox environment could not be maintained, or necrosis when the oxidative insult is to severe.

2.4 Glutathiolation of regulatory proteins as a link between a stimulating oxidative event and reduced cell environment in cell proliferation

During the last two decades the increasing body of evidence reveals that several transcription factors undergo oxidant modification necessary for their activation. For instance, the property of binding DNA and thus regulate gene expression of AP1, NfkB, p53, and SP1 depends on the redox status of cysteinyl thiols in their structures (Sun & Oberley, 1996). Thus, the idea of protein glutathiolation as a regulatory mechanism of importance in cell proliferation came into sight.

Glutathiolation is a protein modification which consists in the covalent union of the tripeptide glutathione to the SH group of the cysteine residue. For a long time this reaction was considered to be a consequence of the equilibrium between protein thiols and GSSG inevitably related to oxidative stress. From this point of view, glutathiolation fulfills two important functions. Firstly, its reversibility enables the preservation of glutathione in the cell and serves as a buffer for the reduction potential; otherwise, GSSG efflux would cause the loss of GSH from the cell, decreasing the reducing capacity which could be recovered only by the synthesis of new GSH (Schafer & Buettner, 2001). Secondly, it provides protection for protein-SH against irreversible modifications and protein damage in response to higher levels of oxidative stress (Dalle-Donne et al., 2007). Interestingly, it was demonstrated that glutathiolation as a posttranslational modification occurs not only during oxidative stress, but also under basal conditions and is involved in regulating distinct transcription factors, such as NF-kB (Pineda-Molina et al., 2001), its inhibitor factor IKK (Reynaert et al., 2006) and c-Jun (Canela et al. 2007). Apparently, the binding capacity of these proteins to DNA or other proteins is modulated by glutathiolation. This relatively recent focus on the implication of glutathiolation modulatory effects on protein function yielded important breakthrough in elucidation of the implication of this modification in various physiological and pathological situations (Giustarini et al. 2004) and raises interesting questions about its possible implications in cell proliferation.

2.4.1 The role of glutathione in DNA synthesis

Among the important roles that GSH plays in cellular physiology, and among the first to be described, was its role in DNA synthesis. The pentose phosphate pathway is a cellular source of NADPH that is involved in reductive biosynthesis. In this process, ribose-5-phosphate is formed and subsequently used for the synthesis of RNA, DNA and nucleotide coenzymes. Apart from the synthesis of nucleotides, NADPH is also required for the formation of amino acids, fatty acids, cholesterol, neurotransmitters and nitric oxide (NO). Furthermore, NADPH is the source of electrons in the process of reduction of ribonucleotides to deoxyribonucleotides catalyzed by the ribonucleotide reductase (Thelander & Reichard, 1979).

The route is initialized by two distinct but complemented systems, the thioredoxin system and the glutaredoxin system. Thioredoxin operates by transferring the electrons to ribonucleotide reductase, and they are supplied by the thioredoxin reductase and NADPH. The glutaredoxin system is initialized by the glutathione reductase, which reduces the GSSG to GSH using the NADPH as source of electrons. GSH is used by the glutaredoxin to provide the reducing power to the ribonucleotide reductase (Zahedi et al., 2009).

The crucial role of glutathione in DNA synthesis has been extensively documented (Thelander & Reichard, 1979; Holmgren, 1976). For instance, Dethlefsen and co-workers (Dethlefsen et al. 1988) showed that glutathione depletion inhibits DNA synthesis in mammary carcinoma cells. In addition, the vital importance of GSH in this process has also been demonstrated in human T lymphocytes (Suthanthiran et al., 1990). As mentioned above GSH is an indispensable requirement in eukaryotes. In contrast, it does not demonstrate the same importance in prokariotes. It has been shown that E. Coli lacking gshA, the rate limiting enzyme in the synthesis of GSH, can grow without GSH supplementation (Greenberg & Demple, 1986; Miranda-Vizuete et al., 1996). On the contrary, in yeast, the depletion of GSH does affect cell proliferation on the level different from DNA synthesis: mutants deficient in GCS after GSH withdrawal arrest cells in G1, whereas a strain with a defect in ribonucleotide reduction arrest cells in S phase (Wang et al., 1997). Since other possible explanations, such as protection against oxidative stress or protection against non-native protein disulfides, have been discarded (Spector el al., 2001), it appears that the essential function of GSH in yeast is related to the redox properties of its thiol group. Consequently, glutathione can be replaced by dithiothreitol, but not with a GSH analog where a thiol group has been substituted by a methyl group (Grant et al., 1996). Since GSH is the reductant for glutaredoxin as explained previously, and glutaredoxin is also essential (Rodriguez-Manzaneque et al., 1999) presumably their vital importance may be interdependent. Then GSH seems to be important in S phase. During the process of DNA replication, errors, such as double-strand breaks (DSBs) that arise from stalled replication forks, require attention by the DNA damage response proteins. Thus, the correct control of DNA synthesis and probably essential molecules, such as GSH, are necessary for the correct DNA processing.

One of the most important proteins involved in DNA damage signaling pathway is the ataxia-telangiectasa mutated protein (ATM). This central signaling protein, mainly for DSBs, is involved in the repairing DNA process necessary after replication stress. Thus cells lacking ATM fail to execute many of the cellular responses to DNA damage (Zhou & Elledge, 2000). In addition, control of ATM responses after DNA replication may be necessary for the correct cell cycle control. In that way, ATM is a central component in the cell cycle regulation. Therefore, patients with ataxia telangiectasia have reduction in DNA synthesis (Painter & Young, 1980). Furthermore, a recent work published by Guo Z. and coworkers describes using a series of elegant experiments how ATM sense the redox changes to modulate their activity (Guo et al, 2010). Interestingly, these authors propose that ATM may regulate global cellular responses to oxidative stress, remarking the essential link between redox control and DNA interacting, remodeling or repairing proteins. In Fanconi anemia for instance, Castillo and coworkers have shown that ATM dependent phosphorylation of FANCD2, one of the main proteins in the Fanconi anemia pathway of DNA repair, is necessary for normal S-phase checkpoint activation after oxidative stress (Castillo et al, 2011).

2.4.2 Regulation of telomerase activity by glutathione

The eukaryotic chromosomes are capped by telomeres, which consist of TTAGGG DNA sequences repeated in tandem, associated with several proteins, which protect the final regions of chromosomes. These structures play an important role in the stability and the complete replication of the chromosomes. Conventional DNA polymerases cannot fully replicate the 3′-end of the lagging strand of linear molecules, and therefore in every cell division telomeric sequences are lost (Komberg, 1969). Telomerase is an important enzyme that ensures the maintenance of normal telomere length. This activity is high in human cancers (Kim et al., 1994), but virtually absent in normal human tissues, except germinal cells (Harley et al., 1990). Telomerase regulation is not completely understood, but its changes are related to both cancer and aging (Sharpless & Depinho, 2004). Studies carried out by Jady et al. show that human telomeres are more accessible during the S-phase (Jady et al., 2006) and that the telomerase assembly with telomeres takes place at this specific moment of the cell cycle (Jady et al., 2006; Tomlison et al., 2006). Telomerase plays a key role in cellular homeostasis, because it maintains the length of the telomeres. This especially important in germinal cells in which it is necessary to keep a normal telomeric length after many cellular divisions. Important contributions about the epigenetic control of telomeres have been reported recently (Koziel et al., 2011). In that way, Maria Blasco has suggested that telomeres are under epigenetic control (García-Cao et al., 2004). Mammalian telomeres and subtelomeric regions are enriched in epigenetic marks that are characteristic of heterochromatin. In addition, histone deacetylase enzymes, such as Sirt6, regulate the telomeric chromatin conformation in order to allow the interaction of WRN protein with these chromosomal regions (Michishita et al., 2008).

There are evidence that point to a role of redox environment in a short term regulation of the activity of this important enzyme. Minamino et al., 2001, using vascular smooth muscle cells, reported that hypoxia up-regulates telomerase activity. Hypoxia is known to lower oxidative stress and thus to increase levels of glutathione. A specific inhibitor of telomerase, 2-[3-(trifluoromethyl) phenyl]isothiazolin-3-one, reacts with a key cysteine residue, which is essential for telomerase activity and must be kept reduced. Consequently, it has been reported that dithiothreitol reverses this inhibition (Hayakawa et al., 1999). Furthermore, antioxidants have been shown to inhibit nuclear export of telomerase reverse transcriptase and thus delay replicative senescence of endothelial cells (Haendeler et al., 2004). In conclusion, a critical cysteine residue must be kept reduced in order to maintain full telomerase activity. It is likely that the glutathione redox potential may be important in this process.

Previous findings of our group showed that telomerase is regulated by the shift in glutathione redox potential within values similar to those found *in* vivo and alterations in telomerase activity are coordinated with changes in critical cell cycle proteins, particularly Id2 and E2F4 (Borras et al., 2004).

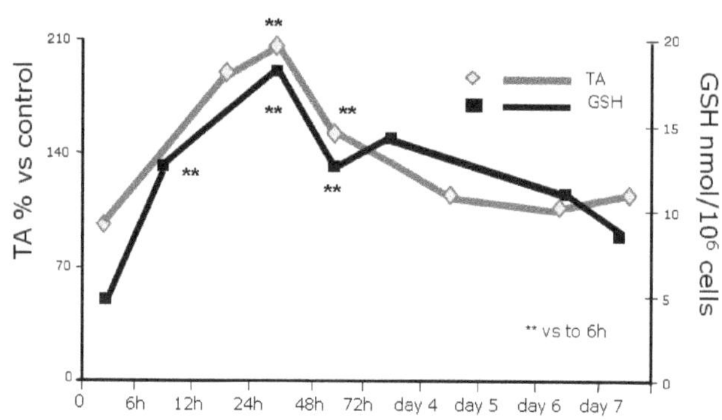

Fig. 1. Reduced glutathione regulates telomerase activity in 3T3 fibroblasts.

Thus, physiological variations in glutathione level induce changes in telomerase activities that are in concordance with changes in cell cycle regulatory proteins. A number of reports have shown similar results. Brown et al., 2007 demonstrated for the first time *in vivo* that high hepatic glutathione levels correlate with increased telomerase activity. Also, the importance of glutathione regulation in telomerase activity has been proved in endothelial progenitor cells (EPC): impairment of antioxidant defences in EPC promoted oxidant mediated apoptosis and telomerase inactivation which subsequently lead to development and/or progression of atherothrombosis (Fujii et al., 2006).

Recent data suggest that telomerase activity is regulated and ordered by telomere structure and telomerase assembly. Experimental evidence suggests that the telomere structure may change in a cell cycle-dependent manner to restrict telomerase activity to S phase (Hug & Ligner, 2006). In addition, telomere structure and specially the telomeric G-overhangs generation are strictly regulated during S phase and prolonged to other cell cycle phases depending on whether are telomeres from the lagging or the leading telomere (Dai et al., 2010). For this to happen, the precise control of the changes not only in telomerase conformation, but in chromatin structure (i.e. in its compactation level) as well, is of vital importance. This finding that telomere length, and, therefore, telomere structure, is tightly regulated in telomerase proficient cells invokes a connection between cell cycle, telomerase and telomere structure (Blasco, 2002). In other words, the mechanism that lies beneath telomerase regulation might be related with the mechanism that control cell proliferation. This opens a highly significant area for exploratory study and the diversity of processes and control mechanisms that could be involved in this phenomenon remain to be elucidated.

3. Compartmentalization of glutathione

3.1 The physiological importance of compartmentalization of glutathione

Pioneer work from Meister, (Meister & Anderson, 1983) correlated GSH synthesis and its degradation throughout the so-called γ-glutamyl cycle, and defined it as a cytosolic processes. The importance of cellular compartmentalization of GSH is two fold, first because it plays an important role in fighting against radical oxygen species (ROS). It is well known that these molecules have a very short half life and exert their action close to the place they were produced. Thus, the presence or absence of GSH could determine the development of localized oxidative damage for the cell structure or metabolic function developed in the vicinity. Secondly, GSH compartmentalization is of vital importance because of its role as a cellular detoxifying agent; it is known that tumours that have high glutathione levels are more resistant to chemotherapy, and the importance of nuclear (Voheringer et al., 1998) and mitochondrial (Benlloch et al. 2005) compartmentalization of GSH has been pointed out.

The overview of compartmentalization of glutathione in mammal cells is a complicated matter. This is due to the presence in the literature of a number of contradictory reports. The reason for the controversy is mainly methodological. Until very recently most reports were mainly based on cell-fractionation techniques. Those techniques appear to be reliable for mitochondrial studies; however their usefulness in nuclear or even endoplasmic reticulum measurements is at least controversial.

3.1.1 Nucleus

Although the role of nuclear GSH in the synthesis of DNA (Thelander & Reichard, 1979) and in protection against oxidative damage or ionizing radiation (Biaglow et al., 1983) is well established, little is known about the concentration of GSH in the nucleus and its regulation. This is due to two main factors. The first is methodological: it is impossible to determine the nuclear concentration of GSH using standard cell fractionation and analytical approaches (for a review see Söderdahl et al., 2003). The second factor is that most, if not all, of the reports share the common view of nuclear GSH distribution in a static situation. Cells are usually studied under steady state conditions *i.e.* when they are confluent (G_0/G_1 phase of the cell cycle). The nuclear membrane dissolves during mitosis and is formed again around newly replicated DNA packed in chromosomes; this spectacular change involves a variety of regulatory mechanisms. Therefore, if the nuclear GSH distribution is studied, the cell cycle physiology should be carefully considered.

The role of GSH in cell cycle regulation has been addressed mainly from the point of view of its overall cellular content. This is surprising since it is in the nucleus where most cell cycle progression events take place. The nucleus changes dramatically during the different phases of cell cycle, and failing to consider the corresponding changes in its redox environment could confer an important disadvantage in elucidating the actual importance of glutathione in the control of cell proliferation.

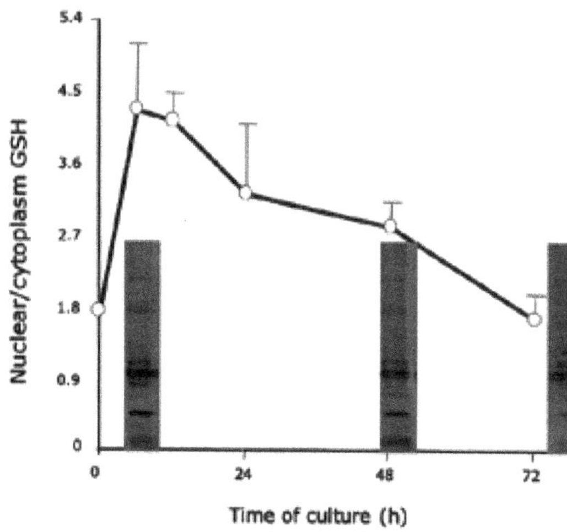

Fig. 2. Modifications of nuclear proteins along the cell cycle.

Our results, in general, are in accordance with the work of Hutter at al, (Hutter et al., 1997), who have studied the redox potential (E) in the normal and malignant cells along the cell cycle. The E of normal cells fluctuates during the cell cycle; for the proliferation to start it has to decrease at least 30mV comparing to its level in the G_0 phase (where the cells are 100% confluent). On the contrary, in cancer cells, the E remains low throughout the complete cell cycle, even at a high cell density (Hutter et al., 1997). Our evaluation of the GSH levels along the cell cycle in different models indirectly confirms these findings.

The work of Hutter et al. was further developed and completed by Hoffman et al. (Hoffman et al., 2008), who proposed recently a novel redox model of cell proliferation. They postulate the existence of a redox switch that helps regulate the proliferation within normal cells; its absence in cancer cells enables the bypass of the restriction point and leads to the loss of the control of cell cycle. The authors offer this model as a base to understand the aberrant cellular proliferation that leads to malignant transformation.

According to "redox model of cell proliferation", in normal cells exist a threshold value (θ) of $E \leq 207 \pm 11$mV which initiates the phosphorylation of different regulatory proteins associated with different phases of the cell cycle and, consequently, cell proliferation. When $E > \theta$ cell enters G1/G0 phase. However, when cancer cells are concerned, Hoffman does not take into account the fluctuations in the E level. In our hands, the increase in GSH level along the cell cycle (before the onset of the proliferation comparing to the GSH level at the final time point) is, indeed, less striking than in 3T3 fibroblasts; two-fold comparing to four-fold, respectively. The author hypothesizes, though, the existence of a reductive limit of -260mV which normal cell could not survive, but would not jeopardise cancer cell.

It was proposed previously that the proliferation occurs within the range of ROS levels, concentrations above or below this range could lead to growth arrest or cell death; hence ROS could act like a dual-edged sword (Davies, 1999).

3.2 Glutathione controls the cell cycle regulatory proteins

3.2.1 Id2 as a redox sensitive protein

The study of the expression of the Id2 along the cell cycle gave further support to this premise. The family of helix-loop-helix proteins denominated Id (inhibitor of DNA binding or inhibitor of differentiation) was demonstrated to be of considerable importance in the regulation of cell growth, differentiation and cancer in many mammalian tissues (Norton, 2000; Yokota & Mori, 2002). Id2, in particular, was shown to disrupt antiproliferative effects of tumour suppressor proteins of the Rb family, thus allowing cell cycle progression (Lasorella et al., 1996). Indeed, the pattern of the Id2 expression detected by Western blotting, confirmed the distribution of the phases of the cell proliferation detected by flow cytometry. This observation was previously published by our group suggesting a redox regulation of this protein (Borras et al., 2004). In addition, the studies of liver regeneration, process that involves DNA synthesis and cell proliferation, gave further support to our findings.

It was demonstrated that when the increase of GSH after partial hepatectomy was prevented, the liver regeneration was delayed and the total liver amount of the DNA was lower than in the control group (Huang et al., 2001). Furthermore, an early increase in Id2 gene has been demonstrated as well as the contribution of Id2 in the control of hepatocyte priming through modulation of c-myc expression (Rodriguez et al., 2006). All these support our notion that Id2 could be an excellent candidate as a protein marker of the redox regulation of cell proliferation in our models.

3.2.2 PCNA as a possible redox sensor in the onset of DNA synthesis

PCNA, a proliferating cell nuclear antigen, is a central protein in both DNA replication and repair. It's a "sliding clamp" that localizes proteins, such as DNA polymerase, to DNA and thus enables the correct DNA replication.

Replication of mammalian genome starts at thousands of origins, called replication foci, which contain PCNA and are activated at different times during S phase. The dynamics of replication foci is still a matter of debate; there are contradictory reports on the organization of the DNA replication sites in diverse cell types attributable to the differences in the technical approach (Dimitrova & Gilbert, 2000; Kennedy et al., 2000). According to Dimitrova, SD and Berezney, R (Dimitrova & Berezney, 2002) there is no fundamental difference in the spatiotemporal organization of the DNA replication in primary, immortalized and malignant mammalian cells. On the contrary, Kennedy's group (Kennedy et al, 2000), observed different patterns of replication foci in primary versus immortalized cell lines, as well as their perinuclear localization in the contact-inhibited cells prior to cell cycle exit (Barbie et al., 2004). Another fundamental question was weather the replication foci are moving along the DNA in the process of the replication, or the DNA is spooling through fixed replication factories. It seems that the important body of evidence is accumulating supporting the fixed-replication-site model (Dimitrova & Gilbert, 2000; Leonhard et al., 2000). The replication machinary bind to DNA, but they are also tethered to an underlying framework called nuclear matrix or skeleton (Leonhardt et al., 2000). Regardless of the discrepancies in their findings, all the authors call attention to the importance of the preserving nuclear architecture in order to guarantee the correct development of the process of DNA replication (Dimitrova & Gilbert, 2000; Barbie et al., 2004; Leonhardt et al., 2000). In addition, it has been shown that chromosome territory organization depends on association with the nuclear skeleton (Leonhardt et al., 2000). More than 20 years ago, Dijkwell et al. (Dijkwell & Wenink, 1986) postulated that the maintenance of the nuclear matrix, especially nuclear lamina, by preserving disulphide bonds depended on the level of nuclear thiols. In accordance to this work, Oleinick et al. (Oleinik et al., 1987) reported that DNA-protein cross links, present at basal level as normal associations of chromosomal loops with the nuclear matrix proteins, can be increased by ionising radiation and removal of intracellular glutathione, and decreased by hydroxyl radical scavengers. The importance of the GSH in cell proliferation could be extrapolated to the safeguarding of the nuclear architecture, providing in that way a proper milieu for the DNA replication. Our results could provide support to the hypothesis of Bellomo et al (Bellomo et al., 1997) that reduced nuclear glutathione may modulate the structural organization of chromatin. It is tempting to speculate that the high nuclear GSH level we observed before (late G1 phase) and at the onset of cell proliferation (S phase) could provide the redox environment that stimulates chromatin decompaction by reducing disulfide bonds.

3.3 Nuclear compartmentalization of glutathione as an important feature of proliferating cell: reduce to replicate

The functional compartmentalization is an obvious characteristic of eukaryotic cell. The organelles, visible by light microscopy, are surrounded by membranes, which, although permitting communication, provide unique and defined environment in each one, which guarantee its accurate function. Probably the most remarkable examples of compartmentalization are oxidative phosphorylation in mitochondria, protein folding in endoplasmic reticulum and, for the purpose of this study the most interesting of all, DNA synthesis. It is interesting to note that, when the first two organelles are concerned, the dependence of their function on the correct GSH level has been thoroughly studied. The high intramitochondrial concentration of GSH is maintained by an active multicomponent transport system "pumping" glutathione from the cytosol into the matrix (Matensson et al., 1990). On the contrary, for the correct folding of proteins into a native structure by disulfide bond formation, the GSH level and the ratio GSH/GSSG in the endoplasmic reticulum is maintained at extremely low level by the limited permeability of the vesicle membrane to GSH (Hwang et al., 1992). However, in the case of nuclear compartmentalization of glutathione the reports were scarce and contradictory over the years. This could be attributed to two main factors: methodological difficulties in measuring nuclear glutathione content and the focus of the research generally limited to confluent cells.

3.4 Modifications of nuclear proteins along the cell cycle

Various studies have demonstrated that the nucleus is more reduced than the cytosol (15mM GSH vs. 11 mM, respectively) (Bellomo et al., 1997; Schafer & Buettner, 2001; Soboll et al., 1995). An important number of nuclear proteins, including transcription factors, require a reduced environment to bind to DNA. More than 62 proteins are involved directly in transcription, nucleotide metabolism, (de)phosphorylation, or (de)ubiquitinylation, which are all essential processes for cell cycle progression (Connour et al., 2004). For instance, it appears that, at the onset of cell proliferation in the early G1 phase, an increase of ROS in the cytoplasm is necessary for the initiation of the phosphorylation cascade mediated by epidermal growth factor (EGF) that, subsequently, activates DNA replication and the cell division (Carpentes & Cohen, 1990). According to Jang and Surh (Jang & Surh, 2003) nuclear GSH may act as a transcriptional regulator of NF-κB, AP-1, and p53 by altering their nuclear redox state. The transcription factor NF-κB is an example of distinct redox-sensitive activation and DNA binding (Hansen et al., 2006); it is activated by various physiological stimuli known to produce ROS; on the contrary, to permit DNA binding, similar to Fos, Jun, and Nrf2, cysteine residue within DNA binding domain must be reduced. Both processes are guaranteed by the adequate redox state of the cytosolic and nuclear environment, respectively.

Interestingly, the nuclear proteins underwent stronger glutathionylation before and at the onset of cell proliferation than at quiescence. It is not surprising if we bear in mind that high level of GSH in the nucleus could provide protection to the proteins against the oxidative threat coming from the cytoplasm at the early phase of cell proliferation, and that glutathiolation, as it is a reversible modification, could be just the way. On the other hand, based on the simplicity of the redox transition from thiol to disulfide and on the fact that the reversibility was energetically favourable, Cotgrave IA and Gerdes RG (Cortgreave & Gerdes, 1998) more than 10 years ago have proposed glutathionylation as a posttranscriptional modification with the regulative finality. They state that it offers "a strong possibility for transducing "oxidative information" from intracellular oxidants via the GSH redox buffer to individual proteins containing "regulatory thiols". Also, recently, this posttranslational modification was proposed as a likely molecular mechanism for redox dependent signalling mediated by GSH (Fratelli et al., 2005). Thus, high level of GSH in the nucleus, observed before and at the onset of cell proliferation, could provide the "GSH redox buffer" necessary for the progressing of oxidant stimulated mitogenesis. It is encouraging to see that the findings of the present study have provided some support to the assumption that a dynamic intracellular redox environment directs the cell proliferation through redox sensitive cell cycle proteins.

4. The depletion of nuclear glutathione hampers the cell cycle progression

With the intention of providing further evidence of the importance of nuclear GSH in the initiation of cell proliferation, we have found ourselves in front of a challenge of depleting nuclear glutathione. A number of reports have focused on the consequences of the depletion of cellular glutathione levels on changes in cellular proliferation (Thomas et al., 1995; Hansen et al., 2006). However, all those reports were performed measuring cellular or total glutathione levels, but there is no information relating cellular proliferation with nuclear glutathione levels. A number of studies have indicated the existence of a nuclear GSH pool that resists depletion after exposure of cells to BSO (Thomas et al., 1995). BSO treatment resulted in the concentration dependent depletion of cytoplasmic GSH, while the depletion of mitochondrial and nuclear pool of GSH required concentrations higher than 100 μM, which induced DNA damage (Green et al., 2006). Spyrou and Holmgren (Spyrou & Holmgren, 1996) showed that inhibition of glutathione synthesis by 0.1 mM BSO was able to decrease GSH synthesis after treatment for 12 hours, but GSH-depleted cells grew as well as control 3T6 cells with no decrease in DNA synthesis. Thus, incubation of cells with low concentration of BSO, although decreases glutathione levels, does not change cell proliferation. On the other hand, Thomas *et al.* (Thomas et al., 1995) showed that non toxic concentrations of N-ethyl maleimide or DEM decreased the GSH level in the nucleus and cytoplasm to a similar extent, whereas the nuclear pool of GSH was much more resistant to BSO depletion.

Based on this findings, we have designed a model to study the effects on the cell proliferation parameters caused by GSH depletion both in the nucleus and the cytoplasm, using 100μM DEM, comparing to the administration of 10 μM BSO when nuclear GSH level is preserved.

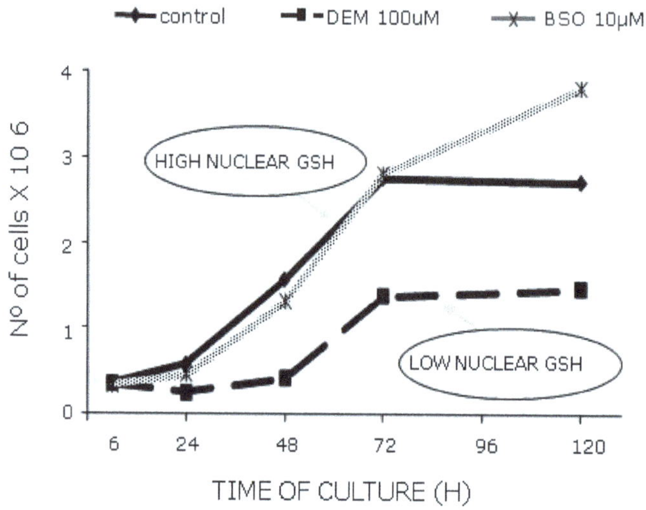

Fig. 3. Changes in cell proliferation caused by GSH depletion.

As reported previously by various authors (Britten et al., 1991; Green et al., 2006; Thomas et al., 1995) nuclear GSH pool was preserved. By contrast, depletion of glutathione levels by DEM induces a marked decrease in nuclear glutathione levels.

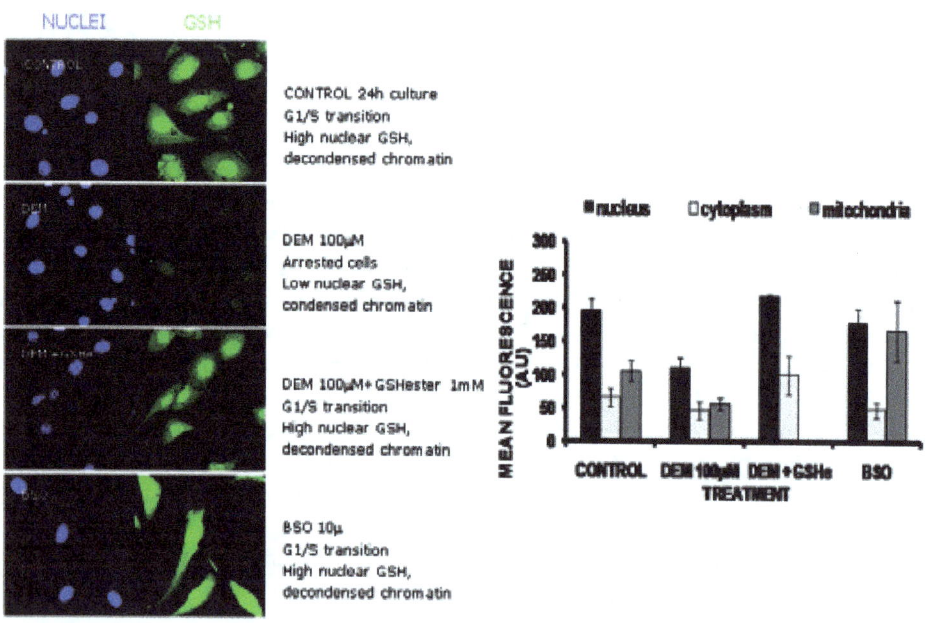

Fig. 4. The depletion of GSH in the nucleus.

The compartmentalization of glutathione depletion could explain the observed differences in the inhibition of cell proliferation. Indeed, our results show that inhibition of glutathione levels by DEM strongly impairs cell proliferation. This difference could be due to the fact that DEM decreases both nuclear and cytosolic glutathione levels in opposition to BSO, which only decreases cytosolic glutathione. It is worth mentioning that the impairment of cell proliferation could not be attributed to the alkylating properties of DEM, since the simultaneous administration of GSHe completely prevented it, nor to the toxicity of the treatment because the cell death was not significantly augmented.

In addition, we have observed the delay in the cell cycle progression caused by DEM, when both nuclear and cytoplasmic GSH was depleted, which is absent in the treatment with BSO when nuclear GSH pool was preserved. Interestingly, Esposito *et al.* (Esposito et al., 2002) showed that direct administration of DEM on the nuclear extracts of COS7 cells induces cell cycle arrest. So, it is daring to speculate that, despite the depletion of cytoplasmic GSH with DEM could not be overlooked, the effect on the cell cycle progression could be attributed to the depletion of the nuclear GSH. Moreover, as Esposito shows, the depletion of nuclear GSH strongly induces a p53-independent accumulation of p21, which causes a cell cycle arrest. In our study, the expression of cell cycle regulatory protein, suggested previously to be under redox control, Id2, was decreased when the level of nuclear GSH was depleted.

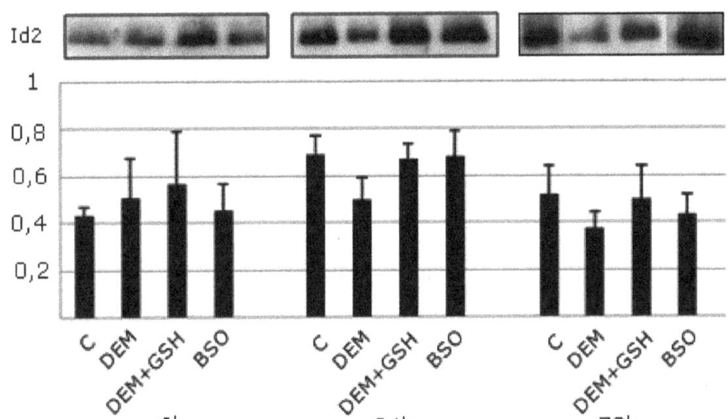

Fig. 5. Nuclear GSH depletion affects Id2 expression.

It has been known that cell proliferation is regulated by a variety of mechanisms working to allow the activation and repression of growth stimulatory genes, one of them being the transcription factors. Previous *in vitro* reports show that the activity of transcription factors is related to its redox environment. In addition, change in the redox potential could induce variations in the activity of those transcription factors. Alterations as small as $\pm$ 15 mV in the redox potential can result in transcription factor translocation and activation or deactivation, depending on the direction of the redox shift (Hutter et al., 1997; Sen & Packer, 1996; Sun & Oberley, 1996). Recently Reddy *et al.* (Reddy et al., 2008) have shown that Nrf2 deficiency leads to oxidative stress and DNA lesions, accompanied by impairment of cell-cycle progression, mainly G(2)/M-phase arrest. Both N-acetylcysteine and glutathione (GSH) supplementation ablated the DNA lesions and DNA damage-response pathways in Nrf2 (-/-) cells; however only GSH could rescue the impaired co-localization of mitosis-promoting factors and the growth arrest. Our results demonstrate for the first time that it is nuclear GSH levels, and not total cellular glutathione levels, that specifically correlate with cellular proliferation. Glutathione is considered essential for survival in mammary cells and other eukaryotic cells, but not prokaryotic cells. However, although a number of important functions have been attributed to GSH, its outstanding role in nucleated, but not in prokaryotic cells, remains unknown. Our results underscore the important role of nuclear glutathione in cell physiology and suggest that manipulation of nuclear GSH levels could be of paramount importance during development and cancer.

5. The occurrence of the glutathione in the nucleus; active transport, de novo synthesis, diffusion or something else

How GSH enters the nucleus and how it is regulated during the different phases of the cell cycle is still a matter of debate. The regulation of such interactions is also unclear. According to Smith and colleagues (Smith et al., 1996), the possible biochemical mechanisms responsible for the turnover of nuclear GSH are the following: 1.GSH may be taken up from the cytoplasm into the nuclei either passively or through energy-dependent processes 2.GSH may be synthesized *de novo* in the nucleus by the enzymes glutamate cysteine ligase and GSH synthetase 3.GSH may function to transport γ-glu-cys-cys.

5.1 ATP dependent sequestration of the GSH to the nucleus

The role of ATP-dependent mechanisms in maintaining the nuclear/cytoplasmic GSH concentration in hepatocytes was demonstrated by Bellomo and co-workers (Bellomo et al., 1997). After 20 min of incubation with the uncoupler protonophore carbonyl cyanide m-chlorophenylhydrazone (CCCP) the nuclear/cytoplasmic GSH gradient disappeared, but the total GSH content remain unchanged. This study was questioned by Briviba et al (Briviba et al., 1993) because of the use of monochlorobimane (BmCl). Despite its high specificity for glutathione this fluorochrome was found to be of no value in the study of cellular GSH distribution; once GSH-BmCl conjugate is formed it demonstrates an increased tendency of nuclear compartmentalization. Indeed, in our study using CMFDA, we have not found an ATP-dependent mechanism of nuclear GSH compartmentalization in 3T3 fibroblasts. Ho and Guenthner, 1997 using nuclear fractions concluded that GSH is taken up by the nucleus by passive diffusion and no evidence for an ATP-dependent mechanism for GSH concentration was observed.

5.2 Nuclear synthesis of glutathione

Glutamate cysteine ligase (GCL) and GSH synthetase activities have been reported in nuclei, and a portion of 4-8% of cell GSH synthetic activity is considered capable of maintaining nuclear GSH levels (Ho and Guenthner, 1997). However, we could not find GCL expression in nuclei of 3T3 fibroblasts. In addition as previously reported BSO, a specific inhibitor of GCL was unable of decreasing nuclear glutathione levels. Thus, at least under our experimental conditions, the possible "de novo" synthesis of nuclear glutathione seems improbable in 3T3 fibroblasts.

5.3 GSH enters nucleus via nuclear pores

The nuclear pore complex is the biochemical machinery that controls the molecular traffic across the nuclear envelope (Feldherr & Akin, 1990; Nigg, 1997). Ions and small hydrophilic

molecules, like glutathione, are considered to move by free and fast diffusion across the nuclear pore (Ribbeck & Gorlich, 2001); nevertheless ion gradients and transnuclear ATP-dependent membrane potential have also been reported (Nigg, 1997). In a series of creative experiments published in early 1990ies, Feldherr CM and Akin D (Feldherr & Akin, 1990; Feldherr & Akin, 1993), shown that permeability of nuclear envelope and nuclear transport were higher in proliferating than in quiescent cells. Reported seven fold reduce in the nuclear transport capacity was induced by the alterations in the characteristics of the pores and not by the changes within the cytoplasm, specifically, the decrease in ATP concentration. One pore forming protein that has been brought into the connection to nuclear glutathione content is Bcl-2. Voehringer and colleagues (Voehringer et al., 1998) showed that over-expression of Bcl-2 recruits GSH to the nucleus. The presence of this protein at the nuclear envelope was demonstrated (Krajewski et al., 1993) and the association with the nuclear pore complexes was suggested. Moreover, Zimmermann et al. (Zimmermann et al., 2007) demonstrated that GSH binds to Bcl-2 in mitochondria, providing a molecular basis for its antioxidant function.
A clear picture emerges showing that the presence of a reduced nuclear environment, probably provided by glutathione, glutaredoxin and thioredoxin mainly, is of paramount importance in the physiology of cell cycle, underscoring the role of oxidative stress in cell proliferation.

6. References

Atzori, L.; Dypbukt, J.M.; Sundqvist, K.; Cotgreave, I.; Edman, C.C.; Moldéus, P. & Grafström, R.C. (1990). Growth-associated modifications of low-molecular-weight thiols and protein sulfhydryls in human bronchial fibroblasts. *Journal of Cellular Physiology*, 143, 1, (April 1990), pp. 165-171, ISSN 0021-9541.

Barbie, D.A.; Kudlow, B.A.; Frock, R.; Zhao, J.; Johnson, B.R.; Dyson, N.; Harlow, E. & Kennedy, B.K. (2004). Nuclear reorganization of mammalian DNA synthesis prior to cell cycle exit. *Molecular and cellular biology*. 24, 2, (January, 2004), pp. 595-607, ISSN 0270-7306.

Benlloch, M.; Ortega, A.; Ferrer, P.; Segarra, R.; Obrador, E.; Asensi, M.; Carretero, J. & Estrela, J.M. (2005). Acceleration of glutathione efflux and inhibition of gamma-glutamyltranspeptidase sensitize metastatic B16 melanoma cells to endothelium-induced cytotoxicity. *Journal of Biological Chemistry*, 280, 8, (February 2005), pp. 6950-6959, ISSN 0021-9258.

Bellomo, G.; Palladini, G. & Vairetti, M. (1997). Intranuclear distribution, function and fate of glutathione and glutathione-S-conjugate in living rat hepatocytes studied by fluorescence microscopy. *Microscopy Research and Technique*. 36, 4, (February 1997), pp. 243-52, ISSN 1059-910X.

Biaglow, J.E.; Varnes, M.E.; Clark, E.P. & Epp, E.R. (1983). The role of thiols in cellular response to radiation and drugs. *Radiation Research*, 95, 3, (September 1983), pp. 437-455, ISSN 0449-3060.

Blasco, M.A. (2002). Telomerase beyond telomeres. *Nature Reviews Cancer*, 2, 8, (August 2002), pp. 627-33, ISSN 1474-175X.

Borrás, C.; Esteve, J.M.; Viña, J.R.; Sastre, J.; Viña, J. & Pallardó, F.V. (2004). Glutathione regulates telomerase activity in 3T3 fibroblasts. *Journal of Biological Chemistry*, 279, 33, (August 2004), pp. 34332-34335, ISSN 0021-9258.

Boyland, E. & Chasseaud L.F. (1969). Glutathione S-aralkyltransferase. *The Biochemical Journal*. 115, 5, (Decembre 1969), pp. 985-991, ISSN 0264-6021.

Britten, R.A.; Green, J.A.; Broughton, C.; Browning, P.G.; White, R. & Warenius H. M. (1991). The relationship between nuclear glutathione levels and resistance to melphalan in human ovarian tumour cells. *Biochemical Pharmacology*, 41, 4, (February 1991) pp. 647-649, ISSN 0006-2952.

Briviba, K.; Fraser, G.; Sies, H. & Ketterer, B. (1993). Distribution of the monochlorobimane-glutathione conjugate between nucleus and cytosol in isolated hepatocytes. *The Biochemical Journal*, 294, Pt 3, (September 1993), pp. 631-633, ISSN 0264-6021.

Brown, K.E.; Meleah Mathahs, M.; Broadhurst, K.A.; Coleman, M.C.; Ridnour, L.A.; Schmidt, W.N. & Spitz, D.R. (2007). Increased hepatic telomerase activity in a rat model of iron overload: a role for altered thiol redox state? *Free Radical Biology Medicine*, 42, 2, (January 2007), pp. 228-235, ISSN 0891- 5849.

Burchill, B.R.; Oliver, J.M.; Pearson, C.B.; Leinbach, E.D. & Berlin, R.D. (1978). Microtubule dynamics and glutathione metabolism in phagocytizing human polymorphonuclear leukocytes. *Journal of Cellular Physiology*, 76, 2, (February 1978), pp. 439-447, ISSN 0021-9541.

Canela, A.; Vera, E.; Klatt, P. & Blasco, M.A. (2007). High-throughput telomere length quantification by FISH and its application to human population studies. *Proceedings of the National Academy of Sciences of the United States of America*, 104, 13 (March 2007), pp.5300-5305, ISSN 0027-8424.

Carpenter, G.& Cohen, S. (1990). Epidermal growth factor. *The Journal of Biological Chemistry*, 265, 14 (May 1990), pp. 7709-7712, ISSN 0021-9258.

Castillo, P.; Bogliolo, M. & Surralles J. (2011). Coordinated action of the Fanconi anemia and ataxia telangiectasia pathways in response to oxidative damage. *DNA Repair(Amst)*. 10, 5 (May 2011), pp. 518-525, ISSN 1568-7864.

Conour, J.E.; Graham, W.V. & Gaskins, H.R. (2004). A combined in vitro/bioinformatic investigation of redox regulatory mechanisms governing cell cycle progression. *Physiological Genomics*, 18, 2 (July 2004), pp. 196-205, ISSN 1094-8341.

Cotgreave, I.A. & Gerdes, R.G. (1998). Recent trends in glutathione biochemistry--glutathione-protein interactions: a molecular link between oxidative stress and cell proliferation? *Biochemical and biophysical research communications*, 242, 1, (January 1998), pp. 1-9, ISSN 0006-291X.

Dai, X.; Huang, C.; Bhusari, A., Sampathi, S.; Schubert, K. & Chai, W. (2010). Molecular steps of G-overhang generation at human telomeres and its function in chromosome end protection. *The EMBO Journal*, 29, 16 (August 2010), pp. 2788-2801, ISSN 0261-4189.

Dalle-Donne, I.; Rossi, R.; Giustarini, D.; Colombo, R. & Milzani, A. (2007). S-glutathionylation in protein redox regulation. *Free Radical Biology Medicine*, 43, 6, (September 2007), pp. 883-898, ISSN 0891-5849.

Davies, K.J. (1999). The broad spectrum of responses to oxidants in proliferating cells: a new paradigm for oxidative stress. *IUBMB Life*, 48, 1, (July 1999), pp. 41-47, ISSN 1521-6543.

De Rey Pailhade, M. (1988). Sur un corps d'origine organique hydrogénant le soufre á froid. *C.R. Acad. Sci.* , 106, pp. 1683-1684, ISSN 1287-4620.

Dethlefsen, L.A.; Lehman, C.M.; Biaglow, J.E. & Peck, V.M. (1988). Toxic effects of acute glutathione depletion by buthionine sulfoximine and dimethylfumarate on murine mammary carcinoma cells. *Radiation Research*, 114, 2, (November 1988), pp. 215-224, ISSN 0449-3060.

Dijkwel, P.A. & Wenink, P.W. (1986). Structural integrity of the nuclear matrix: differential effects of thiol agents and metal chelators. *Journal of cell science*, 84, (August 1986) pp. 53-67, ISSN 0021-9533.

Dimitrova, D.S. & Gilbert, D.M. (2000). Temporally coordinated assembly and disassembly of replication factories in the absence of DNA synthesis. *Nature cell biology*, 2, 10, (October 2000), pp. 686-694, ISSN 1465-7392.

Dimitrova, D.S. & Berezney, R. (2002). The spatio-temporal organization of DNA replication sites is identical in primary, immortalized and transformed mammalian cells. *Journal of cell science*, 115, Pt 21, (November 2002) pp. 4037-4051, ISSN 0021-9533.

Ernst, V.; Levin, D.H. & London, I.M. (1978.) Inhibition of protein synthesis initiation by oxidized glutathione: activation of a protein kinase that phosphorylates the alpha subunit of eukaryotic initiation factor 2. *Proceedings of the National Academy of Sciences of the United States of America*, 75, 9, (September 1978), pp. 4110-4114, ISSN 0027-8424.

Esposito, F., Russo, T. & Cimino, F. (2002). Generation of prooxidant conditions in intact cells to induce modifications of cell cycle regulatory proteins. *Methods in Enzymology*, 352, pp. 258-268, ISSN 0076-6879.

Fratelli, M,; Goodwin, L.O.; Ørom, U.A., Lombardi, S., Tonelli, R., Mengozzi, M. & Ghezzi, P. (2005). Gene expression profiling reveals a signaling role of glutathione in redox regulation. *Proccedings of the National Academy of Science of the United States of America*, 102, 39, (September 2005) pp. 13998-14003, ISSN 0027-8424.

Feldherr, C.M. & Akin, D. (1990). The permeability of the nuclear envelope in dividing and nondividing cell cultures. *The Journal of cell biology*, 111, 1 (July 1990) pp. 1-8 ISSN 0021-9525.

Feldherr, C.M. & Akin, D. (1993). Regulation of nuclear transport in proliferating and quiescent cells. *Experimental cell research*, 205, 1, (March 1993), pp. 179-186, ISSN 0014-4827.

Fujii, H.; Li, S.H.; Szmitko, P.E.; Fedak, P.W. & Verma, S. (2006). C-reactive protein alters antioxidant defenses and promotes apoptosis in endothelial progenitor cells. *Arteriosclerosis, thrombosis, and vascular biology*, 26, 11, (November 2006), pp. 2476-2482 ISSN 1079-5642.

García-Cao, M.; O'Sullivan, R.; Peters, A.H.; Jenuwein, T. & Blasco, M.A. (2004). Epigenetic regulation of telomere length in mammalian cells by the Suv39h1 and Suv39h2 histone methyltransferases. *Nature Genetics*, 36, 1, (January 2004), pp. 94-99, ISSN 1061-4036.

Giustarini, D.; Rossi, R.; Milzani, A.; Colombo, R. & Dalle-Donne, I. (2004). S-glutathionylation: from redox regulation of protein functions to human diseases. *Journal of cellular and molecular medicine*, 8, 2, (April 2004), pp. 201-212, ISSN 1582-1838.

Grant, C.M.; MacIver, F.H. & Dawes, I. W. (1996). Glutathione is an essential metabolite required for resistance to oxidative stress in the yeast Saccharomyces cerevisiae. *Current Genetics*, 29, 6, (May 1996), pp. 511-515, ISSN 0172-8083.

Green, R.M.; Graham, M.; O'Donovan, M.R., Chipman, J.K. & Hodges, N.J. (2006). Subcellular compartmentalization of glutathione: correlations with parameters of oxidative stress related to genotoxicity. *Mutagenesis*, 21, 6, (Novembre 2006), pp. 383-390, ISSN 0267-8357.

Greenberg, J.T. & Demple, B. (1986). Glutathione in Escherichia coli is dispensable for resistance to H2O2 and gamma radiation. *Journal of Bacteriology*, 168, 2, (November 1986), pp. 1026-1029, ISSN 0021-9193.

Guo, Z.; Kozlov, S.; Lavin, M.F.; Person, M.D. & Paull T. (2010)ATM Activation by Oxidative Stress. *Science*. 22, 330, (October, 2010), pp. 517-521 ISSN 0193-4511.

Haendeler, J.; Hoffmann, J.; Diehl, J.F.; Vasa, M.; Spyridopo ulos, I.; Zeiher, A.M. & Dimmeler, S. (2004). Antioxidants inhibit nuclear export of telomerase reverse transcriptase and delay replicative senescence of endothelial cells. *Circulation Research*, 94, 6, (April 2004), pp. 768-775, ISSN 0009-7330.

Halliwell, B. (2007). Oxidative stress and cancer: have we moved forward?. *Biochemical Journal*, 401, 1, (January 2007), pp. 1-11, ISSN 0264-6021.

Hansen, J.M.; Go, Y.M. & Jones, D.P. (2006). Nuclear and mitochondrial compartmentalization of oxidative stress and redox signaling. *Annual Review of Pharmacology and Toxicol*ogy 46, (XXX 2006), pp. 215-234. ISSN 0362-1642.

Harley, C.B.; Futcher, A.B. & Greider, C.W. (1990). Telomeres shorten during ageing of human fibroblasts. *Nature*, 345, 6274, (May 1990), pp. 458-460, ISSN 0028-0836.

Harris, J.W. and Patt, H.M. (1969). Non-protein sulfhydryl content and cell-cycle dynamics of Ehrlich ascites tumor. *Experimental Cell Research*, 56, 1, (July 1969), pp. 134-141, ISSN 0014-4827.

Hayakawa, N.; Nozawa, K.; Ogawa, A.; Kato, N.; Yoshida, K.; Akamatsu, K.; Tsuchiya, M.; Nagasaka, A. & Yoshida, S. (1999). Isothiazolone derivatives selectively inhibit telomerase from human and rat cancer cells in vitro. *Biochemistry*, 38, 35, (August 1999), pp. 11501-11507, ISSN 0006-2960.

Ho, Y.F. & Guenthner, T.M. (1997). Isolation of liver nuclei that retain functional trans-membrane transport. *Journal of Pharmacological and Toxicological Methods*, 38, 3, (Novembre 1997), pp. 163-168, ISSN 1056-8719.

Hoffman, A.; Spetner, L.M. & Burke, M. (2008). Ramifications of a redox switch within a normal cell: its absence in a cancer cell. *Free Radical Biology and Meicine*, 45, 3, (August 2008), pp. 265-268, ISSN 0891-5849.

Holmgren, A. (1976). Hydrogen donor system for Escherichia coli ribonucleoside-diphosphate reductase dependent upon glutathione. *Proceedings of the National Academy of Sciences of the United States of America*, 73, 7, (July 1976), pp. 2275-2279, ISSN 0027-8424.

Hopkins, F. (1929). On glutathione: a reinvestigation. *Journal of Biological Chemistry*, 84, (1929), pp. 269-320, ISSN 0021-9258.

Huang, Z.Z.; Chen, C.; Zeng, Z.; Yang, H., Oh, J.; Chen, L, & Lu, S.C. (2001). Mechanism and significance of increased glutathione level in human hepatocellular carcinoma and liver regeneration. *The Faseb Journal*, 15, 1, (January 2001), pp. 19-21, ISSN 0892-6638.

Hug, N. & Lingner, J. (2006). Telomere length homeostasis. *Chromosoma*, 115, 6, (December 2006), pp. 413-25, ISSN 0009-5915.

Hutter, D.E.; Till, B.G. & Greene, J.J. (1997). Redox state changes in density-dependent regulation of proliferation. *Experimental Cell Research*, 232, 2, (May 1997), pp. 435-438, ISSN 0014-4827.

Hwang, C., A.J. Sinskey, and H.F. Lodish, (1992). Oxidized redox state of glutathione in the endoplasmic reticulum. *Science*, 257, 5076, (September 1992), pp. 1496-1502, ISSN 0193-4511.

Jády, B.E.; Richard, P.; Bertrand, E. & Kiss, T. (2006). Cell cycle-dependent recruitment of telomerase RNA and Cajal bodies to human telomeres. *Molecular Biology of the Cell*, 17, 2, (February 2006), pp. 944-954, ISSN 1059-1524.

Jang, J.H. &. Surh, Y.J. (2003). Potentiation of cellular antioxidant capacity by Bcl-2: implications for its antiapoptotic function. *Biochemical Pharmacology*, 66, 8, (October 2003), pp. 1371-1379, ISSN 0006-2952.

Jones, D.P. (2006). Redefining oxidative stress. *Antioxidants & Redox Signaling*, 8, 9-10, (September-October 2006), pp. 1865-1879, ISSN 1523-0864.

Kennedy BK, Barbie DA, Classon M, Dyson N, Harlow E. (2000). Nuclear organization of DNA replication in primary mammalian cells. *Genes and Development*, 14, 22, (Novembre 2000), pp. 2855-2568, ISSN 0890-9369.

Kim, N.W.; Piatyszek, M.A.; Prowse, K.R.; Harley, C.B.; West, M.D.; Ho, P.L.; Coviello, G.M.; Wright, W.E.; Weinrich, S.L. & Shay, J.W. (1994). Specific association of human telomerase activity with immortal cells and cancer. *Science*, 266, 5193, (December 1994), pp. 2011-2015, ISSN 0036-8075.

Krajewski, S.; Tanaka, S.; Takayama, S.M.; Schibler, M.J.; Fenton, W. & Reed J.C. (1993). Investigation of the subcellular distribution of the Bcl-2 oncoprotein: residence in the nuclear envelope, endoplasmic reticulum, and outer mitochondrial membranes. *Cancer Research*, 53, 19, (October 1993), pp. 4701-4714, ISSN 0008-5472.

Kornberg, A. (1969). Active center of DNA polymerase. *Science*, 163, 874, (March 1969), pp. 1410-1418, ISSN 0036-8075.

Kosower, N.S. & Kosower, E.M. (1978). The glutathione status of cells. *International Review Cytology*, 54, (1978), pp. 109-160, ISNN 0074-7696.

Koziel. J.E.; Fox, M.J.; Steding, C.E.; Sprouse, A.A. & Herbert, B.S. (2011). . Medical genetics and epigenetics of telomerase. *Journal of cellular and molecular medicine*, 15, 3, (March, 2011), pp. 457-467 ISNN 1582-1838.

Lasorella, A.; Iavarone, A. & Israel, M.A. (1996). Id2 specifically alters regulation of the cell cycle by tumor suppressor proteins. *Molecular and cellular biology*, 16, 6, (June 1996), pp. 2570-2578, ISSN 0270-7306.

Leonhardt, H.; Rahn, H.P.; Weinzierl, P.; Sporbert, A.; Cremer, T.; Zink, D. & Cardoso M.C. (2000). Dynamics of DNA replication factories in living cells. *The Journal of Cellular Biology*, 149, 2, (April 2000), pp. 271-280, ISSN 0021-9525.

Martensson, J.; Lai, J.C. & Meister, A. (1990). High-affinity transport of glutathione is part of a multicomponent system essential for mitochondrial function. *Proccedings of the National Academy of Sciences of the United States of America*, 87, 18, (September 1990), pp. 7185-7189, ISSN 0027-8424.

Meister, A. & Anderson, M. E. (1983). Glutathione. *Annual Review of Biochemistry*, 52, (1983), pp. 711-760, ISSN 0066-4154.

Menon, S.G.; Sarsour, E.H.; Spitz, D.R.; Higashikubo, R.; Sturm, M.; Zhang, H. & Goswami, P.C. (2003). Redox regulation of the G1 to S phase transition in the mouse embryo fibroblast cell cycle. *Cancer Research*, 63, 9, (May 2003), pp. 2109-2117 ISSN 1078-0432.

Menon, S.G. & Goswami, P.C. (2007). A redox cycle within the cell cycle: ring in the old with the new. *Oncogene*, 26, 8, (February 2007), pp. 1101-1109, ISSN 0950-9232.

Michishita, E.; McCord, R.A.; Berbe,r E., Kioi, M., Padilla-Nash, H., Damian, M., Cheung, P.; Kusumoto, R., Kawashara, T.L.; Barrett, JC.; Chang, H.Y.; Bohr, V.A.; Ried, T.; Gozani, O. & Chua, K.E. (2008). SIRT6 is a histone H3 lysine 9 deacetylase that modulates telomeric chromatin. *Nature*. 452, 7186, (March 2008), pp. 492-496, ISSN 0028- 0836.

Minamino, T.; Mitsialis, S.A. & Kourembanas, S. (2001). Hypoxia extends the life span of vascular smooth muscle cells through telomerase activation. *Molecular and Cellular Biology*, 21, 10, (May 2001), pp. 3336-3342, ISSN 0270-7306.

Miranda-Vizuete, A.; Rodríguez-Ariza, A.; Toribio, F.; Holmgren, A.; López-Barea, J. & Pueyo, C. (1996). The levels of ribonucleotide reductase, thioredoxin, glutaredoxin 1, and GSH are balanced in Escherichia coli K12. *Journal of Biology Chemistry*, 271, 32, (August 1996), pp. 19099-19103, ISSN 0042-6989.

Nigg, E.A. (1997). Nucleocytoplasmic transport: signals, mechanisms and regulation. *Nature*, 386, 6627, (April 1997), pp. 779-787, ISSN 0028- 0836.

Nkabyo, Y.S.; Ziegler, T.R.; Gu, L.H.; Watson, W.H. & Jones, D.P. (2002). Glutathione and thioredoxin redox during differentiation in human colon epithelial (Caco-2) cells. *American journal of physiology: Gastrointestinal and liver physiology*, 283, 6, (December 2002), pp. G1352-1359, ISSN 0193-1857.

Norton, J.D. (2000). ID helix-loop-helix proteins in cell growth, differentiation and tumorigenesis. *Journal of Cell Science*, 113, Pt 22, (November 2000), pp. 3897-905, ISSN 0021-9533.

Oberley, L.W.; Oberley, T.D. & Buettner, G.R. (1981). Cell division in normal and transformed cells: the possible role of superoxide and hydrogen peroxide. *Medical Hypotheses*, 7, 1, (January 1981), pp. 21-42, ISSN 0306-9877.

Oleinick, N.L.; Chiu, S.M.; Ramakrishnan, N. & Xue, L.Y. (1987). The formation, identification, and significance of DNA-protein cross-links in mammalian cells. *The British Journal of Cancer Supplement*, 8, (June 1987), pp. 135-140, ISSN 0306-9443.

Painter, R. B. & Young, B. R. (1980). Radiosensitivity in ataxia-telangiectasia: A new explanation. *Proceedings of the National Academy of Sciences of the United States of America*, 77, 12 (December 1980), pp. 127315-7317 ISSN 0027-8424.

Pani, G.; Colavitti, R.; Bedogni, B.; Anzevino, R.; Borrello, S. & Galeotti, T. (2000). A redox signaling mechanism for density-dependent inhibition of cell growth. *Journal of Biology Chemistry*, 275, 49, (December 2000), pp. 38891-38899, ISSN 0042-6989.

Pineda-Molina, E.; Klatt, P.; Vázquez, J.; Marina, A.; García de Lacoba, M.; Pérez-Sala, D. & Lamas, S. (2001). Glutathionylation of the p50 subunit of NF-kappaB: a mechanism for redox-induced inhibition of DNA binding. *Biochemistry*, 40, 47, (November 2001), pp. 14134-14142, ISSN 0006-2960.

Post, G.B., Keller, DA.; Connor, K.A. & Menzel, D.B. (1983) Effects of culture conditions on glutathione content in A549 cells. *Biochemical and Biophysical Research Communication*, 114, 2, (July 1983), pp. 737-742, ISSN 0006-291X.

Reddy, N.M.; Kleeberger, S.R.; Bream, .JH.; Fallon, P.G.; Kensler, T.W.; Yamamoto, M. & Reddy, S.P. (2008). Genetic disruption of the Nrf2 compromises cell-cycle progression by impairing GSH-induced redox signaling. *Oncogene*, 27, 44, (October 2008), pp. 5821-5832, ISSN 0950-9232.

Reynaert, N.L.; van der Vliet, A.; Guala, A.S.; McGovern, T.; Hristova, M.; Pantano, C.; Heintz, N.H.; Heim, J.; Ho, Y.S.; Matthews, D.E.; Wouters, E.F. & Janssen-Heininger, Y.M. (2006). Dynamic redox control of NF-kappaB through glutaredoxin-regulated S-glutathionylation of inhibitory kappaB kinase beta. *Proceedings of the National Academy of Sciences of the United States of America*, 103, 35, (August 2006), pp. 13086-13091, ISNN 0027-8424.

Ribbeck, K. & Gorlich, D. (2001). Kinetic analysis of translocation through nuclear pore complexes. *The EMBO Journal*, 20, 6, (March 2001): pp. 1320-1330, ISSN 0261-4189.

Rodriguez, J.L.; Sandoval, J.; Serviddio, G.; Sastre, J.; Morante, M.; Perrelli, M.G.; Martínez-Chantar, M.L.; Viña, J.; Viña, J.R.; Mato, J.M.; Avila, M.A.; Franco, L.; López-Rodas, G.& Torres, L. (2006). Id2 leaves the chromatin of the E2F4-p130-controlled c-myc promoter during hepatocyte priming for liver regeneration. *The Biochemical Journal*, 398, 3, (September 2006) pp. 431-437, ISSN 0264-6021.

Rodríguez-Manzaneque, M.T.; Ros, J.; Cabiscol, E.; Sorribas, A. & Herrero, E. (1999). Grx5 gluta redoxin plays a central role in protection against protein oxidative damage in Saccharomyces cerevisiae. *Molecular and Cellular Biology*, 19, 12, (December 1999), pp. 8180-8190, ISNN 0270- 7306.

Schafer, F.Q. & Buettner, G.R. (2001). Redox environment of the cell as viewed through the redox state of the glutathione disulfide/glutathione couple. *Free Radical Biology Medicine*, 30, 11, (June 2001), pp. 1191-212, ISSN 0891- 5849.

Sen, C.K. & Packer, L. (1996). Antioxidant and redox regulation of gene transcription. *The FASEB Journal*, 10, 7, (May 1996) pp. 709-720, ISSN 0892-6638.

Sharpless, N.E. & DePinho, R. A. (2004). Telomeres, stem cells, senescence, and cancer. *Journal of Clinical Investigation*, 113, 2, (January 2004), pp. 160-168, ISSN 0021-9738.

Sies, H. & Cadenas, E. (1985). Oxidative stress: damage to intact cells and organs. *Philosophical transactions of the Royal Society of London. Series B, Biological sciences*, 311, 1152, (December 1985), pp. 617-631, ISSN 0962-8436.

Sies, H. (1999). Glutathione and its role in cellular functions. *Free Radical Biology Medicine*, 27, 9-10, (November 1999), pp. 916-921, ISSN 0891- 5849.

Smith, J.E. (1977). Elevated erythrocyte glutathione associatd with elevated substrate in high-and low-glutathione sheep. *Biochemica et Biophysica Acta*, 496, 2, (February 1977), pp. 516-520, ISSN 006-3002.

Smith, C.V.; Jones, D.P.; Guenthner, T.M.; Lash, L.H. & Lauterburg, B.H. (1996). Compartmentalization of glutathione: implications for the study of toxicity and disease. *Toxicology and Applied Pharmacology*, 140, 1, (September 1996), pp. 1-12, ISSN 0041-008X.

Soboll, S.; Gründel, S.; Harris, J.; Kolb-Bachofen. V.; Ketterer, B. & Sies, H. (1995). The content of glutathione and glutathione S-transferases and the glutathione peroxidase activity in rat liver nuclei determined by a non-aqueous technique of cell fractionation. *The Biochemical Journal*, 311, Pt 3, (November 1995), pp. 889-894, ISSN 0264-6021.

Söderdahl ,T.; Enoksson, M.; Lundberg, M.; Holmgren, A.; Ottersen, O.P.; Orrenius, S.; Bolcsfoldi, G. & Cotgreave, I.A. (2003). Visualization of the compartmentalization of glutathione and protein-glutathione mixed disulfides in cultured cells. *Faseb Journal*, 17, 1, (January 2003), pp. 124-126, ISSN 0892-6638.

Spector, D.; Labarre, J. & Toledano, M.B. (2001). A genetic investigation of the essential role of glutathione: mutations in the proline biosynthesis pathway are the only suppressors of glutathione auxotrophy in yeast. *Journal of Biology Chemistry*, 276, 10, (March 2001), pp. 7011-7016, ISSN 0042-6989.

Spyrou, G. & Holmgren, A. (1996). Deoxyribonucleoside triphosphate pools and growth of glutathione-depleted 3T6 mouse fibroblasts. *Biochemical and Biophysical Research Communications*, 220, 1, (March 1996), pp. 42-46, ISSN 0006-291X.

Sun, Y. & Oberley, L.W. (1996). Redox regulation of transcriptional activators. *Free Radical Biology Medicine*, 21, 3, (1996), pp. 335-348, ISSN 0891- 5849.

Suthanthiran, M.; Anderson, M.E.; Sharma, V.K. & Meister, A. (1990). Glutathione regulates activation-dependent DNA synthesis in highly purified normal human T lymphocytes stimulated via the CD2 and CD3 antigens. *Proceedings of the National Academy of Sciences of the United States of America*, 87, 9, (May 1990), pp. 3343-3347, ISSN 0027-8424.

Tateishi, N.; Higashi, T.; Shinya, S.; Naruse, A. & Sakamoto, Y. (1974). Studies on the regulation of glutathione level in rat liver. *Journal of Biochemistry*, 75, 1, (January 1974), pp. 93-103, ISSN 0021-9258.

Thelander, L. & Reichard, P. (1979). Reduction of ribonucleotides. *Annual Review Biochemistry*, 48, (1979), pp. 133-158, ISSN 0066-4154.

Thomas, M.; Nicklee, T. & Hedley, D.W. (1995). Differential effects of depleting agents on cytoplasmic and nuclear non-protein sulphydryls: a fluorescence image cytometry study. *British Journal of Cancer*, 72, 1, (July 1995), pp. 45-50, ISSN 0007-0929.

Tomlinson, R.L.; Ziegler, T.D.; Supakorndej, T.; Terns, R.M. & Terns, M.P. (2006). Cell cycle-regulated trafficking of human telomerase to telomeres. *Molecular and Cellular Biology*, 17, 2, (February 2006), pp. 955-965, ISSN 0270- 7306.

Vina, J.; Hems, R. & Krebs, H.A. (1978). Maintenance of glutathione content is isolated hepatocyctes. *Biochemical Journal*, 170, 3, (March 1978), pp. 627-630, ISSN 0264-6021.

Viña, J.; Saez, G.T.; Wiggins, D.; Roberts, A.F.; Hems, R. and Krebs, H.A. (1983). The effect of cysteine oxidation on isolated hepatocytes. *Biochemical Journal*, 212, 1, (April 1983), pp. 39-44, ISSN 0264-6021.

Vina, J. &.Vina, J.R. (1983). Role of gamma glutamil traspeptidase in the regulation of amino acid uptake by mammary gland of the lactating rat., in Functions of glutathione. Biochemical, physiological, Toxicological and clinical aspects, A.L.e. al, Editor. 1983, Raven press New York. p. 23-30, ISBN 10:0890049084.

Viña, J. (1990). Glutathione: Metabolism and Physiological Function. *CRC Press Boston,* ISBN 10:0849332745.

Voehringer, D.W.; McConkey, D.J.; McDonnell, T.J.; Brisbay, S. & Meyn, R.E. (1998). Bcl-2 expression causes redistribution of glutathione to the nucleus *Proceedings of the National Academy of Sciences of the United States of America*, 95, 6, (March 1998), pp. 2956-2960, ISSN 0027-8424.

Wang, P.J.; Chabes, A.; Casagrande, R.; Tian, X.C.; Thelander, L. & Huffaker, T.C. (1997). Rnr4p, a novel ribonucleotide reductase small-subunit protein. *Molecular and Cellular Biology*, 17, 10, (October 1997), pp. 6114-6121, ISSN 0270- 7306.

Yokota, Y. & Mori, S. (2002). Role of Id family proteins in growth control. *Journal of Cellular Physiology*, 190, 1, (January 2002) pp. 21-28, ISSN 0021-9541.

Zahedi, A.V. & Homgren A. (2009). Molecular mechanisms of thioreoxin and glutaredoxin as hydrogen donors for Mammalian S Phase ribonucleotide reductase. *The Journal of Biological Chemistry*, 284, 13, (March 2009), pp. 8233-8240, ISSN 0021-9258.

Ziegler, D.M. (1985). Role of reversible oxidation-reduction of enzyme thiols-disulfides in metabolic regulation. *Annual Review Biochemistry*, 54, (1985), pp. 305-329, ISSN 0066-4154.

Zimmermann, A.K.; Loucks, F.A.; Schroeder, E.K.; Bouchard, R.J.; Tyler, K.L. & Linseman D.A. (2007). Glutathione binding to the Bcl-2 homology-3 domain groove: a molecular basis for Bcl-2 antioxidant function at mitochondria. *The Journal of Biological Chemistry*, 282, 40, (October 2007), pp. 29296-29304, ISSN 0021-9258.

Zhou, B-B.S. & Elledge, S. (2000). The DNA damage response: putting checkpoints in perspective. *Nature*, 408, 6811 (November 2000) pp. 433-439, ISSN 0028-0836.

3

DNA Repair in Pathogenic Eukaryotic Cells: Insights from Comparative Genomics of Parasitic Protozoan

Laurence A. Marchat[1,2], Mavil López-Casamichana[3], Esther Orozco[3] and César López-Camarillo[3]
[1]*Escuela Nacional de Medicina y Homeopatía-IPN, Programa Institucional de Biomedicina Molecular*
[2]*Programa de Doctorado en Biotecnología en Red-IPN*
[3]*Universidad Autónoma de la Ciudad de México, Posgrado en Ciencias Genómicas*
México

1. Introduction

Numerous external and internal DNA damaging agents can affect genetic material to produce single-strand breaks (SSB), double strand breaks (DSB), inter- and intra-strand cross-links in the form of cyclobutane pyrimidine dimers and (6-4)-photoproducts, oxidation and alkylation of bases, or formation of bulky chemical adducts. Cells possess several biological processes that act in a coordinated way to supervise DNA molecules and properly repair DNA lesions to minimize genetic information loss. This DNA repair system, which has been conserved throughout eukaryotes and prokaryotes evolution, includes various pathways that can be classified according to the type of DNA lesion they can restore: i) DSB, the most detrimental lesions of DNA, can be repaired by homologous recombination (HRR) and non-homologous end joining (NHEJ) pathways [Fleck & Nielsen, 2004]; ii) aberrant bases or nucleotides from a single strand DNA can be repaired by base excision repair (BER), nucleotide excision repair (NER) and mismatch repair (MMR) pathways using the complementary strand as template for DNA synthesis. BER mainly restores non-bulky lesions that result from bases alkylation, oxidation or deamination [Krokan et al., 1997]. The main task of NER pathway, which consists in two subpathways: global genome repair (GGR) to remove damage in the overall genome and transcription-coupled repair (TCR) to specifically repair the transcribed strand of active genes, is to eliminate photoproducts produced by ultraviolet (UV) light and other bulky lesions, such as inter- and intra-strand crosslinks [Prakash &Prakash, 2000]. MMR allows the removal of base mismatches and small insertion/deletion loops (IDL) that are formed during the replication process [Marti et al., 2002].

The genome of protozoan parasites is continuously subjected to the effects of antiparasitic drugs and host immune system attacks, which can affect its stability and therefore parasite survival. Thus, efficient DNA maintenance mechanisms are necessary to detect and accurately repair damaged nucleotides. The fully sequenced genome of the four major human pathogens described here provides new insights into parasite biology, including molecular features of

DNA repair mechanisms, and genome evolution. *Entamoeba histolytica* and *Giardia lamblia* (syn. *G. intestinalis, G. duodenalis*) are intestinal parasites that cause diarrheal diseases. *E. histolytica* is responsible for fulminating dysentery, bloody diarrhea, weight loss, fatigue, abdominal pain, which affect 50 million people and provoke 100,000 deaths in developing countries each year. In some cases, *E. histolytica* trophozoites can cross the intestinal wall and use the blood stream to reach different vital organs of the human body, usually the liver (but also the lungs, brain or spleen) to provoke liver abscesses, which can be fatal if untreated [Guo et al., 2007]. *G. lamblia* is another contributor to the enormous burden of diarrheal diseases with over 250 million symptomatic human infections per year worldwide. This anaerobic flagellated protozoa colonises and reproduces in the small intestine of several vertebrates, including human, causing giardiasis, commonly known as Beaver fever, which is characterized by diarrhea, excess gas, stomach or abdominal cramps, upset stomach, and nausea. Additionally, *Giardia* infection has an adverse impact on child linear growth and psychomotor development since the parasite causes iron-deficiency anemia, micronutrient deficiencies and growth retardation associated with diarrhea and malabsorption syndrome [Ankarklev et al., 2010]. Individuals become infected by *E. histolytica* and *G. lamblia* through ingesting or coming into contact with food, soil, or water that have been contaminated by the feces of an infected human or animal. *Plasmodium falciparum* is the protozoan parasite responsible for human malaria, which is one of the most severe infectious diseases with 240 million cases in 2009 and more than 1 million deaths in children each year in Africa alone. The presence of the parasite in red blood cells lead them to stick to blood vessels through a process called cytoadherence, which produce the obstruction of the microcirculation and dysfunction of multiple organs, typically the brain in cerebral malaria. Symptoms usually include fever and headache, in severe cases progressing to coma, and death (Kokwaro, 2009). Trichomoniasis caused by *Trichomonas vaginalis* is the most common nonviral sexually transmitted disease (STD) in the world [WHO, 1995]. It has long been recognized as a frequent cause of vaginitis in women and urethritis in men, but data now link it to cervical cancer and bad pregnancy outcomes [Cotch et al., 1997], as well as to an enhanced risk for human immunodeficiency virus transmission [Sorvillo & Kerndt , 1998]. Here, we combined the use of genomic approaches based on bioinformatic analysis of parasite genome sequence with the review of published reports to perform a comparative description of DNA repair machineries from *E. histolytica, G. lamblia, P. falciparum* and *T. vaginalis*, which cause high morbidity and mortality in many developed and developing countries.

2. DNA repair machineries in pathogenic eukaryotic cells

2.1 Identification of DNA repair machineries

In order to identify amino acids sequences of *E. histolytica, G. lamblia, P. falciparum* and *T. vaginalis* proteins related to DNA repair factors, we performed similarity searches in the Eupath database (http://eupathdb.org/eupathdb/) using the *Saccharomyces cerevisiae* DNA repair proteins from HRR, NHEJ, BER, NER and MMR machineries as probes [reviewed in Lopez-Camarillo et al., 2009]. Putative gene products were selected from BLAST analysis against each parasite database using the Blosum 62 scoring matrix and the following criteria: (i) at least 20% identity and 35% homology to the query sequence and (ii) e-value lower than 0.002, unless a portion of the protein showed a very strong similarity. All sequences, as well as the *E. histolytica* sequences obtained from previous work [López-Camarillo et al., 2009], were then verified by BLAST against *S. cerevisiae* and *Homo sapiens* databases to confirm their identity. Additionally, we also retrieved data from published reports about *G. lamblia*,

P. falciparum and *T. vaginalis* (**Table 1**). The absence of a given sequence in the table indicates that the corresponding gene was not identified in the parasite genome or that the sequence was too divergent to be detected by our *in silico* strategy.

None of the protozoan parasites studied here has the complete DNA repair pathways reported in yeast. HRR is the most conserved pathway suggesting that it is the mayor DSB repair pathway in these protozoan parasites. *E. histolytica, G. lamblia, P. falciparum* and *T. vaginalis* genomes contain most of the RAD52 epistasis group genes, although their functional relevance remains to be determined. Homologs for RAD50, RAD51, MRE11, RAD54 and RPA (lacking the RAD52 interacting domain) have been previously reported in *P. falciparum* [Voss et al., 2002; Malik et al., 2008]. In agreement with its participation in DNA repair, the *PfRad51* gene is overexpressed in the mitotically active schizont stage and in response to methyl methane sulfonate [Bhattacharyya & Kumar, 2003]. In. *T. vaginalis*, RAD50 y MRE11 were previously published as components of the meiotic recombination machinery, although meiosis has not been observed in this organism [Malik et al., 2008]. Ramesh et al. [2005] and Malik et al. [2008] identified the *Rad50/Mre11, Rad52* and *Dmc1 genes* involved in meiotic recombination machinery by HRR in *Giardia.* Intriguingly, *G. lamblia* and *P. falciparum* lack the *nsb1* homologue (*xrs2* in Yeast) that is a component of the MRN complex involved in DSB detection and 3′ ssDNA tails conversion. Recently, we published the *E. histolytica* RAD52 epistasis group involved in HRR [Lopez-Casamichana et al., 2007, 2008]. Interestingly, RT-PCR assays evidenced that some genes were down-regulated, whereas others were up-regulated when DSB were induced by UV-C irradiation, which revealed an intricate transcriptional modulation of *E. histolytica* RAD52 epistasis group related genes in response to DNA damage. Particularly, *Ehrad51* mRNA expression was 16-, 11- and 4-fold increased at 30 min, 3 h and 12 h, respectively. DNA microarrays assays confirmed the activation of *EhMre11, EhRad50,* and *EhRad54* genes at 5 min after DSB induction, suggesting that they represent early sensors of damage in HRR pathway [Weber et al., 2009]. Additionally, the molecular characterization of EhRAD51 showed that the presence of all the functional domains reported in yeast and human homologues. EhRAD51 was upregulated and redistributed from cytoplasm to the nucleus of trophozoites at 3 h after DNA damage and it was able to catalyze specific single-strand DNA (ssDNA) transfer to homologous double strand DNA (dsDNA) forming the three-stranded pairing molecule called D-loop structure, confirming that it is a *bonafide* recombinase in *E. histolytica* [Lopez-Casamichana et al., 2008].

G. lamblia and P. *falciparum* only have three of the eight factors of the NHEJ pathway (including the MNR complex also involved in HRR), which strongly suggest that they preferably use HRR to repair DSB. In contrast, almost all NEHJ pathway factors have been identified in *E. histolytica* and *T. vaginalis,* including the LIF1 ligase, RAD27 nuclease and MRE11/RAD50/NSB1 proteins. However, *E. histolytica* genome does not contain a homologous gene for KU80 subunit [López-Camarillo et al., 2009] and *T. vaginalis* lacks both *ku70* and *ku80* genes [Carlton et al., 2007]. As these proteins form a single KU complex that recognizes DSB sites and recruits other DNA repair factors, our findings could appear contradictory. The absence of conserved KU proteins has also been reported in *Encephalitozoon cunili* [Gill & Fast, 2007] and yeast [Hefferin & Tomkinson, 2005], thus it is possible that these organisms use highly divergent KU proteins to perform the NHEJ pathway.

The other key DNA repair mechanisms represented by BER, NER and MMR pathways operate to repair aberrant bases or nucleotides from a ssDNA using the complementary strand as template for DNA synthesis. As in *E. histolytica* [Lopez-Camarillo et al., 2009], the *G. lamblia* BER pathway appears to be largely incomplete, lacking *apn1, mag1, ogg1, rad10, mus81* and *mms4* genes. Both parasites live under oxygen-limiting conditions and have a highly reduced form of mitocondria called mitosomes [Tovar et al., 1999, 2003]. Then the absence of OGG1 could indicate that they do not suffer oxidative damage to mitochondrial DNA. In contrast, *Plasmodium* Flap endonuclease-1 (PfFEN-1) and Pf DNA Ligase I (PfLigI) have enzymatic activities similar to other species [Gardner et al., 2002; Casta et al., 2008], indicating that BER pathway should be functional in this parasite although several components are lacking.

Most genes involved in NER pathway are represented in *E. histolytica* [Lopez-Camarillo et al., 2009], *G. lamblia, P. falciparum and T. vaginalis* genomes suggesting that this mechanism could be potentially active in these eukaryotic parasites. PfXPB/RAD25, PfXPG/RAD2 and PfXPD/RAD3 have been previously reported in *P. falciparum* [Gardner et al., 2002; Bethke et al., 2007; Casta et al., 2008]. Additionally, the overexpression of *EhDdb1, EhRad23* and *EhRad54* genes after UV-induced DNA damage in *E. histolytica* [Weber et al., 2009] suggested that these genes could be involved in chromatin remodeling complexes as their homologues in human and yeast. *E. histolytica, G. lamblia* and *T. vaginalis* have various *rad3* genes to form the NEF3 complex (RAD2, RAD3, RAD25) of the BER pathway. Particularly, we identified six *rad3* genes and an additional truncated gene in *T. vaginalis*. On the other hand, all the parasites studied here lack almost one of the components of the TFIIH complex subunits (TFB1, TFB2 or TFB3).

As in bacteria, *Drosophila melanogaster, H. sapiens* and many other organisms [Lisby & Rothstein, 2005], *E. histolytica, G. lamblia* [Ramesh et al., 2005], *P. falciparum* [Bethke et al., 2007] and *T. vaginalis* [Malik et al., 2008] have almost all *S. cerevisiae* MMR genes, including the components of the MUTSα (MSH2/MSH6) heterodimer, which strongly suggest that MMR could be an active DNA repair pathway in these parasites. Notably, *E. histolytica* and *P. falciparum* have two *msh2* genes. However, neither *E. histolytica* nor *P. falciparum* present the *msh3* gene that is required for the formation of the MUTSβ (MSH2/MSH3) heterodimer. PfMSH2-1, PfMSH2-2, PfMSH6, PfMLH1 and PfPMS1 proteins potentially participating in MMR have been previously reported in *P. falciparum*. Inhibition of *PfMSH2-2* gene increased mutation rate and microsatellite polymorphism, indirectly demonstrating its relevance in MMR and microsatellite slippage prevention. Moreover, antimalarial drug resistance has been recently related to a defective DNA mismatch repair, mainly in PfMutLα content [Castellini et al., 2011], which demonstrated the relevance of this mechanism for the parasite biology.

Gene name	*E. histolytica*	*G. lamblia*	*P. falciparum*	*T. vaginalis*	*S. cerevisiae*
Homologous recombination repair (HRR) pathway					
rad50	C4M2L7	Q6WD96	C6KSQ6	A2FAD3	P12753
mre11	Q86C23 C4LVX7 C4M8N7*	Q86CI9 A8BR27*	PFA0390w**	A2ECB0	P32829
nbs1	C4M874	-	-	A2DHF7	P33301
rad51	C4M4K4	Q86C21	Q8IIS8 Pf11_0087**	A2FXT7	P25454
rad52	C4M197	Q6WD95	-	-	P06778
rad54 *rad54b*	C4LVM6 C4M7S7	-	Q8IAN4	A2FNE0	P32863
rad51c *rad57*	C4M5L7	-	-	A2GIB8	P38953 P25301

Gene name	*E. histolytica*	*G. lamblia*	*P. falciparum*	*T. vaginalis*	*S. cerevisiae*
rad59	-	-	-	-	Q12223
exo1	C4MBM5	A8BQ11	Q8IBK1	A2E2N7	P39975
rpa1	C4M8G6	-	Q9U0J0 Q8I3A1	A2G5D0	P22336
rpa2	C4LT79	-	-	-	P26754
sgs1	C4M4V5	A8BAJ1 A8B9Y0	Q8I2W7 Q8ILG5	A2DYY2	P35187
rad24	C4M5T7	-	-	A2D9F4	P32641
hpr5	-	-	Q8I3W6	A2F783	P12954
rad17 ddc1 mec3	- - -	- - -	- - -	- A2F0Q2 -	P48581 Q08949 Q02574
Non homologous end joining (NHEJ) pathway					
ku80 *ku70*	C4MBG9 -	- -	- -	- -	P32807 Q04437
lif1	-	-	-	-	P53150
dnl4	C4M5H3	-	-	A2DFX6	Q08387
rad27	C4M6G8	A8B672 D3KG58	Q7K734 Q8IJW1	A2GNP0	P26793
Base excision repair (BER) pathway					
apn1	-	-	Q9BMG7	-	P22936
apn21	-	A8BGE2	O97240	-	P38207
mag1	-	-	-	-	P22134
ogg1	-	-	Q8I2Y2	-	P53397
ntg1	C4M764 C4LYM7	-	Q8II68	A2DS55	P31378
ung1	C4LUV5	A8B632	Q8ILU6	A2GFQ7	P12887
pcna	C4M9R9	A8BIU1	P61074 Q7KQJ9	A2DQV2	P15873
rad1	C4LT01	D3KH96	Q8ID22	A2DS24	P06777
rad10	C4LW01	-	O96136	A2DBF5	P06838
cdc9	C4M5H3	A8BWV4	Q8IES4	A2DFX6	P04819
mus81	-	-	-	A2FKU9	Q04149
mms4	-	-	-	A2DHF7	P38257
Nucleotide excision repair (NER) pathway					
rad2	C4M0V9	-	O96154	A2GNP0	P07276
rad3	C4M8K7 C4M8Q4 C4M6T8	A8BYS3 A8B495	Q8I2H7	A2G2G8 A2E4I6 A2F1W2 A2DDD4 A2E1B9 A2ELX1 A2G2G9*	P06839

Gene name	*E. histolytica*	*G. lamblia*	*P. falciparum*	*T. vaginalis*	*S. cerevisiae*
rad4	-	-	-	-	P14736
rad7	-	-	-	-	P06779
rad14	-	-	-	-	P28519
rad16	-	A8BL62	Q8I4S6	A2D9P9	P31244
rad23	C4MAR5	D3KF29*	Q8IJS8	A2FM19	P32628
rad25	C4MA19	A8BMI7	Q8IJ31	A2DEA8	Q00578
rad26	C4MAR8	A8BK31	-	A2EXQ4	P40352
rad28	-	-	Q8IJ73	A2DZ24	Q12021
ssl1	C4LV67	A8BA50	Q8IEG6	A2ENQ3	Q04673
tfb1	C4LWV8	-	-	-	P32776
tfb2	C4MIG0	-	Q8I4Y8	A2E2N2	Q02939
tfb3	-	D3KH94	Q8I3Y3	-	Q03290
tfb4	C4M9E2	A8B6C2	Q8IDG5	A2EYI3	Q12004
Mismatch repair (MMR) pathway					
mlh1	C4M5R1	-	Q8IIJ0	A2EGR5	P38920
msh2	C4M9J9 B1N4L6	Q6WD97	Q8ILI9 C0H4L8	A2EP54	P25847
msh3	-	-	-	-	P25336
msh6	C4M4T8	A8BC61	Q8I447	A2EA54	Q03834
pms1	C4LW71	A8B4I6	Q8IBJ3	A2G2B4	P14242

Table 1. Comparison of DNA repair machineries from *E. histolytica, G. lamblia, P. falciparum, T. vaginalis* and *S. cerevisiae*. * fragment, ** PlasmoDB database.

2.2 Conservation of DNA repair pathways

To investigate the degree of conservation of DNA repair pathways in protozoan parasites, we next determined the values of Smith-Waterman identity scores between *E. histolytica* proteins and their corresponding orthologues in *G. lamblia, P. falciparum* and *T. vaginalis* by BLAST analysis based in pairwaise sequence alignments and calculated the mean value for each DNA repair machinery (**Fig. 1**). Data of the MNR complex which participate in HRR and NHEJ pathways were included in both mechanisms. DSB repair pathways were generally more conserved than Excision Repair mechanisms. Considering amino acids identity, mean values for HRR and NHEJ pathways were higher in *E. histolytica/P. falciparum* comparison, suggesting that *E. histolytica* machinery was closer to *P. falciparum* than to *G. lamblia* and *T. vaginalis* machineries. The comparison *E. histolytica/G. lamblia* evidenced that HRR is highly conserved between both parasites, whereas components of the other pathways were more divergent. In the case of *E. histolytica/P. falciparum* comparison, NHEJ appeared to be more conserved that HRR, while the identity of HRR and NHEJ factors was very similar in *E. histolytica/T. vaginalis*. In all the parasites, the RAD51 recombinase is the most conserved protein (51%, 58% and 64% when *E. histolytica* protein sequence was compared with *G. lamblia, P. faciparum* and *T. vaginalis* orthologues, respectively), which is consistent with its relevant role in HRR mechanism.

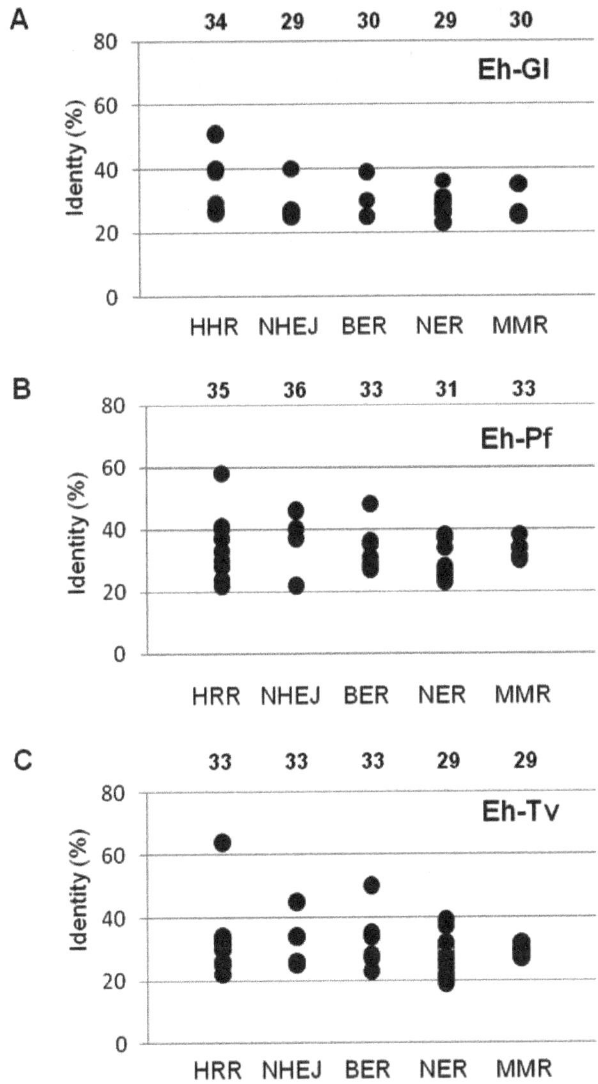

Fig. 1. **Conservation of DNA repair pathways between** *E. histolytica* **and** *G. lamblia* **(A),** *P. falciparium* **(B) and** *T. vaginalis* **(C).** Amino acids sequences from orthologous proteins were compared by Blast and the percentage of identity was determined through pair wise alignment of the most conserved region. Average identity of all pathways is indicated above each graph.

2.3 DNA repair activity in cell free lysates evidences the functionality of DNA repair proteins

Although insights about the activity of DNA repair proteins in protozoa have been mainly obtained from experimental evidence based in heterologous expression and characterization of recombinant proteins, some reports showed that DNA repair activity could be detected in whole cell extracts, supporting the notion that DNA repair pathways already operates *in vivo*. For instance, Haltiwanger et al., (2000) reported the characterization of an AP endonuclease activity in a *P. falciparum* cell free lysate. Authors provide evidence for the presence of class II, Mg^{2+}-dependent and independent AP endonucleases in the extracts. Moreover, they detected that *Plasmodium* AP endonuclease(s) possessed a 3´-phosphodiesterase activity similar to those described in other class II AP endonucleases [Demple et al., 1986]. In a related study, it was reported that a *P. falciparum* lysate contained uracil DNA glycosylase, AP endonuclease, DNA polymerase, flap endonuclease, and DNA ligase activities [Haltiwanger et al., 2000]. In contrast, DNA repair activities in cell lysates have not been detected in *Entamoeba, Giardia* and *Trichomonas* parasites. These data remark the utility of cell free lysates to understand DNA repair pathways, and pointed out to the urgency to investigate endogenous DNA repair activities using whole cell extracts in parasites where no data is available.

3. Functional categorization of *Entamoeba histolytica* DNA repair genes

To define the putative functions of *E. histolytica* DNA repair genes in unrelated DNA repair processes, we investigated the functional diversity of genomic maintenance pathways using Gene Ontology (GO) annotations. Functional related gene groups were predicted by the David bioinformatic resources (http://david.abcc.ncifcrf.gov/gene2gene.jsp), using a functional classification tool which generates a gene-to-gene similarity matrix based in shared functional annotation using over 75,000 terms from 14 functional annotation sources, allowing the classification of highly related genes in functionally related groups. Results from this analysis revealed that a large number of DNA repair genes were miss-annotated in parasites genome databases (43%). However, our analysis clearly showed that the majority of these genes seems to participate in DNA repair related processes. Besides, 57% of genes were predicted to function in DNA repair related process. 11% of genes participates in DNA damage repair, and 18% and 8% have helicase and endonuclease functions, respectively (**Fig. 2**).

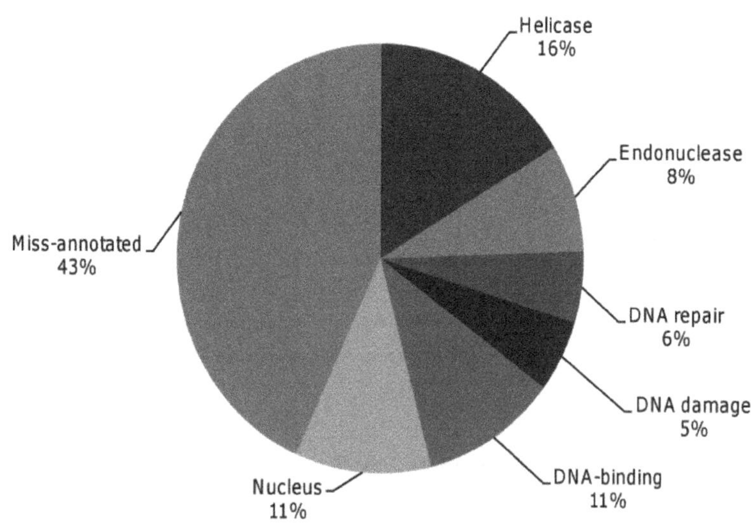

Fig. 2. **Functional categorizations of** *E. histolytica* **DNA repair genes.** Biological processes and molecular functions were determined using David software (http://david.abcc.ncifcrf.gov/gene2gene.jsp). Percentage of genes included in individual categories is given.

4. Duplicated genes: The case of *rad3*

Gene duplicates represent for 8-20% of the genes in eukaryotic cells, and the rates of gene duplication are estimated at between 0.2% and 2% per gene per million years. Gene duplications are one of the major motors in the evolution of genetic systems and may occur in homologous recombination, retrotransposition event, or duplication of an entire chromosome [Zhang, 2003]. Duplicated genes are believed to be a main system for the establishment of new gene functions generating evolutionary novelty [Long & Langley, 1993; Gilbert et al., 1997].

A detailed examination of **Table 1** revealed that several DNA repair genes are duplicated in protozoan parasites, while there is only one gene in yeast. For example, the HRR machinery includes two *rad51* genes in *P. falciparum*, two *rad54* and *mre11* genes in *E. histolytica* [Lopez-Casamichana et al., 2008], two *rpa1* genes in *T. vaginalis*, and two *sgs1* genes in *G. lamblia* and *P. falciparum*. We also identified two *rad27* genes in *P. falciparum* and *G. lamblia* NHEJ pathway, two *E. histolylica ntg1* and *P. falciparum pcna* genes in the BER pathway, as well as two *msh2* genes for the MMR pathway in *E. histolytica* and *P. falciparum*. But the most duplicated gene was the *rad3* gene from the NER mechanism, since there are three genes in *E. histolytica*, two in *G. lamblia* and six in *T. vaginalis*, whereas *P. falciparum* has only one *rad3* gene, alike yeast. Remarkably, gene duplication is evident for many other genes in *T. vaginalis* and reflexes the massive gene expansion inside the large genome of this pathogen [Hartl & Wirth, 2006]. In yeast, the RAD3 protein is involved in mitotic recombination and spontaneous mutagenesis, becoming essential for cell viability in the absence of DNA injury. Furthermore, this protein participates in the repair of UV-irradiated DNA via NER, and constitutes a subunit of RNA polII initiation factor TFIIH [Moriel-Carretero & Aguilera, 2010]. *S. cerevisiae* RAD3 is related to the *H. sapiens* XPD, also known as ERCC2. Defects in human XPD result in a wide range of diseases, including Xeroderma pigmentosum (XP), Cockayne's syndrome, and Trichothiodystrophy characterized by a wide spectrum of symptoms ranging from cancer susceptibility to neurological and developmental defects [Liu et al., 2008].

In order to describe the inferred evolutionary relationships among the most abundant duplicated gene found through the analysis of DNA repair machineries from the human pathogens studied here, we have undertaken a phylogenetic analysis of RAD3 helicase orthologues in *S. cerevisiae*, *E. histolytica*, *T. vaginalis*, *G. lamblia* and *P. falciparum*. We evaluated the minimum evolution of RAD3 proteins through the construction of Neighbor-Joining phylogenetic tree using the *MEGA* version 5.05 [Tamura et al., 2011]. The robustness was established by bootstrapping test, involving 500 replications of the data based on the criteria of 50% majority-rule consensus (**Fig. 3**). Two main branches that came from a common ancestor can be observed. On one branch, *T. vaginalis* RAD3 parologues are clustered into two sister proteins pairs (A2E1B9 and A2ELX1, A2E4I6 and A2DDD4), that have each evolved from the same ancestor. Besides, *E. histolytica* C4M6T8 is closer to *T. vaginalis* A2E4I6 and A2DDD4, than to its own paralogues. The other branch supports *T. vaginalis* A2G2G8 that is closely related to yeast and *P. falciparum* RAD3 proteins that came off the same node. Interestingly, these two organisms only have one *rad3* gene. This branch also includes *E. histolytica* C4M8K7 and C4M8Q4 sister proteins pair. Intriguingly, the two *Giardia* RAD3 proteins have emerged from different nodes and appeared to be more related to orthologues from other species than to each other; particularly, the branch supporting *Giardia* A8B495 also includes *Trichomonas* A2E1B9 and A2ELX1, while *Giardia* A8BYS3 is on the other branch, isolated from the other proteins, such as *Trichomonas* A2F1W2, which suggested that these proteins have evolved early.

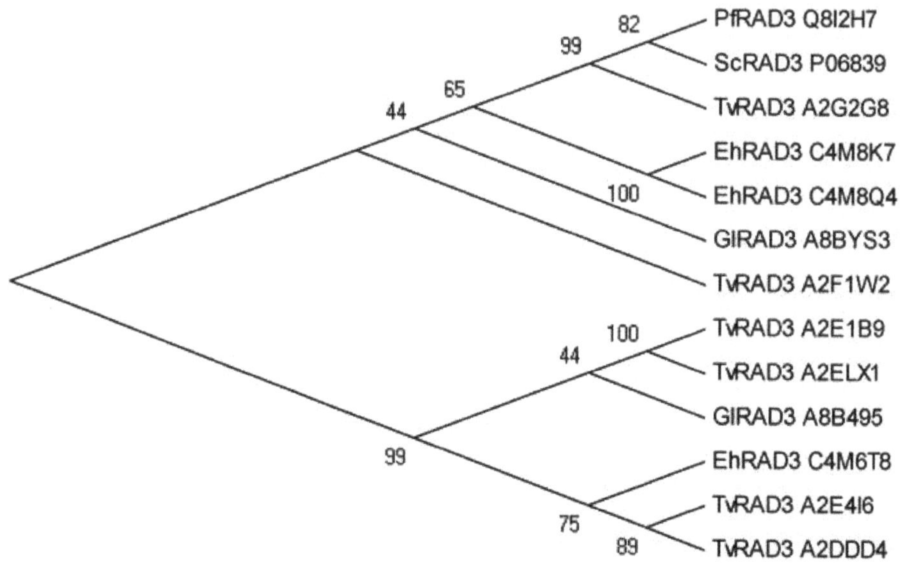

Fig. 3. **Phylogenetic relationships between RAD3 from** *S. cerevisiae, E. histolytica, T. vaginalis, G. lamblia* **and** *P. falciparum***.** The unrooted tree was created with the MEGA 5.05 program using the Neighbor Joining algorithm based on ClustalW. Numbers above the tree nodes indicate the percentage of times that the branch was recovered in 500 replications.

5. Molecular organization of the MNR complex

The MRE11-RAD50-NBS1 (MRN) complex is considered to have an imperative function in DSB repair. This protein complex operates as DSB sensor, co-activator of DSB-induced cell cycle checkpoint signaling, and as a DSB repairs effector in both the HRR and NHEJ pathways [Taylor et al., 2010; Rass et al., 2009]. Additionally, it has also been found to associate with telomeres maintenance at the ends of linear chromosomes. MRE11 and RAD50 orthologues have been reported in all taxonomic Kingdoms. MRE11, RAD50, and XRS2 (the *S. cerevisiae* homologue of vertebrate-specific NBS1) were initially recognized through yeast resistance to DNA damage induced by UV light and X-rays and meiotic recombination studies [Ogawa et al., 1995]. To efficiently perform these functions, this complex has shown particular enzymatic roles. Biochemical experiments have revealed that the phosphoesterase domain of MRE11 works as both a single-and double-stranded DNA endonuclease, besides as 3´-5´ dsDNA exonuclease [D'Amours & Jackson, 2002]. Furthermore, RAD50 and NBS1/Xrs2 are able to promote the activity of MRE11, in an ATP dependent manner [Paul & Gellert, 1998]. ATP binding by RAD50 stimulates the binding of the MR complex to 3´ overhangs and, also, ATP hydrolysis is required to arouse the cleavage of DNA hairpins, inducing modification of endonuclease specificity via DNA relaxing [Paull & Gellert, 1998; de Jager et al., 2002].

In this chapter, we have identified the presence of *Mre11* and *Rad50* genes in the genome of *E. histolytica, T. vaginalis, G. lamblia* and *P. falciparum*. However, all analyzed pathogenic eukaryotic cells, with the exception *of E. histolytica,* lack the *Xrs2* homologue. The absence of a NBS1/Xrs2 homologous sequence in the other parasites might seem antagonistic to the idea of the existence of an active MRN complex. However we cannot discard the possibility that these microorganisms use a very divergent NBS1 protein, or even that this third component could be unessential. In order to initiate the characterization of components of MRN complex in these parasites, we studied the structural and evolutionary relationships between MRE11, RAD50 and NBS1 through PSI-BLAST analysis in comparison to human and yeast orthologues. This program generates a weighted profile from the sequences detected in the first pass of a gapped-BLAST search and iteratively searches the database using this profile as the query, allowing the inclusion of sequences with e-value cut off higher than 0.01 [Alschult et al., 1997]. Using the e-value threshold as a similarity measure, we evidenced a close relation between putative EhMRE11, HsMRE11, ScMRE11, TvMRE11 and PfMRE11. Conversely, GlMRE11 turned out to be less similar to the others, being closer to *E. histolytica* and *T. vaginalis* proteins (**Fig. 4**). On the other hand, analysis of RAD50 orthologues exposed a great conservation of these proteins, since all e-value threshold were <0.0001. As we have previously reported, EhNBS1 is closer to its human homologue than yeast [Lopez-Casamichana et al., 2007].

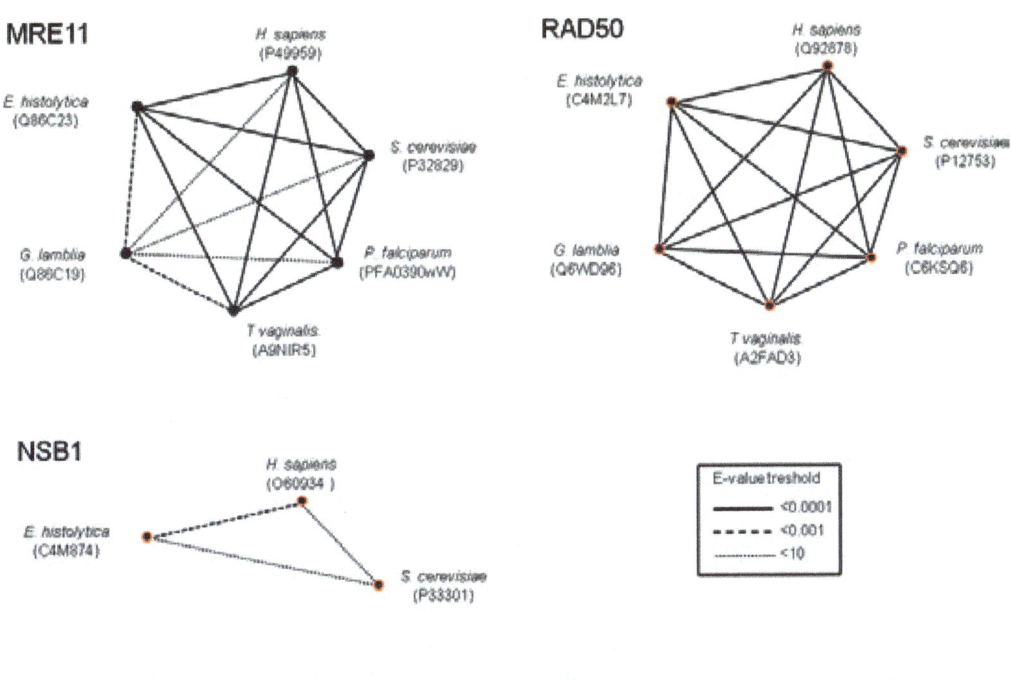

Fig. 4. **Individual protein relationships of MRN complex in pathogenic eukaryotic cells.** Similarity was evaluated through PSI-BLAST analysis. The width of connecting lines indicates similarity level.

To better understand the functionality of MRN complex in these parasites, predicted amino acid sequences of RAD50 and MRE11 were compared through multiple alignment using ClustalW software (http://www.ebi.ac.uk/ clustalw/). Reported functional and structural domains were surveyed using Prosite (http://www.expasy.org/tools/scanprosite/), Pfam (http://www.sanger.ac.uk /Software/Pfam/), SMART (http://smart.emblheidelberg.de/) and Motif Scan (http://myhits.isb-sib.ch/cgi-bin/motifscan) programs. For all studied parasites, our search revealed that the MRE11 orthologues contain the N-terminal Mn2+/Mg2+-dependent nuclease domain including the five conserved phosphoesterase motifs described in yeast protein [Hopkins & Paull, 2008]. Moreover, C-terminal DNA binding domains were also identified [Williams et al., 2007; D'Amours & Jackson, 2002] (**Fig. 5A**).

RAD50 proteins displayed sequence and organizational homology to structural maintenance of chromosome (SMC) family members that control the higher-order structure and dynamics of chromatin. The N-terminal Walker A and C-terminal Walker B nucleotide binding motifs, which associate one with another to form a bipartite ATP-binding cassette (ABC)-type ATPase domain, were predicted [Hopfner et al., 2000; Hopfner et al, 2001]. Furthermore, amino acids flanking Walker motifs form coiled-coil configurations that converge with the cysteine zinc hook (CysXXCys) motif [Hopfner et al., 2002] (**Fig. 5B**). In the interphase of Walker domains, there are two MRE11 binding sites. Formation of the stable MRE11-RAD50 complex is reached by each unit of the MRE11 dimer binding a RAD50 molecule at the intersection of its globular and coiled-coil domains [de Jager et al., 2001a]. Scanning force microscopy experiments have demonstrated that whereas the globular head of the Mre112Rad502 complex links with the ends of linear dsDNA, the two coiled-coil regions of RAD50 are stretchy "arms", and project outward away from the DNA [Hopfner et al., 2002].

The third member of the MRN complex is NBS1 protein that was only detected in *E. histolytica*, but not in *G. lamblia*, *P. falciarum* neither *T. vaginalis*. We have previously reported that EhNBS1 consists of an FHA domain and adjacent BRCT domains at its N-terminus [Lopez-Casamichana et al., 2007]. In *Homo sapiens*, the FHA domain binds phosphorylated threonine residues in Ser-X-Thr motifs present in DNA damage proteins, including CTP1 and MDC1. The BRCT domains in human NBS1 fix Ser-X-Thr motifs when the serine residue is phosphorylated. These phospho-dependent interactions are significant for recruiting repair machineries and checkpoint proteins to DNA DSBs [Lloyd et al., 2009; Williams et al., 2009]. In reconstitution studies, the affinity of MRE11-RAD50 for DNA and its nuclease activity is further enhanced by the addition of NBS1 [Paull & Gellert, 1999].

6. Molecular organization of the RAD51 recombinase

RAD51 recombinase is an essential protein in HRR pathway that catalyzes strand transfer between a broken DNA and its undamaged homologous strand, allowing damaged region to be repaired [Thacker, 2005] Strand exchange reaction is initiated by RAD51-coating of ssDNA released from DSBs, to generate a nucleoprotein filament. This active thread binds the intact dsDNA substrate, searching and locating homologous sequences, and promoting DNA strand exchange in an ATP-dependent manner, forming a heteroduplex structure [Paques & Haber, 1999]. After DNA damage, RAD51 protein has been observed in nuclear complexes forming discrete foci, which are considered as the recombinational DNA repair

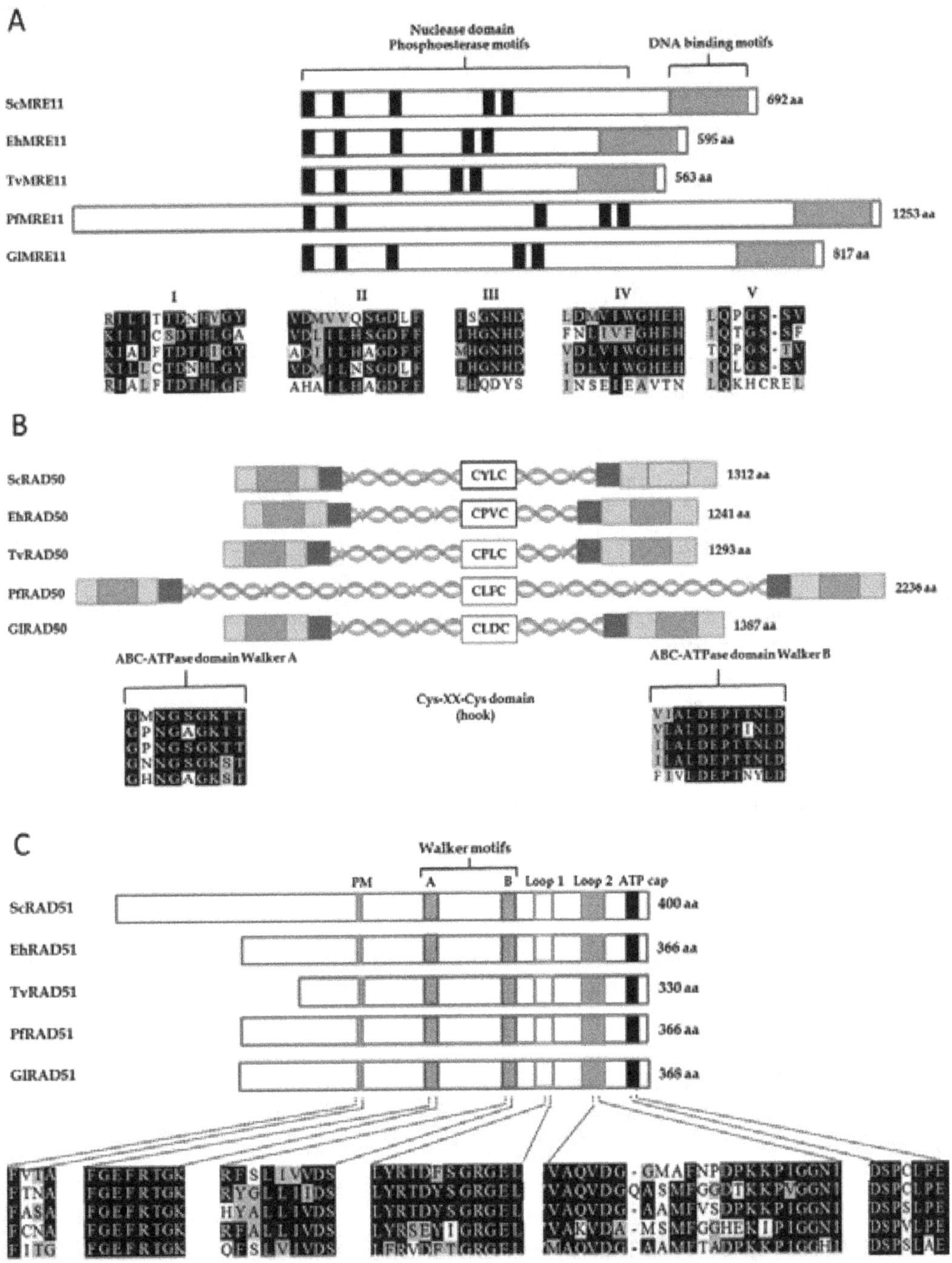

Fig. 5. **Comparison of the amino acids sequence of MRE11, RAD50 and RAD51 proteins of *S. cerevisae E. histolytica, T. vaginalis, P. falciparum* and *G. lamblia.* (A)**. Functional and structural domains of MRE11 proteins. MRE11 phosphoesterase motifs I-V (black

rectangles) and DNA-binding domains (gray rectangles). **(B)**. Functional and structural domains of RAD50 proteins. Walker A (N terminus) and Walker B (C terminus) are marked in the ABC-ATPase domains (gray rectangles), while MRE11-binding sites flank Walker motifs (dark gray rectangles) and the CysXXCys hook domain (white rectangles) are labeled in the coiled-coil central regions. **(C)**. Functional and structural domains of RAD51 proteins. Polymerization motif (PM), as well as Walker A and B motifs, L1 and L2 regions and ATP cap appear as colored rectangles. Boxshade panels: black boxes, identical aa; grey boxes, conserved substitutions.

sites [Tashiro et al., 2000]. RAD51 proteins have been identified in *Trypanosoma brucei* and *Plasmodium falciparum* parasites, which perform HRR to switch the expression of genes encoding surface membrane glycoproteins and generate antigenic variation [Conway et al., 2002; Freitas-Junior et al., 2000]. Furthermore, recombinational rearrangements are responsible for amplification of the multidrug resistance *pfmdr1* gene in *P. falciparum* [Triglia et al., 1991] demonstrating the relevance of HRR to generate genomic versatility and plasticity in protozoan parasites. Molecular analysis and functional assays confirmed that recombinant EhRAD51 is a *bonafide* recombinase that is able to catalyze specific ssDNA transfer to homologous dsDNA forming the three-stranded pairing molecule called D-loop structure. In addition, *E. histolytica RAD51* sequence conserves the typical architecture of RECA/RAD51 family members [Lopez-Casamichana et al., 2008]. Amino acid sequences multiple alignment of RAD51 orthologues from *E. histolytica, S. cerevisae, T. vaginalis, G. lamblia* and *P. falciparum* revealed that all these proteins share functional and structural conserved motifs (**Fig. 5C**). Each of them contains the putative polymerization motif (PM), which tethers individual subunits to form quaternary assemblies in human RAD51 protein [Bell, 2005]. We also identified the ATPase Walker A or phosphate binding loop (P-loop) and Walker B motifs residues, the ssDNA binding loops L1 and L2, as well as the ATP stacking motif or ATP cap at the C terminus, which are essential for nucleofilament assembling and ATP hydrolysis in RAD51/RECA-like recombinases [Shin et al., 2003; Conway et al., 2004].

7. Conclusions

Protozoan parasites are continuously subjected to the effects of antiparasitic drugs and host immune system attacks, which can affect their genome stability and therefore, their survival. In order to maintain the integrity of their DNA molecules, parasites have developed several mechanisms that are efficient to detect and accurately repair damaged nucleotides. Bioinformatic analyses of fully sequenced genomes are useful to identify molecular machineries for DNA repair in protozoan parasites of clinical relevance such as *Entamoeba histolyica, Giardia lamblia, Plasmodium falciparum* and *Trichomonas vaginalis,* which have a world-wide distribution with a high prevalence in developing countries. The computational data presented here provide new information on the evolution of DNA repair proteins and their potential relevance for DNA damage response in these major human pathogens. Future directions would include functional assays, as well as protein expression and protein-protein interactions analysis for the most relevant proteins, in order to contribute to the further elucidation of mechanisms regulating genome integrity in these organisms.

8. Acknowledgments

Genes and predicted protein sequences were obtained from the Eupath database (http://eupathdb.org/eupathdb/) and Uniprot Knowledgebase (http://www.uniprot.org/). This work was supported by UACM (México), CONACyT (México), COFAA-IPN (Mexico), SIP-IPN (Mexico) and European Community grants.

9. References

Alschult, S.F., Madden, T.L., Schaffer, A.A., Zang, J., Zang, Z., Miller, W., Lipman, D.J. (1997). Gapped BLAST and PSI-BLAST: a new generation of protein database search programs. *Nucleic Acid Research*, (September 1997), Vol.25, pp. 3389-3402, ISSN 0305-1048

Ankarklev, J., Jerlstrom-Hultqvist, J., Ringqvist, E., Troell, K., Svard, S.G. (2010). Behind the smile: cell biology and disease mechanisms of Giardia species. *Nature Reviews Microbiology*, Vol.8, (June 2010), pp. 413–422. ISSN: 1740-1526

Bethke, L., Thomas, S., Walker, K., Lakhia, R., Rangarajan, R., Wirth, D. (2007). The role of DNA mismatch repair in generating genetic diversity and drug resistance in malaria parasites. *Molecular and Biochemical Parasitology*, Vol. 155, No. 1, (September 2007), pp. 18–25. ISSN 0166-6851

Bell, C.E. (2005). Structure and mechanism of Escherichia coli RecA ATPase. Molecular Microbiology, Vol.58, No.2, (October 2005, pp.358-366, ISSN 0950-382X

Bhattacharyya, M.K., Kumar, N. (2003). Identification and molecular characterisation of DNA damaging agent induced expression of Plasmodium falciparum recombination protein PfRad51. *International Journal* for *Parasitology*, Vol.33, (October 2002), pp. 1385–1392. ISSN 0020-7519.

Carlton, J.M., Hirt, R.P., Silva, J.C., Delcher, A.L., Schatz, M., Zhao, Q., Wortman, J.R., Bidwell,S.L., Alsmark, U.C., Besteiro, S., et al. (2007). Draft genome sequence of the sexually transmitted pathogen Trichomonas vaginalis. *Science*, Vol. 315, No. 5809, (January 2007), pp. 207-212. ISSN 0036-8075

Casta, L.J., Buguliskis, J.S., Matsumoto, Y., Taraschi, T.F. (2008). Expression and biochemical characterization of the Plasmodium falciparum DNA repair enzyme, flap endonuclease-1 (PfFEN-1). *Molecular and Biochemical Parasitology*, Vol. 157, No. 1, (January 2008), pp. 1-12. ISSN 0166-6851

Castellini, M.A., Buguliskis, J.S., Casta, L.J., Butz, C.E., Clark, A.B., Kunkel, T.A., Taraschi, T.F. (2011). Malaria drug resistance is associated with defective DNA mismatch repair Molecular and Biochemical Parasitology, Vol. 177, No. 2 (June 2010), pp. 143-147. ISSN 0166-6851

Conway, C., Proudfoot, C., Burton, P., Barry, J.D., McCulloch, R. (2002). Two pathways of homologous recombination in Trypanosoma brucei. *Molecular Microbiology*, Vol.45, No.6, (September 2002), pp. 1687-1700, ISSN 0950-382X

Conway, A.B., Lynch, T.W., Zhang, Y., Fortin, G.S, Fung, C.W., Symington, L.S., Rice, P.A. (2004). Crystal structure of a Rad51 filament. *Nature structural & molecular biology*, Vol.11, No.8, (August 2004), pp. 791-796, ISSN 1545-9993

Cotch, M.F., Pastorek, J.G., Nugent, R.P., Hillier, S.L., Gibbs, R.S., Martin, D.H. et al. (1997). Trichomonas vaginalis associated with low birth weight and preterm delivery. The Vaginal Infections and Prematurity Study Group. *Sexually transmitted diseases*, Vol. 4, No.6, (July 1997), pp. 353-360. ISSN0148-5717

D'Amours, D., Jackson, S.P. (2002). The Mre11 complex: at the crossroads of DNA repair and checkpoint signalling. *Nature* Reviews *Molecular Cell Biology,* Vol. 3, (May 2002), pp. 317-327, ISSN 1471-0072

de Jager, M., Dronkert, M.L., Modesti, M., Beerens, C.E., Kanaar, R.,van Gent, D.C. (2001). DNA-binding and strand-annealing activities of human Mre11: implications for its roles in DNA double-strand break repair pathways. *Nucleic Acids Research*, Vol.29, (March 2001), pp. 1317-1325, ISSN 0305-1048

de Jager, M., van Noort, J., van Gent, D.C., Dekker, C., Kanaar, R., Wyman, C. (2001a). Human Rad50/Mre11 is a flexible complex that can tether DNA ends. *Molecular Cell,*), Vol.8, (November, 2001 pp. 1129-113, ISSN 1097-2765

Demple B, Johnson A, Fung D. Exonuclease III and endonuclease IV remove 3' blocks from DNA synthesis primers in H2O2-damaged Escherichia coli. 1986 *Proceedings of the National Academy of Sciences of the United States of America.* Voln 83, No.20, (October 1986), pp. 7731-7735, ISSN 0027-8424

Fleck, O., Nielsen, O. (2004) DNA repair. Journal of Cell Science, Vol. 117, Pt. 4, (February), pp. 515-517, ISSN: 0021-9533

Freitas-Junior, L.H., Bottius, E., Pirrit, L.A., Deitsch, K.W., Scheidig, C., Guinet, F., Nehrbass, U., Wellems, T.E., Scherf, A. (2000). Frequent ectopic recombination of virulence factor genes in telomeric chromosome clusters of P. falciparum. *Nature,* Vol.407, No.6807, (October 2000), pp. 1018-1022, ISSN 0028-0836

Gardner, M.J., Hall, N., Fung, E., White, O., Berriman, M., Hyman, R.W. et al. (2002). Genome sequence of the human parasite Plasmodium falciparum. *Nature,* Vol. 419, No. 6906, (October 2002), pp. 498-511. ISSN 0028-0836

Gilbert, W., de Souza, S. J., Long, M. Y. (1997). Origin of genes. *Proceedings of the National Academy of Sciences of the United States of America,* Vol.94, No.15, (July 1997), pp. 7698-7703, ISSN 0027-8424

Gill, E.E., Fast, N.M. (2007). Stripped-down DNA repair in a highly reduced parasite. *BMC Molecular Biology,* Vol. 8, (March), pp. 24. ISSN 1471-2199

Guo, X., Houpt, E., Petri, W.A.Jr. (2007). Crosstalk at the initial encounter: interplay between host defense and ameba survival strategies. *Current Opinion in Immunology,* Vol.19, (August 2007), pp. 376-384, ISSN 0952-7915

Haltiwanger, B.M., Karpinich, N.O, and Taraschi, T.F. (2000) Characterization of class II apurinic/apyrimidinic endonuclease activities in the human malaria parasite, *Plasmodium falciparum. Biochemical Journal,* Vol. 345, (January 2000), pp. 85-89, ISSN 0264-6021.

Haltiwanger, B.M, Matsumoto Y., Nicolas E., Dianov G.L., Bohr V.A., Taraschi T.F. (2000) DNA base excision repair in human malaria parasites is predominantly by a long-patch pathway. *Biochemistry.* Voln. 39, No. 4, (February 2000), pp. 763-72, ISSN 0006-2960.

Hartl, D.L., Wirth, D.F. (2006), Duplication, gene conversion, and genetic diversity in the species-specific acyl-CoA synthetase gene family of Plasmodium falciparum. *Molecular and Biochemical Parasitology*, Vol.150, No.1, (November, 2006), pp.10-24, ISSN 0166-6851

Hefferin, M.L., Tomkinson, A.E. (2005). Mechanism of DNA double-strand break repair by non-homologous end joining. *DNA Repair (Amsterdam)*, Vol. 4, No. 6, (June 2005), pp. 639-648. ISNN 1568-7864

Hopfner, K.P., Karcher, A., Shin, D.S., Craig, L., Arthur, L.M., Carney, J.P., Tainer, J.A. (2000) Structural biology of Rad50 ATPase: ATP-driven conformational control in DNA double-strand break repair and the ABCATPase superfamily. *Cell*, Vol.101, No.7, (June 2000), pp. 789-800, ISSN 0092-8674

Hopfner, K.P., Karcher, A., Craig, L., Woo, T.T., Carney, J.P., Tainer, J.A. (2001) Structural biochemistry and interaction architecture of the DNA double-strand break repair Mre11 nuclease and Rad50-ATPase. *Cell*, Vol.105, No.4, (May 2011), pp.473-485, ISSN 0092-8674

Hopfner, K.P., Craig, L., Moncalian, G., Zinkel, R.A., Usui, T., Owen, B.A. et al. (2002). The Rad50 zinc-hook is a structure joining Mre11 complexes in DNA recombination and repair. *Nature*, Vol.418, No. 6897, (August 202), pp. 562-566, ISSN 0028-0836

Hopkins, B.B., Paull, T.T. (2008). The P. furiosus mre11/rad50 complex promotes 5′ strand resection at a DNA double-strand break. *Cell*, Vol.135, (October 2008), pp. 250-260, ISSN 0092-8674

Kokwaro, G. (2009). Ongoing challenges in the management of malaria. *Malaria Journal*, Vol.8, Suppl 1, (October 2009), pp. S2. ISSN 1475-2875

Krokan, H.E., Standal, R., Slupphaug, G. (1997). DNA glycosylases in the base excision repair of DNA. *The Biochemistry Journal*, Vol. 325, No.1, (July 1997), pp. 1-16. ISSN 0264-6021

Lisby, M., Rothstein, R. (2005). Localization of checkpoint and DNA repait proteins in eukaryotes. *Biochimie*, Vol.87, No.7, (July), pp. 579589, ISNN 0300-9084

Liu H, Rudolf J, Johnson KA, McMahon SA, Oke M, Carter L, McRobbie AM, Brown SE, Naismith JH, White MF. (2008), Structure of the DNA repair helicase XPD. *Cell*, Vol.133, No.5, (May 2008), pp.801-12, ISSN 0092-8674

Lloyd, J. et al. (2009) A supramodular FHA/BRCT-repeat architecture mediates Nbs1 adaptor function in response to DNA damage. *Cell*, Vol.139, No. , (October 200), pp. 100-111, ISSN 0092-8674

Long, M. Y., Langley, C. H. (1993). Natural selection and the origin of jingwei, a chimeric processed functional gene in Drosophila. *Science*, Vol.260, No.91, (April 1993), pp.91-5, ISSN 0036-8075

López-Camarillo, C., Lopez-Casamichana, M., Weber, C., Guillen, N., Orozco, E., Marchat, L.A. (2009). DNA repair mechanisms in eukaryotes: Special focus in Entamoeba histolytica and related protozoan parasites. *Infection, Genetics and Evolution*, Vol.9, No.6, (December 2008), pp. 1051-1056. ISSN 1567-1348.

López-Casamichana, M., Orozco, E., Marchat, L.A., Lopez-Camarillo, C., (2007). Insights in DNA repair and homologous recombination in Entamoeba histolytica: in silico characterization of EhMRN complex. *Proceedings of the 5th European Congress on Tropical Medicine and International Health,* Monduzzi Editore s.r.l, pp. 7-11 , Medimond, ISBN: 13602276, Italy

López-Casamichana, M., Orozco, E., Marchat, L.A., López-Camarillo, C. (2008). Transcriptional profile of the homologous recombination machinery and characterization of the EhRAD51 recombinase in response to DNA damage in Entamoeba histolytica. *BMC* Molecular Biology, Vol.9, (April 2008), pp.35. ISSN 1471-2199

Malik, S.B., Pightling, A.W., Stefaniak, L.M., Schurko, A.M., Logsdon, J.M. Jr. (2007). An expanded inventory of conserved meiotic genes provides evidence for sex in Trichomonas vaginalis. *PLoS One,* Vol.3, No.8, (August 2007), e2879. ISSN 1932-6203

Marti, T.M., Kunz, C., Fleck, O. (2002). DNA mismatch repair and mutation avoidance pathways. *Journal of Cellular Physiology,* Vol.191, (April 2002), pp. 28-41. ISSN 0021-9541

Moriel-Carretero M, Aguilera A. (2010). Replication fork breakage and re-start: New insights into Rad3/XPD-associated deficiencies. *Cell Cycle,* Vol.9, No.15, (August 2010), pp.2958-62, ISSN 1538-4101

Ogawa, H., Johzuka, K., Nakagawa, T., Leem, S.H., Hagihara, A.H. (1995). Functions of the yeast meiotic recombination genes, MRE11 and MRE2. *Advances in Biophysics,* Vol.31, pp. 67-76. ISSN 0065-227X

Paques, F., Haber, J.E. (1999). Multiple pathways of recombination induced by double-strand breaks in Saccharomyces cerevisiae. *Microbiology and Molecular Biology Reviews,* Vol.63, No.2, (June 1999), pp. 349-404, ISSN 1092-2172

Paull, T.T., Gellert, M. (1999). Nbs1 potentiates ATP-driven DNA unwinding and endonuclease cleavage by the Mre11/Rad50 complex. *Genes & Development,* Vol.13, No.10, (May 1999). pp. 1276-1288. ISSN 0890-9369

Paull, T.T., Gellert, M. (1998). The 30 to 50 exonuclease activity of Mre11 facilitates repair of DNA double-strand breaks. *Molecular Cell,* Vol. 1, (June 1998), pp. 969-979, ISSN 1097-2765

Prakash, S., Prakash, L. (2000). Nucleotide excision repair in yeast. *Mutation Research,* Vol.451, No.1-2, (June 2000), pp. 13-24. ISSN 1383-5742

Ramesh, M.A., Malik, S.B., Logsdon, J.M.Jr. (2005). A phylogenomic inventory of meiotic genes: evidence for sex in Giardia and an early eukaryotic origin of meiosis. *Current Biology,* Vol.15, (January 2005), pp. 185-191. ISSN 0960-9822

Rass, E., Grabarz, A., Plo, I., Gautier, J., Bertrand, P. , Lopez, B.S. (2009). Role of Mre11 in chromosomal nonhomologous end joining in mammalian cells. *Nature Structural & Molecular Biology,* Vol.16, (August 2009), pp. 819-824, ISSN 1545-9985

Shin, D.S., Pellegrini, L., Daniels, D.S., Yelent, B., Craig, L., Bates, D. et al. (2003). Full-length archaeal Rad51 structure and mutants: mechanisms for RAD51 assembly and control by BRCA2. *EMBO Journal,* Vol.22, (September 2003), pp. 4566-4576, ISSN 0261-4189

Sorvillo, F., Kerndt, P. (1998). Trichomonas vaginalis and amplification of HIV-1 transmission. *The Lancet*, Vol.351, (January 1998), pp. 213-214. ISSN 0140-6736

Tamura, K., Peterson, D., Peterson, N., Stecher, G., Nei, M., Kumar, S. (2011). MEGA5: Molecular Evolutionary Genetics Analysis using Maximum Likelihood, Evolutionary Distance, and Maximum Parsimony Methods. *Molecular Biology and Evolution* (submitted), *ISSN 0737-4038*

Tashiro, S., Walter, J., Shinohara, A., Kamada, N., Cremer, T. (2000). Rad51 accumulation at sites of DNA damage and in postreplicative chromatin. *Journal of Cell Biology*, Vol.150, No.2, (July 2000), pp. 283-291, INSS 1540-8140

Taylor, E.M., Cecillon, S.M., Bonis, A., Chapman, J.R., Povirk, L.F., Lindsay,H.D. (2010). The Mre11/Rad50/Nbs1 complex functions in resection-basedDNA end joining in Xenopus laevis. *Nucleic Acids Research*, Vol.38, (November 2009), pp. 441–454, ISSN 0305-1048

Thacker, J. (2005). The RAD51 gene family, genetic instability and cancer. *Cancer Letters*, 2005 Mar 10;Vol. 219, No. 2, (March 2005), pp. 125-135, ISSN 0304-3835

Tovar, J., Leon-Avila, G., Sanchez, L.B., Sutak, R., Tachezy, J., et al. (2003). Mitochondrial remnant organelles of Giardia function in iron-sulphur protein maturation. *Nature*, Vol. 426, No. 6963, (November 2003), pp. 172-176; ISSN 0028-0836

Tovar J, Fischer A, Clark CG. (1999). The mitosome, a novel organelle related to mitochondria in the amitochondrial parasite Entamoeba histolytica. *Molecular Microbiology*, Vol. 32, No. 5, (June 1999), pp. 1013-1021. ISSN: 0950-382X

Triglia, T., Foote, S.J., Kemp, D.J., Cowman, A.F. (1991). Amplification of the multidrug resistance gene pfmdr1 in Plasmodium falciparum has arisen as multiple independent events. *Molecular and Cellular Biology*, Vol.11, No.10, (October 2010), pp. 5244-5250, ISSN 0270-7306

Voss, T.S., Mini, T., Jenoe, P., Beck, H.P. (2002). Plasmodium falciparum possesses a cell cycle-regulated short type replication protein A large subunit encoded by an unusual transcript. *The* Journal *of Biological* Chemistry, Vol.277, No.20, (May 2002), pp. 17493-17501. ; ISSN 0021-9258

Weber, C., Marchat, L.A., Guillen, N., López-Camarillo, C. (2009). Effects of DNA damage induced by UV irradiation on gene expression in the protozoan parasite Entamoeba histolytica. *Molecular* & Biochemical *Parasitology*, Vol. 164, No. 2, (April 2009), pp. 165-169. ISSN 0166-6851

World Health Organization (WHO). (1995). Global Programme on AIDS Report 1995. Geneva: WHO; 1995. An overview of selected curable sexually transmitted diseases

Williams, R.S., Dodson, G.E., Limbo, O., Yamada, Y., Williams, J.S., Guenther, G. et al. (2009). Nbs1 flexibly tethers Ctp1 and Mre11-Rad50 to coordinate DNA double-strand break processing and repair. *Cell*, Vol.139, No.1, (October 2009), pp. 87-99, ISSN 0092-8674

Williams, R.S., Williams, J.S., Tainer, J.A. (2007). Mre11-Rad50-Nbs1 is a keystone complex connecting DNA repair machinery, double-strand break signaling, and the chromatin template. *Biochemistry and Cell Biology*, Vol.85, (August 2007), pp. 509-520, ISSN 0829-8211

Zhang, J. (2003). Evolution by gene duplication: an update. *Trends in Ecology & Evolution*, (June 2003) Vol. 18, No. 6, pp.292-298, ISSN 0169-5347

4

Role for PKCδ on Apoptosis in the DNA Damage Response

Kiyotsugu Yoshida
Medical Research Institute, Tokyo Medical and Dental University, Tokyo, Japan

1. Introduction

Genotoxic stress induces cell cycle arrest, DNA repair, and apoptotic cell death. The decision by cells either to repair DNA lesions and continue through the cell cycle or to undergo apoptosis is relevant to the incidence of mutagenesis and, subsequently, carcinogenesis. In this regard, incomplete repair of DNA damage prior to replication or mitosis can result in the accumulation of heritable genetic changes. Therapeutic anti-cancer treatments that use genotoxic agents must strike a balance between induction of repair and apoptosis in order to maximize the therapeutic effect. However, the nature of the cellular signaling response that determines cell fate such as survival or death is far from being understood. Certain insights have been derived from the finding that diverse isozymes of the protein kinase C (PKC) family are activated in response to DNA damage. PKC-mediated signaling pathway modulates destiny of cells following genotoxic insults (Yoshida 2007a, Yoshida 2008a). In particular, recent studies have shown that certain isozyme of PKC controls function of the p53 tumor suppressor in induction of cell cycle arrest, DNA repair, and apoptosis. In the past 10 years, understanding the molecular mechanisms of apoptosis mediated by PKC has advanced considerably, and the primary focus of this review is to provide an overview of PKC and p53, its mode of action and its physiological role in DNA damage-induced apoptosis.

2. Protein kinase C

The protein kinase C (PKC) family of serine-threonine kinases was first described as a calcium-activated, phospholipid-dependent serine/threonine protein kinase (Takai et al. 1977). PKC is activated diacylglycerol (DAG) hydrolyzed from phosphatidylinositol (PI) by phospholipase C (PLC) under a different cell-signaling system (Nishizuka 1984, Nishizuka 1988, Nishizuka 1992, Nishizuka 1995). It has attracted attention as an intracellular receptor for tumor-promotor phorbol esters, such as 12-O-tetradecanoyl-13-phorbol acetate (TPA) (Niedel et al. 1983). Although PKC had been recognized as a protein kinase, subsequent studies have revealed that it belongs to a family of serine/threonine-specific protein kinases and is activated by diverse stimuli and participates in various cellular processes, such as growth, differentiation, apoptosis, and cellular senescence (Casabona 1997, Clemens et al. 1992, Goodnight et al. 1994, Hofmann 1997, Hug and Sarre 1993, Nishizuka 1984, Nishizuka 1988, Nishizuka 1992, Nishizuka 1995). PKC consists of at least 11 isozymes (α, βI, βII, γ, δ, ε, ζ, η, θ, ι/λ and μ) with selective tissue distribution, activators, and substrates. PKC isozymes have been categorized into three groups: i) the classical/conventional PKCs (cPKCs: α, βI, βII γ), which are calcium dependent and activated by DAG; ii) the novel PKCs (nPKCs: δ, ε, θ, μ), which are calcium-independent and activated by DAG; and iii) the atypical PKCs (aPKCs: ζ, λ), which are calcium-independent and not activated by DAG (Casabona 1997, Goodnight et al. 1994, Hug and Sarre 1993, Nishizuka 1988, Nishizuka 1992, Nishizuka 1995). The cell-specific expression and subcellular localization of individual PKC isozymes indicate important isozyme-specific functions. To elucidate these functions, it should be necessary to study the individual features of each isozyme, such as expression, post-translational modification, substrate specificity, subcellular localization and signaling cross-talk with other proteins. Moreover, the involvement of a PKC isozyme in a signaling pathway resulting in a specific cellular response can be investigated by diverse distinct methods such as overexpression or inhibition of enzyme.

3. PKC and apoptotic cell death upon genotoxic insults

Novel PKCδ, θ, and μ are substrates for the effector caspase-3, and proteolytic activation of these novel PKCs has been associated with cell death (Datta et al. 1997, Emoto et al. 1995, Endo et al. 2000). However, recent studies have shown that PKC acts upstream of caspases to regulate cell death. For example, PKC activators enhanced caspase activation, whereas an inhibitor of PKC prevented caspase activation in response to DNA damage (Basu et al. 2001). In particular, studies with PKCδ-/- mice suggest that PKCδ plays pivotal roles in the regulation of cell proliferation and apoptosis (Humphries et al. 2006, Leitges et al. 2001). PKCδ is activated by a variety of stimuli including ionizing radiation, anti-cancer agents, reactive oxygen species (ROS), ultraviolet radiation, growth factors and cytokines (Carpenter et al. 2002, Chen et al. 1999, Denning et al. 1996, Konishi et al. 2001, Reyland et al. 1999, Yoshida and Kufe 2001, Yoshida et al. 2002). Molecular mechanisms such as tyrosine phosphorylation and proteolytic cleavage by caspase-3 are of importance to understand the pro-apoptotic role for PKCδ activation. PKC isozymes have been implicated in the growth factor signal transduction pathway (Nishizuka 1992). By contrast, activation of PKCδ inhibits cell cycle progression and down-regulation of PKCδ is linked to tumor promotion, suggesting that PKCδ may have a negative effect on cell survival (Lu et al. 1997, Watanabe et al. 1992). In many cases, the growth-inhibitory effects of PKCδ have been linked to changes in the expression of factors that influence cell cycle progression. Furthermore, PKCδ plays a pivotal role in the genotoxic stress response leading to apoptosis in various cell types (Brodie and Blumberg 2003, Reyland 2007, Yoshida 2007a). In addition, cells derived from PKCδ-/- mice were shown to be defective in mitochondria-dependent apoptosis (Humphries et al. 2006, Leitges et al. 2001). These findings thus support our proposition of a pro-genotoxic role for PKCδ. PKCδ is activated in response to diverse cellular stimuli by various processes, including membrane translocation (Joseloff et al. 2002, Wang et al. 1999), protein-protein interaction (Benes et al. 2005), tyrosine phosphorylation (Denning et al. 1996, Kaul et al. 2005), and proteolytic cleavage (Emoto et al. 1995, Ghayur et al. 1996, Yoshida 2007a, Yoshida et al. 2003). The translocation of PKCδ to discrete subcellular compartments and/or proteolytic cleavage can be induced by numerous stimuli, such as ceramide, TNFα, UV irradiation, ionizing radiation, oxidative stress, and etoposide (DeVries et al. 2002, Majumder et al. 2000, Matassa et al. 2001, Reyland et al. 1999, Yamaguchi et al. 2007b, Yoshida 2007a, Yoshida et al. 2006a, Yoshida et al. 2002, Yoshida et al. 2003, Yoshida et al. 2006b). Importantly, recent studies have shown that genotoxin-induced PKCδ activation is in part dependent upon Ataxia telangiectasia mutated (ATM) (Yoshida et al. 2003). Whereas ATM activates c-Abl, and c-Abl activates PKCδ, a potential explanation is that DNA damage induces an ATM→c-Abl→PKCδ pathway (Yoshida 2007b, Yoshida and Miki 2005, Yoshida et al. 2005). Alternatively, ATM may directly activate PKCδ in the DNA damage response. In either case, nuclear targeting of PKCδ is pre-requisite for ATM-mediated full activation of PKCδ.

4. Nuclear translocation of PKCδ in the apoptotic responses

Translocation of PKCδ into the nucleus has been demonstrated in various cells (Blass et al. 2002, DeVries et al. 2002, DeVries-Seimon et al. 2007, Eitel et al. 2003, Scheel-Toellner et al. 1999, Yoshida et al. 2003, Yuan et al. 1998). Recent study showed that PKCδ translocates to nucleus after exposure of cells with 1-β-D-arabinofuranosylcytosine (ara-C) (Yoshida et al. 2003). Moreover, pretreatment with PKCδ inhibitor, rottlerin, attenuates nuclear targeting of PKCδ (Yoshida et al. 2003), suggesting that its kinase activity is required for nuclear translocation. A putative nuclear localization signal has been identified at the C-terminus of the catalytic domain of PKCδ (DeVries et al. 2002). Numerous PKCδ targets and substrates, including the p53 tumor suppressor, are nuclear proteins that function in induction of apoptosis.

5. Role for p53 in response to DNA damage

The tumor suppressor protein p53 plays a central role in mediating stress and DNA damage-induced cell cycle arrest and apoptosis (Vogelstein et al. 2000). The p53 protein controls normal responses to DNA damage and other forms of genotoxic stress and is an indispensable element in maintaining genomic stability (Vogelstein et al. 2000). In fact, *p53* is the most frequently mutated gene in human cancers (Nigro et al. 1989). The level of p53 protein is mostly undetectable in normal cells but rapidly increases in response to a variety of stress stimuli. The mechanism by which the p53 protein is stabilized is not completely understood, but post-translational modification plays a crucial role (Shieh et al. 1997). Mutations in the *p53* gene are frequently correlated with generation of human cancers; however, the p53 pathway can be also derailed by diverse oncogenic molecules (Oren et al. 2002). The *p53* gene knocked-out mice develop tumors with an increased rate (Donehower et al. 1992). It is reasonable that many agents may inhibit the p53 pathway as part of the road toward tumor promotion. However, mechanisms for action of many chemical agents that promote tumor development have not been elucidated. With the central role of p53 in mind, agents that promote tumor formation might block the p53 pathway. Importantly, p53 is regulated primarily via post-translational modifications, especially phosphorylation, and the accumulation of p53 is the first step following cellular stress (Oren 1999). The *mdm2* gene is a transcriptional target of p53, and once synthesized, the MDM2 protein can bind to p53 at its NH2 terminus leading to its rapid degradation through the ubiquitin proteasome-mediated pathway (Kubbutat and Vousden 1998, Oren 1999, Ryan et al. 2001). Upon DNA damage, p53 is phosphorylated at multiple sites at the NH2 terminus, thereby inhibiting MDM2 binding (Burns and El-Deiry 1999, Canman et al. 1998, Kubbutat and Vousden 1998, Oren 1999, Ryan et al. 2001, Siliciano et al. 1997). As a result, p53 degradation stops and p53 accumulates. p53 can also be phosphorylated at its COOH-terminal regulatory domain, which influences its DNA binding

(Meek 1998). In this context, constitutive phosphorylation of p53 by PKC at its COOH-terminal domain can lead to its degradation through ubiquitin proteasome-mediated pathway (Chernov et al. 2001). Moreover, treatment with PKC inhibitors, such as H7 or bisindolylmaleimide I, prohibited COOH-terminal phosphorylation of p53 and increased accumulation of p53 without any effect on the formation of the p53-MDM2 complex (Chernov et al. 2001). However, PKC inhibitors were incapable of p53 accumulation in human papilloma virus-positive HeLa cells (Chernov et al. 2001, Chernov et al. 1998).

6. PKCδ regulation of p53

The p53 tumor suppressor is activated following genotoxic stress. Transactivation of p53 target genes dictates cell cycle arrest and DNA repair or apoptosis. Accumulating studies have demonstrated that PKCδ regulates p53 expression at the transcriptional and post-translational levels.

6.1 Control at the transcription

Recent reports document that PKCδ transactivates expression of *p53* at the transcriptional level (Abbas et al. 2004, Liu et al. 2007, Yoshida 2008a). The tumor-promoting phorbol ester 12-O-tetradecanoylphorbol-13-acetate (TPA) hinders DNA damage-induced up-regulation of p53 by down-regulating PKCδ. TPA initiates tumor formation in a variety of mice and tissue culture models, and this has been correlated with the down-regulation of PKC (Hansen et al. 1990). TPA initially induces and then diminishes the activity of the diacylglycerol-dependent PKC isoforms (Fournier and Murray 1987, Hansen et al. 1990). Previous studies showed that the tumor-promoting activities of TPA are mediated at least in part by down-regulating PKCδ (Lu et al. 1997). Moreover, transgenic mice over-expressing PKCδ were resistant to tumor promotion by TPA (Reddig et al. 1999). In this regard, previous studies implied that TPA can inhibit the DNA damage-mediated induction of p53 (Magnelli et al. 1995). Moreover, other studies with protein kinase inhibitors suggested that PKCδ regulates the p53 signalsome pathway (Ghosh et al. 1999). Regulation of p53 upon stress most commonly occurs by inhibiting ubiquitination and degradation of the p53 protein. In contrast, repression of p53 by inhibiting PKCδ is caused by the prevention of p53 synthesis, not augmented degradation of p53 protein. Inhibiting PKCδ blocks both basal transcription of the human *p53* gene and initiation of transcription from the human *p53* promoter. The DNA damage-elicited increase in *p53* accumulation is drastically inhibited by pre-treatment with TPA. In addition, the PKCδ inhibitor, rottlerin, is also able to block the DNA damage-mediated induction of *p53*. More importantly, pre-treatment of cells with TPA or treatment with rottlerin results in the inhibition of basal *p53* transcription. In this regard, accumulation of *p53* could not be achieved by any means, including proteasome inhibition, after TPA or rottlerin treatment, since *p53* transcription is hindered. Thus, the tumor-suppressing effects for PKCδ are mediated at least in part through activating *p53* transcription. Suppression of the *p53* promoter has been implied as a mechanism for tumor promotion (Raman et al. 2000, Stuart et al. 1995). Damaged genes in tumor cells are generally the mechanistic drivers toward oncogenesis. However, abrogation of endogenous genes, specifically tumor suppressors, may be also a crucial regulatory mechanism for tumor promotion. In this context, agents that interfere with the activity of PKCδ may inhibit p53 responses.

Recent study also demonstrated that PKCδ induces the promoter activity of p53 via the p53 core promoter element (CPE-p53) and that such induction is enhanced after DNA damage. Upon genotoxic insults, PKCδ is activated and interacts with the death-promoting transcription factor Btf (Bcl-2-associated transcription factor) to co-occupy CPE-p53. Inhibition of PKCδ decreases the affinity of Btf to CPE-p53, thereby reducing *p53* expression. Concomitant with these results, abrogation of Btf-mediated *p53* transcription by RNA interference leads to repression of p53-mediated apoptosis in response to genotoxic stress. These findings demonstrate that activation of *p53* transcription by PKCδ induces p53-dependent apoptosis following DNA damage (Liu et al. 2007).

6.2 Control at the post-translation

Recent study demonstrated that both PKCδ and IKKα, but not IKKβ, are targeted to the nucleus after oxidative stress (Yamaguchi et al. 2007a, Yamaguchi et al. 2007b). PKCδ interacts with and activates IKKα. Significantly, upon exposure to oxidative stress, PKCδ-mediated IKKα activation does not contribute to NF-κB activation; rather, nuclear IKK controls transcription activity of p53 by phosphorylation on Ser20. These findings indicate a novel mechanism in which the PKCδ→IKKα signaling pathway contributes to ROS-induced p53 activation. Recent studies have also demonstrated that phosphorylation of p53 at Ser46 induces p53AIP1 expression, resulting in the commitment to the apoptotic cell death (Matsuda et al. 2002, Oda et al. 2000, Taira et al. 2007, Yoshida 2008b). Furthermore, upon genotoxic stress, p53DINP1 is induced and then recruits a kinase(s) to p53, which specifically phosphorylate Ser46 (Okamura et al. 2001). We initially found that PKCδ is associated with Ser46 phosphorylation (Yoshida et al. 2006a). This phosphorylation was required for the interaction of PKCδ to p53. Importantly, p53DINP1 associated with PKCδ in response to anti-cancer agents. In concert with these findings, PKCδ potentiates p53-dependent apoptotic cell death by Ser46 phosphorylation. Taken together, PKCδ controls p53 to induce apoptosis in the cellular response to DNA damage (Yoshida et al. 2006a). Of note, our subsequent studies have demonstrated that another kinase DYRK2 plays a major and direct role on apoptosis induction by phosphorylating p53 at Ser46 in response to DNA damage (Taira et al. 2007, Taira et al. 2010). We also recently found that PKCδ regulates MDM2 expression independently of p53. Given that *Mdm2* mRNA change was detected in p53-proficient, but not deficient cells, PKCδ affected Mdm2 at the post-translational level. In this context, treatment of proteasome inhibitor MG132 restored Mdm2 expression to the steady-state level. Moreover, PKCδ inhibited Mdm2 ubiquitination in p53-deficient cells and loss of PKCδ resulted in an increase in Mdm2 proteasomal degradation. P300/CBP-associated factor (PCAF), an ubiquitin ligase 3 for Mdm2, was observed to participate in Mdm2 ubiquitination by PKCδ inhibition and PCAF silencing rescued Mdm2 diminution. We thus conclude that PKCδ regulates Mdm2 expression distinctively of p53 pathway by affecting Mdm2 ubiquitination and maintenance of Mdm2 expression by PKCδ is important to ensure normal genotoxic cell death response in human cancer cells (Hew et al. 2011).

7. Future perspective

PKCδ plays a pivotal role in the control of apoptotic cell death in response to a diverse array of stress stimuli. Thus PKCδ is a pro-apoptotic kinase activated by multiple mechanisms, including subcellular translocation and proteolysis. The proteolytic activation of PKCδ is also important not only in activating the downstream apoptotic cascade including p53, but also in amplifying upstream caspase signaling. Most of the studies mentioned above suggest that the role of PKCδ in the induction of apoptosis is tightly associated with its caspase-dependent cleavage and the regulation of p53. However, functional regulation of p53 by PKCδ remains largely unclear. In this regard, thorough investigation coupled with PKCδ and p53 should be enhanced from multiple views. In the encounter with genotoxic insults, ATM controls various cellular responses, such as cell cycle arrest, transcription, DNA repair, and apoptosis. In this context, DNA damage-induced PKCδ is modulated under ATM, suggesting the notion that establishment of the ATM→PKCδ→p53 signaling cascade provides new mechanistic light on how PKCδ functions as the pro-apoptotic kinase in the nucleus (Figure 1) (Yoshida 2007a, Yoshida 2008a). While dysregulation of the PKCδ signalsome confers resistance to anticancer drugs (Meinhardt et al. 1999), there is little

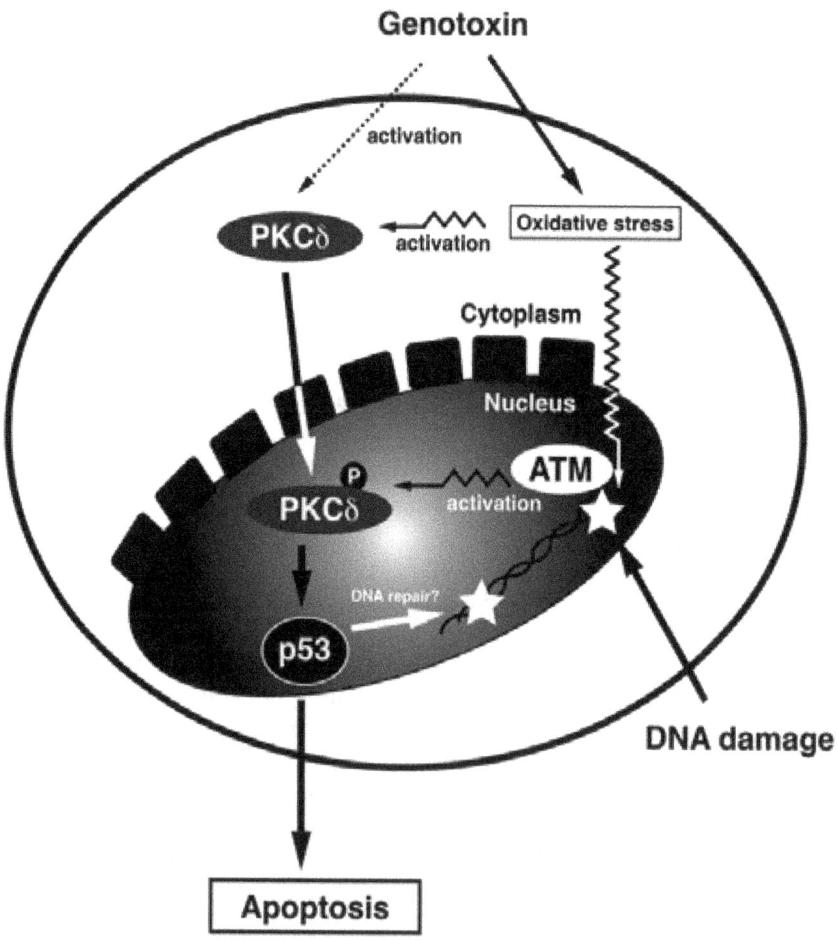

Fig. 1. A hypothetical schema for nuclear targeting of PKCδ in response to DNA damage. Following DNA damage, PKCδ translocates from the cytoplasm into the nucleus. In addition, some genotoxic stress also exerts cytoplasmic oxidative stress to activate PKCδ. In the nucleus, PKCδ is activated by ATM, then induces apoptosis (or DNA repair) in a p53-dependent manner.

understanding of how the PKCδ signaling pathway is influenced when cancer cells acquire resistance to chemotherapeutic drugs. Considering the importance of PKCδ in genotoxic stress-induced apoptosis, a thorough understanding of how it controls apoptosis should benefit cancer therapeutic potentials. Finally, novel PKCδ-based therapy may be used in combination with other agents to confer synergism and prevent the development for drug resistance.

8. References

Abbas, T., White, D., Hui, L., Yoshida, K., Foster, D. A., Bargonetti, J. (2004). Inhibition of human p53 basal transcription by down-regulation of protein kinase Cdelta. J Biol Chem 279:9970-7.

Basu, A., Woolard, M. D., Johnson, C. L. (2001). Involvement of protein kinase C-delta in DNA damage-induced apoptosis. Cell Death Differ 8:899-908.

Benes, C. H., Wu, N., Elia, A. E., Dharia, T., Cantley, L. C., Soltoff, S. P. (2005). The C2 domain of PKCdelta is a phosphotyrosine binding domain. Cell 121:271-80.

Blass, M., Kronfeld, I., Kazimirsky, G., Blumberg, P. M., Brodie, C. (2002). Tyrosine phosphorylation of protein kinase Cdelta is essential for its apoptotic effect in response to etoposide. Mol Cell Biol 22:182-95.

Brodie, C., Blumberg, P. M. (2003). Regulation of cell apoptosis by protein kinase c delta. Apoptosis 8:19-27.

Burns, T. F., El-Deiry, W. S. (1999). The p53 pathway and apoptosis. J Cell Physiol 181:231-9.

Canman, C. E., Lim, D. S., Cimprich, K. A. et al. (1998). Activation of the ATM kinase by ionizing radiation and phosphorylation of p53. Science 281:1677-9.

Carpenter, L., Cordery, D., Biden, T. J. (2002). Inhibition of protein kinase C delta protects rat INS-1 cells against interleukin-1beta and streptozotocin-induced apoptosis. Diabetes 51:317-24.

Casabona, G. (1997). Intracellular signal modulation: a pivotal role for protein kinase C. Prog Neuropsychopharmacol Biol Psychiatry 21:407-25.

Chen, N., Ma, W., Huang, C., Dong, Z. (1999). Translocation of protein kinase Cepsilon and protein kinase Cdelta to membrane is required for ultraviolet B-induced activation of mitogen-activated protein kinases and apoptosis. J Biol Chem 274:15389-94.

Chernov, M. V., Bean, L. J., Lerner, N., Stark, G. R. (2001). Regulation of ubiquitination and degradation of p53 in unstressed cells through C-terminal phosphorylation. J Biol Chem 276:31819-24.

Chernov, M. V., Ramana, C. V., Adler, V. V., Stark, G. R. (1998). Stabilization and activation of p53 are regulated independently by different phosphorylation events. Proc Natl Acad Sci U S A 95:2284-9.

Clemens, M. J., Trayner, I., Menaya, J. (1992). The role of protein kinase C isoenzymes in the regulation of cell proliferation and differentiation. J Cell Sci 103 (Pt 4):881-7.

Datta, R., Kojima, H., Yoshida, K., Kufe, D. (1997). Caspase-3-mediated cleavage of protein kinase C theta in induction of apoptosis. J Biol Chem 272:20317-20.

Denning, M. F., Dlugosz, A. A., Threadgill, D. W., Magnuson, T., Yuspa, S. H. (1996). Activation of the epidermal growth factor receptor signal transduction pathway stimulates tyrosine phosphorylation of protein kinase C delta. J Biol Chem 271:5325-31.

DeVries, T. A., Neville, M. C., Reyland, M. E. (2002). Nuclear import of PKCdelta is required for apoptosis: identification of a novel nuclear import sequence. EMBO J 21:6050-60.

DeVries-Seimon, T. A., Ohm, A. M., Humphries, M. J., Reyland, M. E. (2007). Induction of apoptosis is driven by nuclear retention of protein kinase C delta. J Biol Chem 282:22307-14.

Donehower, L. A., Harvey, M., Slagle, B. L. et al. (1992). Mice deficient for p53 are developmentally normal but susceptible to spontaneous tumours. Nature 356:215-21.

Eitel, K., Staiger, H., Rieger, J. et al. (2003). Protein kinase C delta activation and translocation to the nucleus are required for fatty acid-induced apoptosis of insulin-secreting cells. Diabetes 52:991-7.

Emoto, Y., Manome, Y., Meinhardt, G. et al. (1995). Proteolytic activation of protein kinase C delta by an ICE-like protease in apoptotic cells. EMBO J 14:6148-56.

Endo, K., Oki, E., Biedermann, V. et al. (2000). Proteolytic cleavage and activation of protein kinase C [micro] by caspase-3 in the apoptotic response of cells to 1-beta -D-arabinofuranosylcytosine and other genotoxic agents. J Biol Chem 275:18476-81.

Fournier, A., Murray, A. W. (1987). Application of phorbol ester to mouse skin causes a rapid and sustained loss of protein kinase C. Nature 330:767-9.

Ghayur, T., Hugunin, M., Talanian, R. V. et al. (1996). Proteolytic activation of protein kinase C delta by an ICE/CED 3-like protease induces characteristics of apoptosis. J Exp Med 184:2399-404.

Ghosh, J. C., Suzuki, K., Kodama, S., Watanabe, M. (1999). Effects of protein kinase inhibitors on the accumulation kinetics of p53 protein in normal human embryo cells following X-irradiation. J Radiat Res (Tokyo) 40:23-37.

Goodnight, J., Mischak, H., Mushinski, J. F. (1994). Selective involvement of protein kinase C isozymes in differentiation and neoplastic transformation. Adv Cancer Res 64:159-209.

Hansen, L. A., Monteiro-Riviere, N. A., Smart, R. C. (1990). Differential down-regulation of epidermal protein kinase C by 12-O-tetradecanoylphorbol-13-acetate and diacylglycerol: association with epidermal hyperplasia and tumor promotion. Cancer Res 50:5740-5.

Hew, H. C., Liu, H., Miki, Y., Yoshida, K. (2011). PKCdelta regulates Mdm2 independently of p53 in the apoptotic response to DNA damage. Mol Carcinog.

Hofmann, J. (1997). The potential for isoenzyme-selective modulation of protein kinase C. FASEB J 11:649-69.

Hug, H., Sarre, T. F. (1993). Protein kinase C isoenzymes: divergence in signal transduction? Biochem J 291 (Pt 2):329-43.

Humphries, M. J., Limesand, K. H., Schneider, J. C., Nakayama, K. I., Anderson, S. M., Reyland, M. E. (2006). Suppression of apoptosis in the protein kinase Cdelta null mouse in vivo. J Biol Chem 281:9728-37.

Joseloff, E., Cataisson, C., Aamodt, H. et al. (2002). Src family kinases phosphorylate protein kinase C delta on tyrosine residues and modify the neoplastic phenotype of skin keratinocytes. J Biol Chem 277:12318-23.

Kaul, S., Anantharam, V., Yang, Y., Choi, C. J., Kanthasamy, A., Kanthasamy, A. G. (2005). Tyrosine phosphorylation regulates the proteolytic activation of protein kinase Cdelta in dopaminergic neuronal cells. J Biol Chem 280:28721-30.

Konishi, H., Yamauchi, E., Taniguchi, H. et al. (2001). Phosphorylation sites of protein kinase C delta in H2O2-treated cells and its activation by tyrosine kinase in vitro. Proc Natl Acad Sci U S A 98:6587-92.

Kubbutat, M. H., Vousden, K. H. (1998). Keeping an old friend under control: regulation of p53 stability. Mol Med Today 4:250-6.

Leitges, M., Mayr, M., Braun, U. et al. (2001). Exacerbated vein graft arteriosclerosis in protein kinase Cdelta-null mice. J Clin Invest 108:1505-12.

Liu, H., Lu, Z. G., Miki, Y., Yoshida, K. (2007). Protein kinase C delta induces transcription of the TP53 tumor suppressor gene by controlling death-promoting factor Btf in the apoptotic response to DNA damage. Mol Cell Biol 27:8480-91.

Lu, Z., Hornia, A., Jiang, Y. W., Zang, Q., Ohno, S., Foster, D. A. (1997). Tumor promotion by depleting cells of protein kinase C delta. Mol Cell Biol 17:3418-28.

Magnelli, L., Cinelli, M., Chiarugi, V. (1995). Phorbol esters attenuate the expression of p53 in cells treated with doxorubicin and protect TS-P53/K562 from apoptosis. Biochem Biophys Res Commun 215:641-5.

Majumder, P. K., Pandey, P., Sun, X. et al. (2000). Mitochondrial translocation of protein kinase C delta in phorbol ester-induced cytochrome c release and apoptosis. J Biol Chem 275:21793-6.

Matassa, A. A., Carpenter, L., Biden, T. J., Humphries, M. J., Reyland, M. E. (2001). PKCdelta is required for mitochondrial-dependent apoptosis in salivary epithelial cells. J Biol Chem 276:29719-28.

Matsuda, K., Yoshida, K., Taya, Y., Nakamura, K., Nakamura, Y., Arakawa, H. (2002). p53AIP1 regulates the mitochondrial apoptotic pathway. Cancer Res 62:2883-9.

Meek, D. W. (1998). Multisite phosphorylation and the integration of stress signals at p53. Cell Signal 10:159-66.

Meinhardt, G., Roth, J., Totok, G., Auner, H., Emmerich, B., Hass, R. (1999). Signaling defect in the activation of caspase-3 and PKCdelta in human TUR leukemia cells is associated with resistance to apoptosis. Exp Cell Res 247:534-42.

Niedel, J. E., Kuhn, L. J., Vandenbark, G. R. (1983). Phorbol diester receptor copurifies with protein kinase C. Proc Natl Acad Sci U S A 80:36-40.

Nigro, J. M., Baker, S. J., Preisinger, A. C. et al. (1989). Mutations in the p53 gene occur in diverse human tumour types. Nature 342:705-8.

Nishizuka, Y. (1984). The role of protein kinase C in cell surface signal transduction and tumour promotion. Nature 308:693-8.

Nishizuka, Y. (1988). The molecular heterogeneity of protein kinase C and its implications for cellular regulation. Nature 334:661-5.

Nishizuka, Y. (1992). Intracellular signaling by hydrolysis of phospholipids and activation of protein kinase C. Science 258:607-14.

Nishizuka, Y. (1995). Protein kinase C and lipid signaling for sustained cellular responses. FASEB J 9:484-96.

Oda, K., Arakawa, H., Tanaka, T. et al. (2000). p53AIP1, a potential mediator of p53-dependent apoptosis, and its regulation by Ser-46-phosphorylated p53. Cell 102:849-62.

Okamura, S., Arakawa, H., Tanaka, T. et al. (2001). p53DINP1, a p53-inducible gene, regulates p53-dependent apoptosis. Mol Cell 8:85-94.

Oren, M. (1999). Regulation of the p53 tumor suppressor protein. J Biol Chem 274:36031-4.

Oren, M., Damalas, A., Gottlieb, T. et al. (2002). Regulation of p53: intricate loops and delicate balances. Biochem Pharmacol 64:865-71.

Raman, V., Martensen, S. A., Reisman, D. et al. (2000). Compromised HOXA5 function can limit p53 expression in human breast tumours. Nature 405:974-8.

Reddig, P. J., Dreckschmidt, N. E., Ahrens, H. et al. (1999). Transgenic mice overexpressing protein kinase Cdelta in the epidermis are resistant to skin tumor promotion by 12-O-tetradecanoylphorbol-13-acetate. Cancer Res 59:5710-8.

Reyland, M. E. (2007). Protein kinase Cdelta and apoptosis. Biochem Soc Trans 35:1001-4.

Reyland, M. E., Anderson, S. M., Matassa, A. A., Barzen, K. A., Quissell, D. O. (1999). Protein kinase C delta is essential for etoposide-induced apoptosis in salivary gland acinar cells. J Biol Chem 274:19115-23.

Ryan, K. M., Phillips, A. C., Vousden, K. H. (2001). Regulation and function of the p53 tumor suppressor protein. Curr Opin Cell Biol 13:332-7.

Scheel-Toellner, D., Pilling, D., Akbar, A. N. et al. (1999). Inhibition of T cell apoptosis by IFN-beta rapidly reverses nuclear translocation of protein kinase C-delta. Eur J Immunol 29:2603-12.

Shieh, S. Y., Ikeda, M., Taya, Y., Prives, C. (1997). DNA damage-induced phosphorylation of p53 alleviates inhibition by MDM2. Cell 91:325-34.

Siliciano, J. D., Canman, C. E., Taya, Y., Sakaguchi, K., Appella, E., Kastan, M. B. (1997). DNA damage induces phosphorylation of the amino terminus of p53. Genes Dev 11:3471-81.

Stuart, E. T., Haffner, R., Oren, M., Gruss, P. (1995). Loss of p53 function through PAX-mediated transcriptional repression. EMBO J 14:5638-45.

Taira, N., Nihira, K., Yamaguchi, T., Miki, Y., Yoshida, K. (2007). DYRK2 is targeted to the nucleus and controls p53 via Ser46 phosphorylation in the apoptotic response to DNA damage. Mol Cell 25:725-38.

Taira, N., Yamamoto, H., Yamaguchi, T., Miki, Y., Yoshida, K. (2010). ATM augments nuclear stabilization of DYRK2 by inhibiting MDM2 in the apoptotic response to DNA damage. J Biol Chem 285:4909-19.

Takai, Y., Kishimoto, A., Inoue, M., Nishizuka, Y. (1977). Studies on a cyclic nucleotide-independent protein kinase and its proenzyme in mammalian tissues. I.

Purification and characterization of an active enzyme from bovine cerebellum. J Biol Chem 252:7603-9.

Vogelstein, B., Lane, D., Levine, A. J. (2000). Surfing the p53 network. Nature 408:307-10.

Wang, Q. J., Bhattacharyya, D., Garfield, S., Nacro, K., Marquez, V. E., Blumberg, P. M. (1999). Differential localization of protein kinase C delta by phorbol esters and related compounds using a fusion protein with green fluorescent protein. J Biol Chem 274:37233-9.

Watanabe, T., Ono, Y., Taniyama, Y. et al. (1992). Cell division arrest induced by phorbol ester in CHO cells overexpressing protein kinase C-delta subspecies. Proc Natl Acad Sci U S A 89:10159-63.

Yamaguchi, T., Kimura, J., Miki, Y., Yoshida, K. (2007a). The deubiquitinating enzyme USP11 controls an IKKalpha -p53 signaling pathway in response to TNFalpha. J Biol Chem 282:33943-8.

Yamaguchi, T., Miki, Y., Yoshida, K. (2007b). Protein kinase C delta activates IkappaB-kinase alpha to induce the p53 tumor suppressor in response to oxidative stress. Cell Signal 19:2088-97.

Yoshida, K. (2007a). PKCdelta signaling: Mechanisms of DNA damage response and apoptosis. Cell Signal 19:892-901.

Yoshida, K. (2007b). Regulation for nuclear targeting of the Abl tyrosine kinase in response to DNA damage. Adv Exp Med Biol 604:155-65.

Yoshida, K. (2008a). Nuclear trafficking of pro-apoptotic kinases in response to DNA damage. Trends Mol Med 14:305-13.

Yoshida, K. (2008b). Role for DYRK family kinases on regulation of apoptosis. Biochem Pharmacol 76:1389-1394.

Yoshida, K., Kufe, D. (2001). Negative regulation of the SHPTP1 protein tyrosine phosphatase by protein kinase C delta in response to DNA damage. Mol Pharmacol 60:1431-8.

Yoshida, K., Liu, H., Miki, Y. (2006a). Protein Kinase C delta regulates Ser46 phosphorylation of p53 tumor suppressor in the apoptotic response to DNA damage. J Biol Chem 281:5734-40.

Yoshida, K., Miki, Y. (2005). Enabling death by the Abl tyrosine kinase: mechanisms for nuclear shuttling of c-Abl in response to DNA damage. Cell Cycle 4:777-9.

Yoshida, K., Miki, Y., Kufe, D. (2002). Activation of SAPK/JNK signaling by protein kinase Cdelta in response to DNA damage. J Biol Chem 277:48372-8.

Yoshida, K., Wang, H. G., Miki, Y., Kufe, D. (2003). Protein kinase Cdelta is responsible for constitutive and DNA damage-induced phosphorylation of Rad9. EMBO J 22:1431-41.

Yoshida, K., Yamaguchi, T., Natsume, T., Kufe, D., Miki, Y. (2005). JNK phosphorylation of 14-3-3 proteins regulates nuclear targeting of c-Abl in the apoptotic response to DNA damage. Nat Cell Biol 7:278-85.

Yoshida, K., Yamaguchi, T., Shinagawa, H., Taira, N., Nakayama, K. I., Miki, Y. (2006b). Protein kinase C delta activates topoisomerase IIalpha to induce apoptotic cell death in response to DNA damage. Mol Cell Biol 26:3414-31.

Yuan, Z. M., Utsugisawa, T., Ishiko, T. et al. (1998). Activation of protein kinase C delta by the c-Abl tyrosine kinase in response to ionizing radiation. Oncogene 16:1643-8.

5

The Influence of Individual Genome Sensitivity in DNA Damage Repair Assessment in Chronic Professional Exposure to Low Doses of Ionizing Radiation

Mirta Milić[1], Ružica Rozgaj[1], Vilena Kašuba[1], Ana Marija Jazbec[2], Patrizia Hrelia[3] and Sabrina Angelini[3]

[1]*Institute for Medical Research and Occupational Health, Mutagenesis Unit, Zagreb*
[2]*Faculty of Forestry, University of Zagreb, Zagreb,*
[3]*Department of Pharmacology, University of Bologna, Bologna,*
[1,2]*Croatia*
[3]*Italy*

1. Introduction

During their working and living activities, humans are constantly exposed to different environmental genotoxic agents. Biological consequences of the exposure are accumulation of different mutations and DNA damage that can lead to disruption of genetic material. Numerous endogenous genotoxic agents can also cause DNA damage. Loss of normal cell function can cause cell death or can result in different health disorders, including teratogenic and cancerogenic effects (Jeggo & Lavin, 2009). There is an increasing concern about mutagenic and cancerogenic effects of genotoxic agents and their influence on individuals who are exposed to them by accident, or by living/working lifestyle (Au, 1991; Carrano & Natarajan, 1988; Kassie et al., 2000).

Exposure to ionising radiation, as a well known genotoxic agents (Balasem & Ali, 1991; Erexon et al., 1991; Fenech et al., 1990; He et al., 2000; Jeggo & Lavin, 2009), can leed to different DNA damage, such as oxidative damage, base and sugar modification in DNA, apurinic/apirimidinic places, single/double strand chromosomal breaks, adduct creation, inter/intra DNA cross linking and other types of damage (Hall & Giaccia, 2006). Numerous studies deal with ionising radiation exposure of individuals who are chronically professionally exposed to low doses (Andreassi, 2009; Au, 1991; Carrano & Natarajan, 1988; Kassie et al., 2000). The results showed the increase in chromosomal damage during chronically low dose exposure (Barquinero et al., 1993; Boutcher, 1985; Cardoso et al., 2001; Jha, 1991; Nowak & Jankowski, 1991), but without confirmed relationship between the received dose and the intensity of DNA damage (Bolus, 2001; Coates et al., 2004; Morgan, 2003; Mothersill et al., 2000, 2001; Seymour & Mothersill, 2000). The influence of chronically low dose exposure has been considered mutagenic and cancerogenic (Fachini et al., 2009). Although it is possible to estimate the influence of absorbed dose and the effect on the exposed individuals, consequences of continuous low dose exposure are still a great topic of researches.

The medical stuff represents the best investigated group of professionals exposed to low levels of ionising radiation (UNSCEAR, 2000). During their work, all the employees wear dosimeters (film, TLD or electronic ones) that are analysed on monthly bases. In addition, they are under regular medical control.

Duration and the intensity of exposure to low doses of ionising radiation have significantly decreased over the last decades. The results of analysed dosimeters showed that the received doses are significantly below the regulatory threshold of 20 mSv per year, sometimes even under the dosimeters detection abilities (Kubelka et al., 2011).

Persons employed in emergency medical units and nuclear medicine workers are exposed to higher doses and show higher DNA damage than workers in diagnostic radiology departments (Sari-Minodier et al., 2007).

Andreassi et al. (2009) reported higher amount of DNA damage among interventional cardiologists when compared to clinical cardiologists. Epidemiological researches have shown the connection between the amounts of accumulated doses and the risk of tumour developing (Berrington et al., 2001; Maitre et al., 2003; Wang et al., 2002; Yoshinaga et al., 1999). Cardisi et al. (2005) reported the relationship between exposure to low doses of ionising radiation and cancer in study that involved 400 000 nuclear industry workers.

Today's general opinion is that initial event in radiation carcinogenesis is un/ missrepaired double strand break of DNA molecule, which is a major lesion that leads to developing of chromosomal abnormalities and genetic mutations (Little, 2000).

Accidental or therapeutical acute exposure to ionising radiation can cause different cytogenetic damage, including higher amount of micronuclei (small amount of chromatin in the shape of small nuclei in cytoplasm that was not divided into two new nuclei after first cell division) and chromosomal aberrations (single /double strand breaks of chromosome, inter/intra chromosomal exchange, dicentrics, acentrics, etc.). Recently, different biomarkers are used for monitoring of people occupationally exposed to chronical low doses of ionising radiation. The use of combined biomarkers can offer better assessment and health care of those individuals. With them a phenomenon of adaptive response has been observed. This response can be seen after the first adapting dose of ionising radiation is received (mostly under 10 cGy). After exposure to higher, so called challenging dose, above 100 cGy, those individuals show lower amount of DNA damage when compared to those who did not receive the first, adapting dose. There is also evidence that the amount of dose received can influence the adaptive response (Gourabi & Mozdarani, 1998). A great variability in DNA damage response to ionising radiation exposure of cell lines *in vitro* and individuals *in vivo* have been reported (Bosi & Olivieri, 1989; Shadley & Wiencke, 1989). Adaptive response has been shown also in persons after clinical, environmental or working exposure (Barquinero et al., 1993, 1995, 1996; Monsieurs et al., 2000; Padovani et al., 1995; Szumiel, 1998; Tedeschi et al., 1995, 1996). Individual differences in DNA repair genes can also influence on this response (Milić, 2010).

Molecular mechanisms of adaptive response are still not clear. It has been considered that it depends on the synthesis and/or protein expression, especially those involved in DNA repair mechanism (Boothman et al., 1989; Ikushima, 1989, 1996; Robson et al., 1999; Wolf et al., 1989, 1996; Youngblom et al., 1989). Early induction response (Okayasu et al., 2000;

Stecca & Gerber, 1998), changes in gene expression, gene transcription regulation are also related with adaptive response. Mutations in genes involved in DNA repair can cause DNA missrepair, chromosome endings fusion, fusion of unprotected telomere ends and double strand breaks after exposure to ionising radiation (Bailey et al., 2004; Bailey & Goodwin, 2004; Sasaki et al., 2002).

The accuracy of any risk assessment, especially low dose exposures, depends on both the resolution of the method, and the baseline data obtained in well-selected controls. Alkaline comet assay (single-cell gel electrophoresis, SCGE) is an easy-to-use, quick and very sensitive method for detecting primary DNA strand breaks, that is, direct DNA damage within single cells (Tice et al., 1990; Collins, 2004) and can be applied to proliferating and non proliferating cells (Kassie et al., 2000) to determine DNA damage as a result of endogenous factors, lifestyle (Hoffman & Speit, 2005), and occupational or environmental exposure (Valverde et al., 1999).

After relaxation, DNA can be seen as a comet during electrophoresis due to strand breaks (Singh, 2000). The advantages of this technique are sensitivity, reproducibility, easy to use, low expences. It is a rapid method and the amount of sample necessary for the analysis is very small. Comet assay enables analysis of any sort of cells, whether it is plant, animal or human origin, no matter are those single cells from the cell culture or from the tissue. Due to the short-time performance of this technique (it is possible to have results after few hours), it has become well accepted in investigation of different genotoxic agents both *in vitro* and *in vivo* conditions (Betti et al., 1994; Kassie et al., 2000; Kruszewski et al., 1998; McKelvey-Martin et al., 1993; Wojewodzka et al., 1998).

In this method, single cells are embedded into so called agarosis sandwich. Cytoplasm and membranic cell structures are lysed with high concentrated EDTA solution (ethylenediaminetetraacetic acid) and detergents, causing total cell DNA to be free. There are two comet assay protocols, whether alkaline or neutral denaturation is used.

Neutral version enables detection of double stranded DNA breaks (Olive et al., 1990). Under alkaline conditions, single stranded breaks, alkaline labile sites (AP, parts of DNA that can break easily in alkaline solutions), DNA-DNA and DNA protein crosslinking can be detected. Alkaline labile sites are apurinic and apirimidinic DNA bases that can break easily when exposed to alkaline conditions (Singh et al., 1988). After alkaline/neutral denaturation, the cells undergo electrophoresis. Concerning the high molecular weight of the entire DNA molecule, DNA can not pass through the agarose pores towards the anode. Only the small, damaged fragments can pass through. During electrophoresis, the velocity of those fragments that are caused by single or double chromosome breaks depends on their molecular weight. The smaller they are, the faster they get (Plappert et al., 1995). After electrophoresis, the slides are stained with fluorescent dye (usually ethidium bromide). Epifluorescent microscope is used for single cells analysing. Undamaged cells have round shape, while damaged one are similar to the shape of the comet. The mostly used parameters of comet assay are the tail length (TL), percentage of DNA in tail (TI) and the tail moment (TM). Tail length (usually expressed in micrometers) is measured from the centre of the comet head till the end of the comet tail (that is the distance of the fragments from the major DNA that have travelled through the gel during electrophoresis). It is proportional with DNA damage and with length of the fragments (Singh et al., 1988; Tice et al., 1990). TI is measured with computer programme for comet assay analysis. The amount of the damage is estimated based on the ratio of DNA percentage in head and in tail of a comet. Some researchers prefer tail moment as the most reliable marker of DNA damage, because it combines measurements of tail length and percentage of DNA in tail (Ashby et al., 1995; Hellman et al., 1995; 1997; Mc Kelvey-Martin et al., 1998). Collins (2004) emphasizes the advantage of TI considering that the percentage of the tail DNA reflects the real DNA damage. Comet assay can also detect apoptotic and necrotic cells. Apoptotic cells show small comet head, and most of DNA is spread in tail in the shape of a cloud (Fairbairn et al., 1995; Olive, 1999). Comet assay is also a valuable technique to study the kinetics of primary DNA damage. It enables to estimate the DNA damage level immediately after the exposure, even when the exposure included very small dose in very short exposure period (Tice et al., 1990; Plappert et al., 1995). Fast repair can represent a problem in DNA damage evaluation in populations occupationally exposed to low doses of ionising radiation and therefore the development of sensitive methods is necessary for those experiments. Most of the primary DNA damage is repaired 30 minutes after the exposure to ionising radiation (Frankenberg-Schwager, 1989), and 2 hours after the exposure to dose of 2 Gy, most of the damaged DNA is totally repaired (Plappert et al., 1997).

Polymorphism by definition is expression of different phenotypes in the same species due to the change/s in genotype. They usually include loss (deletion) of small or bigger part of DNA molecule, insertion of specific number of nucleotides or repetition of di-, three-, or oligonucleotides in variant number. The number or repeating differs among individuals.

Variations in human genome are usually caused by variations in DNA sequence, that is based on the change of only one nucleotide (one from the four nucleotides; A-adenine, T-thymine, C-cytosine or G-guanosine is replaced by the other) usually known as SNP polymorphism (*single nucleotide polymorphism*). Among almost 15 million of SNPs in human genome, 50.000 to 100. 000 of them can change the function or gene expression.

The connection of the change in only one nucleotide (that happens once in every 1000nucleotides in human genome) with the complex aetiology of malignant diseases is poorly investigated (Bonassi et al., 2005). More than 7 millions of well known SNPs in human genome appear with the allelic frequency higher than 5% of the entire population (Hinds et al., 2005). More than 70% of SNPs in human population have the frequency less than 5 % and those SNPs are called rare SNPs (Shastry, 2009). The results of new experiments have shown the connection between gene polymorphisms and risk association with disease developing (Norpa, 2004), especially in polymorphisms of DNA repair genes and folic acid metabolism. Polymorphisms can lead to different gene expression (decreased or increased) and through this process can influence on cell repair mechanisms (Hung et al., 2005; Parl, 2005; Weiss et al., 2005; Kotsopoulos et al., 2007). Variations in DNA repair capacity have been also observed among healthy individuals (Setlow, 1983).

Among 130 genes involved in DNA repair mechanisms, 80 of them are carriers of more than 400 SNPs (Mohrenweiser et al., 2003). DNA damage and repair correlate with the radiation sensitivity and are important in radiation protection and radiotherapy (Ross et al., 2000). Due to individual variations, some persons have higher sensitivity when compared with general population (Berwick, 2000). It has been estimated that 10 -15 percent of healthy people have phenotype that shows decreased possibility for successful DNA damage repair (Mohrenweiser & Jones, 1998; Hu et al., 2002a). Higher risk of mutations, genome instability and malignant tumours have been observed among persons with decreased DNA repair capacity (Berwick & Vineis, 2000; Chen et al., 2002; Collins & Harrington, 2002; Divine et al., 2001; Hou et al., 2002; Kumar et al., 2003; Sturgis et al., 1999; Winsey et al., 2000).

The connection between ionising radiation and SNPs in gene involved in DNA repair has been described by several authors (Aka et al., 2004; Hu et al., 2001; Lunn et al., 2000; Touil et al., 2002). There is an increased interest for exploring of SNPs of genes that are part of biological response to ionising radiation and connecting them with clinical sensibility. Those SNPs could be used for an estimation of exposure to ionising radiation (Andreassen, 2005).

Determination of high risk population on the basis of genetic polymorphism could help in tumour prevention. The influence of polymorphisms can be crucial in the exposure to low doses of ionising radiation (Boffetta et al., 1999).

2. Materials and methods

This study included 126 subjects, 70 medical workers occupationally exposed to low doses of ionising radiation (gastroenterologists, cardiologists, anaesthesiologists, surgeons, radiologists, radiology technicians, nurses) of both gender (45 females, 25 men; mean age was 40 years, from 20-60 years old) and 56 individuals in control group who were not exposed to neither ionising radiation nor to chemical mutagens (14 women and men; mean age 40 years, from 23 to 60 years old) (Table 1).

	Control group	Exposed group
Subjects (No.) F/M	56 14/42	70 45/25
Age±SD (Min-Max)	40.53±10.92 (23-60)	40.27±10.8 (20-60)
Smoking, Y/N	16/40	31/39
Alcohol, Y/N	35/21	21/49
Years of exposure±SD (Min-Max)	-	12.22±8.65 (1-38)

Table 1. Characteristics of the control and exposed group considering the gender, age, years of exposure, smoking status and alcohol consumption.

The examinees were informed of the study scope and experimental details, have filled a standardised questionnaire designed to obtain relevant information on the current health status, medical history, and lifestyle, and gave their written consent, submitted and approved by the local Ethics Committee. The questionnaire included data on the exposure to possible confounding factors: smoking, alcohol consumption, use of medicines, contraceptives, severe infections, or viral diseases over the past six months, vitamin intake, recent vaccinations, presence of known inherited genetic disorders and chronic diseases, family history of cancer, exposure to diagnostic X-rays. Subjects with history of previous radio- or chemotherapy were not included. Exposed group was under regular film dosimetry and the dose received did not exceed 20mSv/year (data not shown).

Two millilitres of venous blood was stored in heparinised vacutainers for comet assay and assessment of DNA repair kinetics and stored at +4°C before further procedure. Detailed protocol is described before (Milić et al., 2010). Five millilitres of venous blood was stored in vacutainers with EDTA (ethylenediaminetetraacetic acid) at -20°C until further DNA isolation (Milić et al., 2010). Blood samples were irradiated with 60Co (Alcyon, CGR-MeV, France). The doses used were 2 and 4 Gy, with the same distance from the source (80 cm). Irradiation field was 15 x 15 cm^2. After irradiation, samples were kept at + 4°C to prevent the repair of the damage. Details are also described before (Milić et al., 2010).

2.1 Comet assay

Alkaline version of comet assay (Singh et al., 1988) with small modifications was used. Detailed procedure is described elsewhere (Milić, 2010; Milić et al., 2010). The slides were marked and stored at +4°C till the beginning of the irradiation. Control samples were put into cold lysis solution immediately after preparation and left there for 24 hours at +4°C (Milić, 2010). Irradiated blood gel samples were incubated at 37°C in serum free RPMI 1640 medium. Zero samples were immediately immersed into lysis solution. DNA repair kinetics was measured at 0, 15, 30, 60 and 120 minutes after exposure, and additional 24 hours for samples irradiated with the dose of 4 Gy. Specific measure points were based on the results of other researches (Singh et al., 1988; Price, 1993; Tice, 1995). The 2 Gy dose was a standard daily dose in radiotherapy, while the 4 Gy dose was chosen as a ″challenging″ dose for the exposed group. After the repair, slides were vertically placed into cold lysis solution at 4°C, overnight. Protein denaturation and DNA unwinding were done at 4°C in denaturation buffer (1 mM Na2EDTA and 300 mM NaOH) (pH 13.0) for 20 minutes. Horizontal electrophoresis in fresh cold denaturation buffer was done at 300 mA and 25 V for 20 minutes. The slides were washed in neutralisation buffer (0.4 M Tris-HCl, pH 7.5) three times. Slides were stained with 50 μL of ethidium bromide solution (20 $\mu g mL^{-1}$, Sigma) (per slide), covered with cover slip and kept in container, in the dark conditions at 4°C.

The procedure was done under dimmed light, in order to avoid additional DNA damage caused by the exposure to the normal light. Each slide was examined using a 250x magnification fluorescence microscope (Zeiss, Germany) equipped with an excitation filter of 515-560 nm and a barrier filter of 590 nm. A total of 200 comets per sample and per interval were scored (100 from each of two replicate slides). Comets were randomly captured at a constant depth of the gel, avoiding the edges of the gel, occasional dead cells and superimposed comets. Using a black and white camera, the microscope image was transferred to a computer-based image analysis system (Comet Assay II, Perceptive Instruments Ltd., U.K.). To avoid the variability, one well-trained scorer scored all comets. Three parameters of DNA damage were analysed: tail length (TL, presented in micrometres), tail DNA (TI, %) and tail moment (TM).

2.2 DNA isolation

Genomic DNA was isolated from peripheral lymphocytes according to modified protocol by Daly et al. (1996) or according to protocol for genomic DNA lymphocyte isolation from QUIAGEN (mini KIT). DNA was purified with two times centrifugation at 4°C, 500 μL of 70 percent ethanol added every time. The pellet was dried overnight at room temperature and diluted in 100 µL of TE buffer (10mM Tris–HCl, pH 7.4; 1 mM EDTA, pH 8.0). Purity and concentration of DNA was specified by spectrophotometric method (NanoDrop ND- 1000 spectrophotometer, NanoDrop Technologies, Thermo Scientific, Wilmington, USA). Samples were diluted till concentration of 10 ng μL^{-1} and kept at -20 °C till amplification. Specific polymorphisms were determined: in BER- (base excision repair) APE1- (apurinic/apirimidinic endonuclease, Asp148Glu), hOGG1 (human 8-oxoguanine DNA glycosylase, Ser326Cys), XRCC1 (X-ray repair cross-complementing protein-group 1, Arg194Trp); in NER- (nucleotide excision repair) XPD (Xeroderma pigmentosum-group D, Lys751Gln; DSBR- (double-strand-break repair) XRCC3 (X-ray repair cross-complementing protein-group 3, Thr241Met), PARP1 (poly (ADP-ribose) polymerase 1, Val762Ala); in DRR- (direct reversal repair) MGMT (O6-methylguanine-DNA methyltransferase, Leu84Phe) Genotyping was performed by either Real Time PCR (polymerase chain reaction) with Taqman assay, or after electrophoresis and fluorescence visualisation, DNA samples were cut with restriction enzymes.

2.3 Polymerase chain reaction-RFLP

In a total volume of 10 ml, 10 ng of genomic DNA was amplified for each sample. Compounds for the reaction mixture are given in Table 2.

PCR reaction was completed in six steps: (I) incubation at 94 °C (2 min) for Taq DNA polymerase activation; (II) incubation at 94 °C (30 s) for denaturation of double stranded DNA; (III) incubation at specific temperature that depended on the specific gene (30 s), for hybridisation of primers (Table 3); (IV) incubation at 72 °C (30 s) for DNA synthesis. Steps No.2 to No. 4 were repeated for 34 times. After that there were steps: (V) incubation at 72 °C (5 min) and (VI) incubation at 10 °C.

Reaction mixture	Stock solution	Final concentration for PCR reaction
(DMSO)	(1x)	(for XRCC3-0.05x)
reH_2O	1x	0.64x (for XRCC3-0.59x)
10X BUFFER	10x	1.00 x
$MgCl_2$	50 mM	2.00 mM
dNTP	1.25 mM	0.11 mM
Primer F	20 µM	0.30 µM
Primer R	20 µM	0.30 µM
DNA polymerase (Platinum Taq, Invitrogen)	5 U μl^{-1}	0,03 U μl^{-1}

Table 2. Compounds for PCR-RFLP reaction (10 µl of reaction mixture (9 µl of Master Mix and 1 µl of DNA sample).

GENE	rs	PCR method	primers	°C	Restriction enzyme
XPD ex 23 or ERCC2	rs13181 [Aag > Cag; Lys751Gln]	RFLP (Angelini et al., 2005)	F CCC CTC TCC CTT TCC TCT GTT R GCT GCC TTC TCC TGC GAT TA	61	PstI (37 °C, overnight) CTGCA*G G*ACGTC HOwt-29,244bp; HE-29,63,181,244bp; HOSNP-29,63,181bp
XPD10	rs1799793 [Gac > Aag; Asp312Asn]	Real Time TaqMan assay C_3145050_10	none	none	none
XRCC1 ex10	rs861539 [aCg > aTg; Trp194Arg]	RFLP (Angelini et al., 2005) RT TaqMan assay C_622564_10	F GCC CCT CAG ATC ACA CCT AAC R CAT TGC CCA GCA CAG GAT AA	61	MspI (37 °C, overnight) C*CGG GGC*C WT-161, 53 bp; HE-241, 161, 53 bp; SNP-214 bp
XRCC3 ex7	rs861539 [aCg > aTg; Thr241Met]	RFLP (Angelini et al., 2005)	F GCT CGC CTG GTG GTC ATC R CTT CCG CAT CCT GGC TAA AAA	60	Hin1 II/NIa III (37 °C, overnight)
hOGG1, ex4	rs1052133 [tCc > tGc; Ser326cys]	RFLP (Godderis et al., 2006) RT TaqMan assay C_3095552_1	F CCCAACCCCAGTGGATTCTCATTGC R GGTGCCCCATCTAGCCTTGCGGCCCTT	60	SatI/ Fnu4HI (37 °C, overnight) GC*NGC CGN*CG HOwt-214,20pb; HE-214,165,49,20pb; HOSNP-165,49,20pb
PARP1	-	RT TaqMan assay	Real time	none	none
APE1	rs1130409 [gaT > gaG; Asp148Glu]	RFLP (Hu et al., 2002) RT TaqMan assay C_8921503_10	F CTGTTTCATTTCTATAGGCTA R AGGAACTTGCGAAAGGCTTC	57	BfaI (37 °C, overnight) (Asp/Asp 164bp, Asp/Glu 164,144,20bp; Glu/Glu-144,20bp)
MGMT C/T	rs12917, Leu84Phe	RT TaqMan assay	Real time	none	none

Table 3. Gene, forward and reverse primers, method used for determination of polymorphism, hybridisation temperature, restriction enzymes and the DNA fragments.

After PCR reaction, DNA products were cut with specific restriction enzymes (Fermentas, Vilnius, Litva) that have cut DNA samples on specific places and have given different DNA fragments in order to recognize which samples were homozygote wild type, heterozygote and polymorphic homozygotes. Treatment with restriction enzymes was performed at 37 °C in a period of 3 hours or overnight (due to the specification of specific restriction enzyme used in the reaction). Enzymes, time intervals of cutting, the temperature for those enzymes and the resulting DNA fragments after the cutting are given in Table 3. After electrophoresis that lasted 30 minutes at 200 V, PCR products were analysed on 10%-polyacrilamid gel (Bio-Rad, Hercules, USA).

Genotype results were regularly confirmed by random repetition of the samples.

PCR products were also amplified with Real-Time PCR (Real-Time PCR ABI Prism 7300 thermocycler, Applied Biosystems, Foster City, USA) with TaqMan allelic discrimination assay (Applera, Foster City, USA). Allelic determination was done by their software. Compounds for the Real-Time PCR mixture is shown in Table 4. Forty cycluses were performed for division between VIC and FAM fluorescence stain. The intensity of those stains is selecting the samples into three categories (Angelini et al., 2005).

Ingredients	Volume/µl
TaqMan Master Mix	6.5
reH_2O	5.33
Specific primers for every gene	0.65
DNA sample	0.5

Table 4. Compounds for Real Time PCR reaction. Steps in Real Time PCR-a were: (I) 95 °C (10 min); (II) 92 °C (15 s); and (III) 60 °C (10 min).

3. Results

DNA repair kinetics after the exposure to gamma radiation of 2 and 4 Gy was measured on a group of 126 subjects, 70 medical workers and 56 controls (Figure 1).

The groups differed in average age, gender, smoking status and alcohol consumption. The mean values for both groups did not significantly differ, although inter-individual differences were notable. In control group higher level of DNA damage compared to exposed group was observed, but without statistical difference. The repair dynamic was the same in both groups.

After genotyping, heterozygotes and polymorphic homozygotes were grouped together to evaluate polymorphic allele appearance. Number of individuals carrying particular gene is given in Table 5. Frequency of genotyping did not differ from expected Hardy-Weinberg equilibrium.

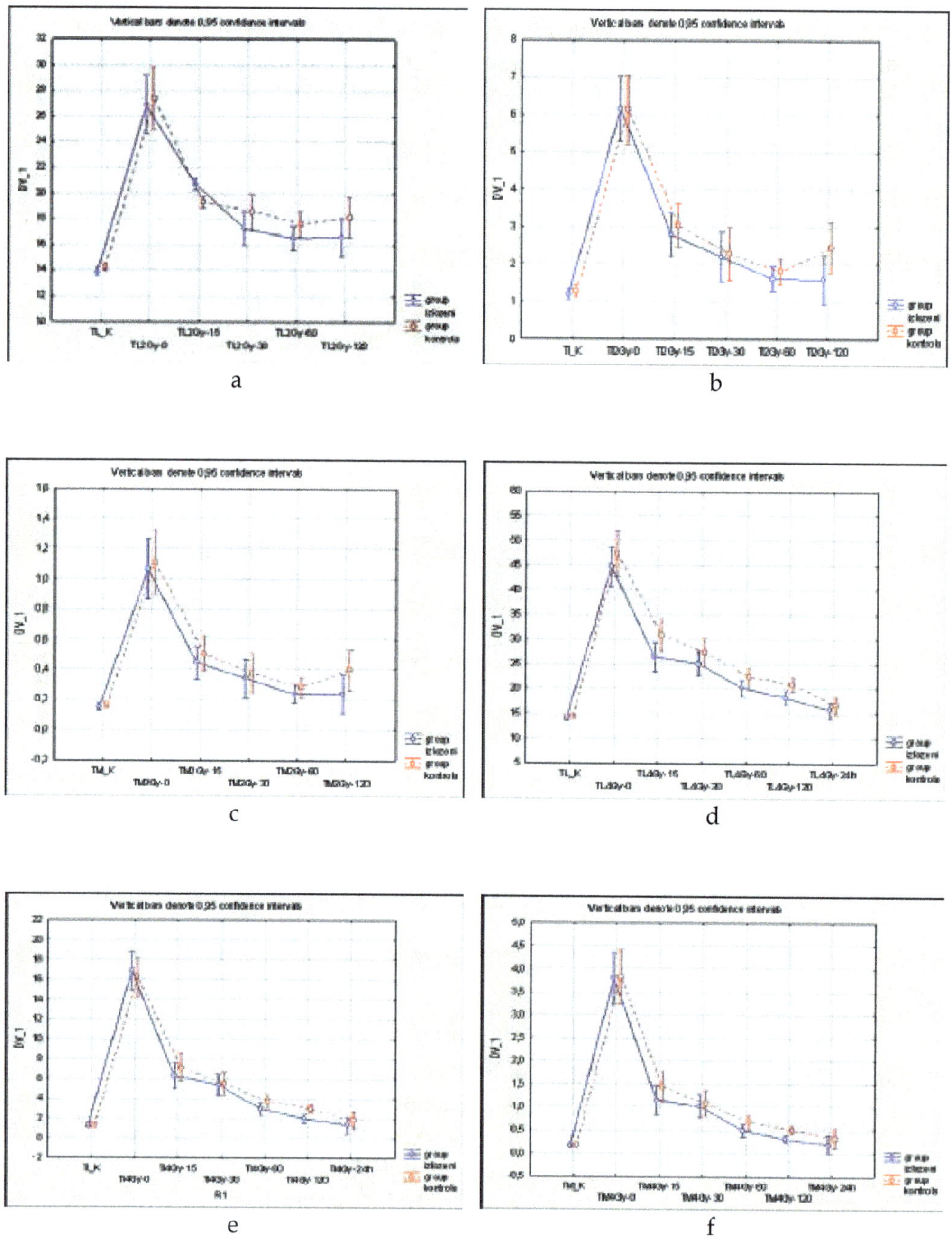

Fig. 1. Graphical results of DNA repair. Red colour - control group; blue - exposed group. a- TL after 2 Gy irradiation, b-TI after 2 Gy, c-TM after 2 Gy, d- TL after 4 Gy irradiation, e- TI after 4 Gy, f- TM after 4 Gy.

Gene	Group (WT/HE/SNP)	Control (WT/HE/SNP)	Exposed (WT/HE/SNP)
XPD 23	42/58/26	15/33/8	27/25/18
XPD 10	43/63/20	17/33/6	26/30/14
XRCC1	47/67/12	22/25/9	25/42/3
PARP1	83/37/6	33/18/5	50/19/1
HOGG1	78/43/5	42/14/0	36/29/5
APE1	43/57/26	19/27/10	24/30/16
MGMT C/T	87/34/5	39/16/1	48/18/4
XRCC3	45/61/20	23/26/7	22/35/13

Table 5. Number of individuals in three genotyping groups for all genes (WT-homozygote wild type, HE-heterozygote, SNP-polymorphic homozygote).

Variable	st	χ^2	p
XRCC1	1	0.1697	0.6804
hOGG1	1	7.3298	**0.0068**
APE2	1	0.0018	0.9665
XPD21	1	0.6372	0.4247
PARP2	1	2.1624	0.1414
MGMT C/T	1	0.0167	0.8971
XRCC3	1	1.6433	0.1999
smoking	1	1.7174	0.19
sex	1	13.2499	**0.0003**

Table 6. Results of χ2-test in the exposed and control group compared to genotype frequency, smoking and gender.

The differences between exposed and control group were analysed by χ2-test. Significant difference was found for hOGG1 gene and for gender (Table 6). Observed difference between smokers and non smokers was insignificant.

Multivariate regression analysis was used to estimate the influence of smoking, gender, age, years of exposure and genotypes on comet assay parameters immediately after and 120 minutes after exposure to 2 Gy and after 24 hours for the dose of 4 Gy.

Immediately after irradiation with the 2 Gy dose, exposed group had significantly lower amount of DNA damage than control group. Individuals with polymorphic variants of XRCC3 gene had higher TL than their homozygotes. Polymorphic variants of hOGG1 gene had higher TI than homozygotes. Polymorphic variants of hOGG1 gene had significantly higher TM than their homozygotes.

Tail length values significantly differed between the two groups both immediately after and also 120 minutes after irradiation with 2 Gy. Polymorphic variants of APE1 and XPD10 genes had higher TI and TM compared to homozygotes 120 min after irradiation with 2 Gy, and polymorphic variants of MGMT C/T and XRCC3 genes had significantly lower TI and TM than homozygotes (Table 7).

Variable	PE	SE	Parc R^2	F	p
Log TL-2 Gy-0'					
Group	-0.10669	0.04189	0.0468	6.49	0.0124
XRCC3	0.09351	0.04390	0.0312	4.54	0.0357
MTR	0.07742	0.04335	0.0291	3.19	0.0772
Log TI-2 Gy-0'					
hOGG1	0.14426	0.07300	0.0509	3.91	0.0376
Log TM-2 Gy-0'					
TS	0.16398	0.10332	0.1157	2.52	0.0243
hOGG1	0.16083	0.09018	0.0776	3.18	0.0223
Log TL-2 Gy-120'					
Group	0.00069854	0.00019567	0.0914	12.74	0.0006
XPD 10	0.00037667	0.00020220	0.0274	3.47	0.0655
XRCC3	0.00031641	0.00020077	0.0220	2.48	0.1183
TI-2 Gy-120'					
Group	0.16440	0.04433	0.0004	13.75	0.1012
APE1	0.08068	0.04704	0.0896	2.94	0.0217
XPD10	0.09252	0.04627	0.0484	4.0	0.0239
MGMT C/T	-0.07375	0.04608	0.1128	2.56	0.0217
XRCC3	-0.09915	0.04763	0.0401	4.33	0.0262
TM-2 Gy-120'					
Group	0.48944	0.12713	0.0002	14.82	0.1075
APE1	0.23214	0.13490	0.0885	2.96	0.0217
XPD10	0.26994	0.13268	0.0447	4.14	0.0247
MGMT C/T	-0.20599	0.13216	0.1224	2.43	0.0204
XRRC3	-0.29847	0.13659	0.0313	4.77	0.0289

Table 7. Results of *stepwise* procedure in multivariate regression analysis for three comet assay parameters as a depended variable in the entire population immediately after radiation with 2 Gy dose and 120 minutes after irradiation (only the statistically significant results are shown in the Table).

Immediately after 4 Gy irradiation, multivariate regression analysis showed influence of smoking on TL. Polymorphic variants of SHMT1 genes had lower TL than their homozygotes. Gender had significant influence on TI. Polymorphic variants of SHMT1 and PARP1 genes had lower TI and TM when compared to their homozygotes.

Polymorphic variants of APE1 gene showed positive correlation with TL 24 hours after radiation with 4 Gy. Polymorphic variants of MGMT C/T gene had lower TL than homozygotes.

With the increase of age, significant increase in TI was measured 24 hours after exposure to 4 Gy. Polymorphic variants of PARP1 gene had lower values of TI than homozygotes. Age has shown positive correlation with TM. Lower values for TM were observed among polymorphic variants of PARP1 gene when compared to homozygotes (Table 8).

Variable	PE	SE	Parc R^2	F	p
TL-4 Gy-0'					
Smoking	4.10520	2.19325	3.50	0.0642	0.0267
SHMT1	-3.74806	2.11391	3.14	0.0793	0.0297
TI-4 Gy-0'					
Gender	1.37561	0.94228	2.13	0.1475	0.0199
SHMT1	-1.65022	0.95455	2.99	0.0870	0.0294
PARP1	-1.63931	1.02226	2.57	0.1120	0.0257
TM-4 Gy-0'					
SHMT1	-0.14041	0.07716	3.31	0.0718	0.0304
PARP1	-0.13713	0.08267	2.75	0.1003	0.0260
TL-4 Gy-24h					
Gender	0.00036220	0.00017016	4.53	0.0361	0.0468
MTR	0.00047723	0.00017978	7.05	0.0094	0.0499
APE1	0.00036597	0.00018268	4.01	0.0483	0.0329
MGMT C/T	-0.00034719	0.00017942	3.74	0.0562	0.0359
TI-4 Gy-24h					
Gender	0.11087	0.04594	5.82	0.0180	0.0390
Age	0.00387	0.00203	3.63	0.0601	0.0376
TS	-0.07933	0.05406	2.15	0.1461	0.0741
MTHFR4	0.09859	0.04499	4.80	0.0313	0.0372
PARP1	-0.10466	0.04861	4.64	0.0342	0.0267
TM-4 Gy-24h					
Gender	2.03821	0.60467	11.36	0.0011	0.0869
Age	0.05384	0.02783	3.74	0.0565	0.0349
MTHFR4	1.59011	0.62442	6.48	0.0127	0.0635
MTR	0.97502	0.62696	2.42	0.1238	0.0224
PARP1	-1.21130	0.67510	3.22	0.0765	0.0313

Table 8. Results of *stepwise* procedure in multivariate regression analysis for three comet assay parameters as a depended variable in the entire population immediately after radiation with 4 Gy dose and 24 hours after irradiation (only the statistically significant results are shown in the Table).

3.1 Discussion

Development of new methods in genotoxicology, especially on molecular level, has greatly improved the knowledge and understanding of processes that follow after the organism was exposed to ionising radiation. In the same time, better radiation protection, that includes more sophisticated handling of radiation sources, better education of personnel who are operating on those sources, precise dosimetry and the use of protection equipment have reduced health risk in specific population occupationally exposed to ionising radiation. Recent investigations in the field of radiation protection have focused on individual differences in radiosensitivity. It has been shown that DNA repair capability is regulated with different mechanisms that include great number of genes involved directly or indirectly in the repair process.

DNA damage kinetics of primary damage can give us first information about the level of the damage. Estimation of damage after exposure to low doses of ionising radiation is possible in a very short time period (Olive et al., 1990, 1995; Tice et al., 1990). Most of the DNA breaks can be repaired during 30 minutes from the exposure to ionising radiation (Frankenberg-Schwager, 1989), and two hours from the exposure, almost all the damage is repaired (Plappert et al., 1997). Since the repair is so quick, estimation of DNA damage represents a major problem in studies of occupationally exposed professionals and demands developing of sensitive methods for detecting the level of DNA damage after exposure to low doses of ionising radiation.

In this study the influence of gene polymorphisms on DNA repair after exposure to 2 and 4 Gy of gamma radiation was investigated. The analysis of comet assay parameters did not give consistent results. Immediately after the irradiation with the dose of 2 Gy, values for tail intensity, which is recently considered the most reliable parameter for DNA damage estimation (Collins, 2004), were higher than the values of other authors for the same dose (Cornetta et al., 2006). The exposed and control group also had significantly higher TL and TM for all observed time intervals when compared to the control values before irradiation in both groups. On the other hand, TI significantly decreased after 30 minutes from the exposure. After 60 minutes from the exposure, the values did not significantly differ from the control values before irradiation in both control and exposed group. Those results were different that the ones found by Cornetta et al. (2006) during DNA repair assessment after the exposure to the dose of 2 Gy. They have shown that even after 60 minutes from the exposure, TI were still significantly higher than before radiation. The differences in significance in TL and TI in our research showed different sensitivity of those two parameters. Tail length values implicate the existence of small DNA fragments that have created comet tail shape during electrophoresis and showed the length of travelling of small fragments from the nucleus. On the other hand, TI show the amount of damaged DNA in comet tail. Damaged DNA can be seen as small DNA fragments or relaxed DNA loops from the comet head created during electrophoresis. Tail moment shows the ratio of DNA in comet tail. Our results have shown that most of the DNA damage has been repaired during 30 minutes from the exposure to 2 Gy. The amount of the unrepaired damage did not significantly differ from the amount of the damage in samples that were not irradiated, but were also investigated in DNA repair process. The results showed that TI was better marker of DNA damage than TL. Those findings are in agreement with results of Kumaravel & Jha (2006), who have also estimated the reliability of comet assay parameter after the exposure of peripheral blood samples to gamma irradiation with the doses of 0, 1, 2, 4 and 8 Gy. Besides the fact that TI and TM showed greater reliability for DNA damage estimation, they have also showed strong correlation with the received dose of irradiation.

After 4 Gy irradiation, the values for all three parameters in both control and exposed groups were higher than after irradiation with 2 Gy. Tail length values in irradiated samples were significantly higher than non-irradiated samples for the time periods of 0, 15, 30, 60 and 120 minutes, but not after 24 hours for both exposed and control group.

Values for TI and TM in irradiated samples were significantly different from the values of non-irradiated samples for time period of 0, 15, 30 and 60 minutes, suggesting that most of DNA damage has been repaired during that period, although the values measured 120 minutes and 24 hours after the exposure did not reach the values before the exposure in exposed and control group. The results indicate the existence of small amount of DNA damage that is still present even after 24 hours from the exposure, independently of the dose level. The results could be explained by the difference in the repair of single stranded and double stranded DNA breaks. Single stranded DNA breaks are usually formed after the exposure to gamma or X-ray (90 %), while only small part of damage is created by double stranded breaks (10 %) (Cornetta et al., 2006). The repair of double stranded breaks after the exposure to ionising radiation usually lasts 12 or 16 hours (Vodicka et al., 2004), that is considerably longer than the repair of single stranded breaks. The amount of unrepaired damage in this experiment did not statistically differ from the control values before irradiation for both control and the exposed group. The difference between exposed and nonirradiated samples was higher for 2 Gy dose. The existence of small amount of unrepaired damage shows the importance of assessment of exposure to ionising radiation, especially to low doses and suggesting possible accumulation of primary, unrepaired damage that can lead to permanent damage and genome instability.

When the unrepaired amount of damage was compared, the results are implicating the existence of adaptive response in professionally exposed individuals to low doses of ionising radiation. Adaptive response in human lymphocytes has been described by other authors (Olivieri & Bosi, 1990; Sankaranarayanan et al., 1989; Shadley &Wolff, 1987; Wiencke et al., 1986; Wolff et al., 1990; Wolff, 1992, 1996). Aka et al. (2004) reported the existence of residual damage in tail intensity 60 and 120 minutes after the exposure to dose of 2 Gy. In their experiment, tail intensity values were also higher in the control group than the exposed one.

According to our results, despite the difference in the amount of damage, kinetics of repair after the exposure to both doses was similar to the one for the nonirradiated group. Unexpectedly, the difference between control and exposed group was significantly higher after 2 Gy than after 4 Gy exposure. These results were not in agreement with Wojcik et al. (1996) who claimed that kinetics of repair was faster in the exposed group. Aka et al. (2004) used comet assay for DNA repair assessment in human lymphocytes of male nuclear power plant workers and also for the control group (N=31). After the exposure, there was not significantly different repair kinetics between exposed and control group. Our results were comparable, indicating that healthy persons use the same repair mechanism, no matter if they are professionally exposed to ionising radiation or not. High standard deviation, also seen in the results of other author (DeMeo et al., 1991; Maluf et al., 2001; Maluf, 2004; Tice, 1995), implicated on the influence of interindividual differences. Since the comet assay measures primary DNA damage after the exposure, those results can be a marker of different gene activity. Besides the gene activity, the DNA repair can be influenced by the smoking status, gender, age and years of occupational exposure.

Smoking can also cause DNA damage when heavy and non heavy smokers were compared (Maluf et al., 2001; Maluf, 2004). Marcon et al. (2003) showed that heavy smokers can repair DNA damage after the exposure to 2 Gy faster than non smokers or non- heavy smokers. Olivieri et al. (1984) and Shadley (1994) suggested the existence of adaptive response that protects lymphocytes from oxidative damage. Smokers also showed lower levels of oxidised pyrimidinic bases in lymphocytes when compared to non-smokers (Berasati et al., 2001). Touil et al. (2002) showed that chemicals from the smoke can create covalent bonds between DNA and proteins, that can result with lower migration of DNA during electrophoresis, showing false results, that is lower damage. Cebulska et al. (2007) showed negative influence of smoking on the efficiency of DNA repair in lymphocytes. On the other hand, Rzeszowska-Wolny et al. (2005) did not find significant correlation between smoking and DNA damage and DNA repair after the irradiation of human lymphocytes with the dose of 2 Gy. Our results also did not show the influence of smoking on DNA repair of primary damage, except for the tail length after the exposure to 4 Gy dose. The results are similar to Aka et al. (2004) on nuclear power plant workers.

It is still not clear whether the basal damage differ due to gender. Dusinska et al. (2004a) did not find the difference in creation of strand breaks, nor in the amount of DNA damage sensitive to action of specific enzymes such as endonuclease III, or FPG enzyme or alkali labile sites, although male had lower DNA damage after the treatment with hydrogen peroxide (Dusinska et al., 2004a, b). Bajpayee et al. (2002) showed that healthy men have more basal damage in lymphocytes than women. Our results showed that difference was only seen after the 4 Gy dose, where women had higher values for DNA damage in all three parameters observed in comet assay immediately after and 24 hours after the irradiation. There was not similar number of male and female, and that could also influence the results. Trzeciak et al. (2008) showed that there are differences in the amount of damage and the repair rate after the exposure of whole blood sample to 6.3 Gy dose. But most of the experiments did not show the gender influence on DNA repair capacity (Muller et al., 2001, 2002; Rajaee-Behbahani et al., 2001; Marcon et al., 2003).

Age influence was not seen in this experiment. That is in agreement with other authors (Betti et al., 1994; Frenzili et al., 1997). Rzeszowska-Wolny et al. (2005) did not show the influence of sex on DNA damage level and DNA repair by the comet assay after the exposure to 2 Gy dose. Maluf et al. (2001) showed positive correlation of age and DNA repair in the exposed group. Singh et al. (1988) described positive correlation between the age and DNA damage in non-smokers.

Although former results showed the existence of radio adaptive response, our results did not confirm the relationship between primary DNA damage and adaptive response. Few authors have also shown lower DNA damage levels after the repeated exposure to ionising radiation (Sankaranarayanan et al., 1989; Wang et al., 1991; Ikushima, 1992; Domingues et al., 1993).

APE1 gene is involved in BER repair. Polymorphism in exon 5 is connected with hypersensitivity during the exposure to ionising radiation (Au et al., 2006). Results are in agreement with Au et al. (2006). There was positive correlation of polymorphic variants and DNA damage level 120 minutes after the exposure to 2 Gy.

Polymorphic variants of hOGG1 gene showed positive correlation with TI and TM measured immediately after the exposure to the dose of 2 Gy. The results are in agreement with Aka et al. (2004) who showed the connection between polymorphic variants of hOGG1 Ser326Cys with lower capability of repair of oxidative DNA damage in the exposed, but not in the control group measured 60 and 120 minutes after the exposure to 2 Gy. After 120 minutes from the exposure, 71 % of individuals with high level of DNA damage had polymorphic variant of hOGG1 gene. Cornetta et al. (2006) did not show the influence of hOGG1 polymorphism on DNA damage.

Goode et al. (2002)) showed the connection between polymorphic variants of hOGG1 with higher risk of lung, head and neck cancer. hOGG1 and XRCC1 are involved in the same

repair pathway, while hOGG1 cuts oxidised base, XRCC1 together with ligase closes the break. Aka et al. (2004) and Matullo (2003) have described their connection. On the other hand, Cornetta et al. (2006), did not show significant difference between XRCC1, hOGG1 and XPC polymorphisms and DNA damage level measured 30 minutes from the exposure to 2 Gy dose. Yamane et al. (2004) showed that homozygotes differ for 2 fold factor in cutting of 8-oxodeoxiguanosine when compared to heterozygote.
XRCC1 polymorphism did not show the influence on DNA damage and repair, but polymorphic variants had lower levels of DNA damage for all three parameters measured. The results are not in agreement to those of Cornetta et al. (2006). Tail intensity values after the exposure to 2 Gy dose, immediatelly after, 30 minutes and 60 minutes after, homozygotes and polymorphic variants showed significant differences.
The two most common SNP polymorphisms in XPD gene are in exons 10 and 23. The results of studies of those polymorphisms are inconsistent. Naccarati et al. (2006) observed fewer number of single strand breaks in polymorphic homozygotes compared to heterozygotes and wild type of homozygotes. Similar results state Vodicka et al. (2004), analyzing chromosome aberrations frequency. Polymorphic XPD23 gene variants did not influence primary DNA damage, while polymorphic XPD10 gene variants showed positive correlation in all three comet assay parameters 120 min after exposure to 2 Gy of gamma radiation.
Polymorphic variants of XRCC3 in the exposed group had highest values for DNA damage. There was also positive correlation of polymorphic variants with TL immediately after the exposure to 2 Gy and negative correlation with TI and TL 120 minutes from the exposure to 2 Gy dose. Aka et al. (2004) did not find the correlation with primary damage, probably because this gene is involved in double strand breaks repair. PARP1 is important for integrity of chromosome ends and is involved in maintaining the integrity of BER and NHEJ repair. Our results showed negative correlation between polymorphic variants and TI values measured immediately after the exposure to 4 Gy and with TM values measured 24 hours after the exposure to 4 Gy.
MGMT C/T variants have higher risk of glioma (Liu et al., 2009), but there are no investigations that are connecting it with ionising radiation. In our study polymorphic variants have shown negative correlation with DNA damage level measured 120 minutes after the exposure to 2 Gy.

4. Conclusion

The results indicate that in addition to individual gene polymorphisms, the influence of combinations of polymorphic genes to DNA damage and repair should be tested.

5. Acknowledgment

This study was partly supported by the Ministry of Science, Education and Sports of the Republic of Croatia (grant number 0022-0222148-2137).

6. References

Aka, P.; Mateuca, R.; Buchet, J.P.; Thierens, H. & Kirsch-Volders, M. (2004) Are genetic polymorphisms in OGG1, XRCC1 and XRCC3 genes predictive for the DNA strand break repair phenotype and genotoxicity in workers xx)posed to low dose ionising radiations? *Mutat Res* 556: 169-181.

Andreassen, C.N. (2005) Can risk of radiotherapy-induced normal tissue complications be predicted from genetic profiles? *Acta Oncologica* 44: 801-815.

Andreassi, M.G.; Foffa, I.; Manfredi, S.; Botto, N.; Cioppa, A. & Picano, E. (2009) Genetic polymorphisms in XRCC1, OGG1, APE1 and XRCC3 DNA repair genes, ionizing radiation exposure and chromosomal DNA damage in interventional cardiologists. *Mutat Res* 666(1-2): 57-63.

Angelini, S.; Kumar, R.; Carbone, F.; Maffei, F.; Forti, G.C.; Violante, F.S.; Lodi, V.; Curti, S.; Hemminki, K. & Hrelia, P. (2005) Micronuclei in humans induced by exposure to low level of ionizing radiation: influence of polymorphims in DNA repair genes. *Mutat Res* 570: 105-117.

Ashby, J.; Tinwell, H.; Lefevre, P.A. & Browne, M.A. (1995) The single cell gel electrophoresis assay for induced DNA damage (comet assay): measurement of tail length and moment. *Mutagenesis* 10(2): 85-90.

Au, W.W. (1991) Monitoring human populations for effects of radiation and chemical exposures using cytogenetic techniques. *Occup Med* 4:597-611.

Au WW (2006) Heritable susceptibility factors for te development of cancer. *J Radiat Res* 47B: 13-17

Bailey, S. & Goodwin, E. (2004) DNA and telomeres: beginnings and endings. *Cytogenet Genome Res* 104: 109-115.

Bailey, S.; Cornforth, M.; Ullrich, R. & Goodwin, E. (2004) Dysfunctional mammalian telomeres join with DNA double-strand breaks. *DNA Repair* 3: 349-357.

Bajpayee, M.; Dhawan, A.; Parmar, D.; Pandey, A.K.; Mathur, N. & Seth, P.K. (2002) Gender-related differences in basal DNA damage inlymphocytes of a healthy Indian population using the alkaline Comet assay. *Mutat Res* 520: 83-91.

Balasem, A,N. & Ali, A.S.K. (1991) Establishment of dose-response relationships between doses of Cs137 gamma-rays and frequencies of micronuclei in human peripheral blood lymphocytes. *Mutat Res* 259:133–138.

Barquinero, J.F.; Barrios, L.; Caballin, M.R.; Miro, R.; Ribas, M.; Subias, A. & Egozcue, J. (1993) Cytogenetic analysis of lymphocytes from hospital workers occupationally exposed to low levels of ionizing radiation. *Mutat Res* 286: 275–279.

Barquinero, J.F.; Barrios, L.; Caballin, M.R.; Miro, R.; Ribas, M.; Subias, A. & Egozcue, J. (1995) Occupational exposure to radiation induces an adaptive response in human lymphocytes. *Int J Radiat Biol* 67 (2): 187-191.

Barquinero, J.F.; Barrios, L.; Caballin, M.R.; Miro, R.; Ribas, M.; Subias, A. & Egozcue, J. (1996) Decreased sensitivity to the cytogenetic effects of bleomycin in individuals occupationally exposed to ionizing radiation. *Mutat Res* 354:81-86.

Berasati Nia, A.; Van Schooten: F.J.; Schilderman, P.A.E.L.; De Kok, T.M.C.M.; Haenen, G.R.; Van Herwijnen, M.H.M.; Van Agen, E.; Pachen, D. & Kleinjans, J.C.S. (2001) A multi-biomarker approach to study the effects of smoking on oxidative DNA damage and repair and antioxidative defence mechanisms. *Carcinogenesis* 21: 395-401.

Berrington, A.; Darby, S.C.; Weiss, H.A. & Doll, R. (2001) 100 years of observation on British radiologists: mortality from cancer and other causes 1897–1997. *Br J Radiol* 34 74: 507–519.

Berwick, M. & Vineis, P. (2000) Markers of DNA repair and susceptibility to cancer in humans: An epidemiological review. *J Natl Cancer Inst* 91: 874-897.

Berwick, M. (2000) Gene-environment interaction in melanoma. *Forum Geneva* 10: 191- 200.

Betti, C.; Davini, T.; Gianessi, L.; Loprieno, N. & Barale, R. (1994) Microgel electrophoresis assay (comet test) and SCE analysis in human lymphocytes from 100 normal subjects. *Mutat Res* 307: 323-333.

Boffetta, P.; Caporaso, N.; Cuzick, J.; Lang, M.; Vineis, P.; Malats, N. & D'Errico, A. (1999) Metabolic polymorphisms and susceptibility to cancer. IARC Publications, 44 Lyon, France.

Bolus, N.E. (2001) Basic review of radiation biology and terminology. *J Nucl Med Technol* 46 29(2): 67-73. Review.

Bonassi, S.; Ugolini, D.; Kirsch-Volders, M.; Stromberg, U.; Vermeulen, R. & Tucker, J.D. (2005) Human population studies with cytogenetic biomarkers: review of the literature and future prospectives. *Environ Mol Mutagen* 45: 258–270.

Boothman, D.A.; Bouvard, I. & Hughes, E.N. (1989) Identification and characterisation of X-ray-induced proteins in human cells. *Cancer Res* 49 (11): 2871-2878.

Bosi, A. & Olivieri, G. (1989) Variability of the adaptive response to ionizing radiations in humans. *Mutat Res* 211(1): 13-17.

Boutcher, S. & Haas, T. (1985) External radiation doses to nuclear medicine technologists from procedures using 99mTc radiopharmaceuticals. *Can J Radiogr Radiother Nucl Med* 16: 161–165.

Cardisi, E.; Vrijheid, M.; Blettner, M.; Gilbert, E.; Hakama, M.; Hill, C.; Howe, G.; Kaldor, D.; Muirhead, C.R.; Schubauer-Berigan, M.; Yoshimura, T.; Bermann, F.; Cowper, G.; Fix, J.; Hacker, C.; Heinmiller, B.; Marshall, M.; Thierry-Chef, I.; Utterback, D.; Ahn, ,Y.O.; Amoros, E.; Ashmore, P.; Auvinen, A.; Bae, J.M.; Bernar Solano, J.; Biau, A.; Combalot, E.; Deboodt, P.; Diez Sacristan, A.; Eklof, M.; Engels, H.; Engholm, G.; Gulis, G.; Habib, R.; Holan, K;, Hyvonen, H.; Kerekes, A.; Kurtinaitis, J.; Malker, H.; Martuzzi, M.; Mastauskas, A.; Monnet, A.; Moser, M.; Pearce, M.S.; Richardson, D.B.; Rodriguez-Artalejo, F.; Rogel, A.; Tardy, H.; Telle-Lamberton, M.; Turai, I.; Usel, M. & Veress, K. (2005) Risk of cancer after low doses of ionising radiation: retrospective cohort study in 15 countries. *Br Med J* 331: 77–80.

Cardoso, R. S.; Takahashi-Hyodo, S.; Peitl Jr, P.; Ghilardi-Neto, T. & Sakamoto-Hojo, E.T. (2001) Evaluation of chromosomal aberrations, micronuclei, and sister chromatid exchanges in hospital workers chronically exposed to ionizing radiation. *Teratog Carcinog Mutagen* 21: 431–439.

Carrano, A.V. & Natarajan, A.T. (1988) Considerations for population monitoring using cytogenetic techniques. ICPEMC publication 14. *Mutat Res* 204: 379–406.

Cebulska-Wasilewska, A.; Pawłyk, I.; Panek, A.; Wiechec,´ A.; Kalina, I.; Popov, T.; Georgieva, T. & Farmer, P.B. (2007) Exposure to environmental polycyclic aromatic hydrocarbons: influences on cellularsusceptibility to DNA damage (sampling Kosice and Sofia). *Mutat Res* 620: 145–154.

Chen, S.; Tang, D.; Xue, K.; Xu, L.; Ma, G.; Hsu, Y. & Cho, S.S. (2002) DNA repair gene XRCC1 and XPD polymorphisms and risk of lung cancer in a Chinese population. *Carcinogenesis* 23: 1321-1325.

Coates, P.J.; Lorimore, S.A. & Wright, E.G. (2004) Damaging and protective cell signalling in the untargeted effects of ionizing radiation. *Mutat Res* 568: 5-20.

Collins, A. & Harrington, V. (2002) Repair of oxidative DNA damage: assessing its contribution to cancer prevention. *Mutagenesis* 17: 489-493.

Collins, A.R. (2004) The Comet Assay for DNA damage and repair: Principles, applications and limitations. *Mol Biotechnol* 26: 249-261.

Cornetta, T.; Festa, F.; Testa, A. & Cozzi, R. (2006) DNA damage repair and genetic polimorphisms: assessment of indivisual sensitivity and repair capacity. *Int J Radiation Oncology Biol Phys* 66 (2): 537-545.

Daly, A.K.; Steen, V.M.; Fairbrother, K.S. & Idle, J.R. (1996) CYP2D6 multiallelism. *Meth Enzymol* 272: 199–210.

DeMeo, M.; Laget, M.; Castegnaro, M. & Dumenil, G. (1991) Genotoxic activity of potassium permanganate in acidic solutions. *Mutat Res* 260: 295-306.

Divine, K.K.; Gilliland, F.D.; Crowell, R.E.; Stidley, C.A.; Bocklage, T.J.; Cook, D.L. & Belinsky, S.A. (2001) The XRCC1 399 glutamine allele is a risk factor for adenocarcinoma of the lung. *Mutat Res* 461: 273-278.

Domingues, I; Panneerselvam, N.; Escalza, P.; Natarajan, A.T. & Cortes, F. (1993) Adaptive response to radiation damage in human lymphocytes conditioned with hydrogen peroxide as measured by the cytokinesis-block micronucleus technique. *Mutat Res* 301: 135–141.

Dusinska, M.; Collins, A.; Kazimirova, A.; Barancokova, M.; Harrington, V.; Volkovova, K.; Staruchova, M.; Horska, A.; Wsolova, L.; Kocan, A.; Petrik, J.; Machata, M.; Ratcliffe, B. & Kyrtopoulos, S. (2004a) Genotoxic effects of asbestos in humans. *Mutat Res* 553: 91–102.

Dusinska, M.; Kazimirova, A.; Barancokova, M.; Horska, A.; Burghardtova, K.; Volkovova, K.; Staruchova, M.; Wsolova, L. & Collins, A.R. (2004b) Does occupational exposure to mineral fibres cause DNA or chromosome damage? *Mutat Res* 553: 103–110.

Erexon, G.L.; Kligerman, A.D.; Bryant, M.F.; Sontag, M.R. & Halperin, E.C. (1991) Induction of micronuclei by X-radiation in human, mouse and rat peripheral blood lymphocytes. *Mutat Res* 253: 193–198.

Fachini, A.L.; Mello, S.S.; Sandrin-Garcia, P.; Junta, C.M.; Ghilardi-Netto, T.; Donadi, E.A.; Da Silva, G.A.; Elza, P. & Sakamoto-Hojo, T. (2009) Gene expression profiles in radiation workers occupationally exposed to ionizing radiation. *J Radiat Res* 50: 61–71.

Fairbairn, D.W.; Olive, P.L.; O´Neill, K.L. (1995) The comet assay: a comprehensive review. *Mutat Res* 339: 37-59.

Fenech, M.; Denham, J.; Francis, W. & Morley, A.A. (1990) Micronuclei in cytokinesis blocked lymphocytes of cancer patients following fractionated partial-body radiotherapy. *Int J Radiat Biol* 57: 373–383.

Frankenberg-Schwager, M. (1989) Review of repair kinetics for DNA damage induced in eukaryotic ce,lls in vitro by ionizing radiation. *Radiother Oncol* 14: 307-320.

Frenzili, G.; Betti, C.; Davini, T.; Desideri, M.; Fornai, E.; Gianessi, L.; Maggiorelli, F.; Paoletti, P. & Barale, R. (1997) Evaluation of DNA damage in leukocytes of ex smokers by single cell gel electrophoresis. *Mutat Res* 375: 117-123.

Goode E.L-; Ulrich C.M. & Potter J.D. (2002) Polymorphisms in DNA repair genes and associations with cancer risk. *Cancer Epidemiol Biomarkers Prev* 11: 1513–1530.

Gourabi, H. & Mozdarani, H. (1998) A cytokinesis-blocked micronucleus study of the radioadaptive response of lymphocytes of individuals occupationally exposed to chronic doses of radiation. *Mutagenesis* 13(5): 475-480.

Hall, E.J. & Giaccia, A.J. (2006) Radiobiology for the Radiologist. 6th edn. Lippincott Williams & Wilkins, Philadelphia

He, J.L.; Chen, W.L.; Jin, L.F. & Jin, H.Y. (2000) Comparative evaluation of the in vitro micronucleus test and comet assay for the detection of genotoxic effects of X-ray radiation. *Mutat Res* 469:223–231.

Hellman, B.; Vaghef, H. & Bostrom, B. (1995) The concepts of tail moment and tail inertia in the single cell gel electrophoresis assay. *Mutat Res* 336: 123-131.

Hellman, B.; Vaghef, H.; Friis, L. & Edling, C. (1997) Alkaline single cell gel electrophoresis of DNA fragments in biomonitoring for genotoxicity: an introductiory study on healthy human volunteers. *International Archives of Occupational and Environmental Health* 69: 185-192.

Hinds, D.A.; Stuve, L.L.; Nilsen, G.B.; Halperin, E.; Eskin, E.; Ballinger, D.G.; Frazer, K.A. & Cox, D.R. (2005) Whole genome patterns of common DNA variation in three human populations. *Science* 307: 1072-1079.

Hoffmann H. & Speit G. (2005) Assessment of DNA damage in peripheral blood of heavy smokers with the comet assay and the micronucleus test. *Mutat Res* 581:105-14.

Hou, S.M.; Falt, S.; Angelini, S.; Yang, K.; Nyberg, F.; Lambert, B. & Hemminki, K. (2002) The XPD variant alleles are associated with increased aromatic DNA adduct level and lung cancer risk. *Carcinogenesis* 23: 599-603.

Hu, J.J.; Smith, T.R.; Miller, M.S.; Mohrenweiser, H.W.; Golden, A. & Case, L.D. (2001) Amino acid substitution variants of APE1 and XRCC1 genes associated with ionizing radiation sensitivity. *Carcinogenesis* 22: 917–922.

Hu, J.J.; Mohrenweiser, H.W.; Bell, D.A.; Leadon, S.A. & Miller, M.S. (2002a) Symposium overview: genetic polymorphisms in DNA repair and cancer risk. *Toxicol Appl Pharmacol* 185: 64–73.

Hu, J.J.; Smith, T.R.; Miller, M.S.; Lohman, K. & Case, L.D. (2002b) Genetic regulation of ionizing radiation sensitivity and breast cancer risk. *Environ Mol Mutagen* 39: 208-215.

Hu, Z.; Ma, H.; Chen, F.; Wei, Q. & Shen, H. (2005) XRCC1 polymorphisms and cancer risk: a meta-analysis of 38 case-control studies. *Cancer Epidemiol Biomarkers Prevent* 14:1810–1818.

Hung, R.J.; Hall, J.; Brennan, P. & Boffetta, P. (2005) Genetic polymorphisms in the base excision repair pathway and cancer risk: a HuGE review. *Am J Epidemiol* 162(10): 21 925-942.

Ikushima, T. (1989) Radio-Adaptive Response: Characterization of a cytogenetic repair induced by low-level ionizing radiation in cultured Chinese hamster cells. *Mutat Res* 227 (4): 241-246.

Ikushima, T. (1992) Radio-adaptive response: involvement of induction of specific gene expression by low doses of ionizing radiation. In: Sugahara T, Sagan L, Aoyama T(ed.) Low Dose Irradiation and Biological Defence Mechanisms. Elsevier Science Publishers BV, Amsterdam, 255–263.

Ikushima, T.; Aritomi, H. & Morisita, J. (1996) Radioadaptive Response: Efficient repair of radiation-induced DNA damage in adapted cells. *Mutat Res* 358(2):193-198.

Jeggo, P. & Lavin, M.F. (2009) Cellular radiosensitivity: how much better do we understand it? *Int J Radiat Biol* 85:1061-1081.

Jha, A.N. & Sharma, T. (1991) Enhanced frequency of chromosome aberrations in workers occupationally exposed to diagnostic X-rays. *Mutat Res* 260: 343–348.

Kassie, F.; Parzefall, W. & Knasmuller, S. (2000) Single cell gel electrophoresis assay: new technique for human biomonitoring studies. *Mutat Res* 463: 13–31.

Kotsopoulos, J.; Chen, Z.; Vallis, K.A.; Poll, A.; Ainsworth, P. & Narod, S.A. (2007) DNA repair capacity as a possible biomarker of breast cancer risk in female BRCA1 mutation carriers. *Br J Cancer* 96:118–125.

Kruszewski, M.; Wojewodzka, M.; Iwanenko, T.; Collins, A.R. & Szumiel, I. (1998) Application of the comet assay for monitoring DNA damage in workers exposed to chronic low-dose irradiation: II. Base damage. *Mutat Res* 416: 37–57.

Kubelka, D.; Sviličić, N.; Kralik, I.; Belamarić, N.; Faj, D.; Novosel, N.; Vukić, V. & Tečić Z. (2011) .Analiza učinkovitosti i usklanenosti s EU propisima zakonodavstva kojim se regulira radiološka i nuklearna sigurnost [Analysis of efficacy and conformity with the EU acquis communautaire of the radiation protection and nuclear safety legislative; *in Croatian*]. In: Krajcar Bronić I, Kopjar N, Milić M, 1 Branica G, editors. Proceedings of the 8th Symposium of the Croatian Radiation Protection Association; 13-15 Apr 2011; Krk, Croatia. Zagreb: Denona; p. 31-37.

Kumar, R.; Hoglund, L.; Zhao, Ch.; Forsti, A.; Snellman, E. & Hemminki, K. (2003) Single nucleotide polymorphisms in the XPG gene: determination of role in DNA repair and breast cancer risk. *Int J Cancer* 103: 671-675.

Kumaravel, T.S. & Jha, A.N. (2006) Reliable Comet assay measurements for detecting DNA damage induced by ionising radiation and chemicals. *Mutat Res* 605: 7-16.

Little, J.B. (2000) Radiation carcinogenesis. *Carcinogenesis* 21: 397–404.

Liu, Y.; Scheurer, M.E.; El-Zein, R.; Cao, Y.; Do, K.A.; Gilbert, M.; Aldape, K.D.; Wei, Q.; Etzel, C. & Bondy, M.L. (2009) Association and interactions between DNA repair gene polymorphisms and adult glioma. *Cancer Epidemiol Biomarkers Prev* 18(1): 204-214

Lunn, R.M.; Helzlsouer, K.J.; Parshad, R.; Umbach, M.D.; Harris, E.L.; Sanford, K.K. & Bell D.A. (2000) XPD polymorphisms: effects on DNA repair proficiency. *Carcinogenesis* 21: 551–555.

Maitre, A.; Colonna, M.; Gressin, C.; Menegoz, F. & de Gaudemaris, R. (2003) Increased incidence of haematological cancer among physicians in a University Hospital. *Int Arch Occup Environ Health* 76: 24–28.

Maluf, S. & Erdtmann, B. (2001a) Genomic instability in Down syndrome and Fanconi anemia assessed by micronucleus analysis and single-cell gel electrophoresis. *Cancer Genet Cytogenet* 124: 71–75.

Maluf, S.W.; Passos, D.F.; Bacelar, A.; Speit, G. & Erdtmann, B. (2001b) Assessment of DNA damage in lymphocytes of workers exposed to X-radiation using the micronucleus test and the comet assay. *Environ Mol Mutagen* 38: 311–315

Maluf, S.W. (2004) Monitoring DNA damage following radiation exposure using cytokinesis-block micronucleus method and alkaline single-cell gel electrophoresis. *Clinica Chimica Acta* 347: 15-24.

Marcon, F.; Andreoli, C.; Rossi, S.; Verdina, A.; Galati, R. & Crebelli, R. (2003) Assessment of individual sensitivity to ionizing radiation and DNA repair efficiency in a healthy population. *Mutation Research* 541: 1–8.

Matullo, G.; Peluso, M.; Polidoro, S.; Guarrera, S.; Munnia, A.; Krogh, V.; Masala, G.; Berrino, F.; Panico, S.; Tumino, R.; Vineis, P. & Palli, D. (2003) Combination of DNA repair gene single nucleotidepolymorphisms and increased levels of DNA adducts in a population-based study. *Cancer Epidemiol. Biomarkers Prev* 12: 674–677

McKelvey-Martin, V.J.; Green, M.H.L.; Schmezer, P.; Pool-Zobel, B.L.; De Me´o, M.P. & Collins, A. (1993) The single cell gel electrophoresis assay (comet assay): a European review. *Mutat Res* 288: 47–63.

McKelvey-Martin, V.J.; Ho, E.T.S.; McKeown, S.R.; Johnston, S.R.; McCarthy, P.J.; Rajab, N.F. & Downes, C.S. (1998) Emerging applications of the single cell gel electrophoresis (Comet) assay. I. Management of invasive transitionalcell human bladder carcinoma. II. Fluorescent in situ hybridization Comets for the identification of damaged and repaired DNA sequences in individual cells. *Mutagenesis* 13: 1–8.

Milić, M.; Rozgaj, R.; Kašuba, V.; Kubelka, D.; Angelini, S. & Hrelia, P. (2010) DNA repair genes and radiation sensitivity. *Arh Hig Rada Toksikol* 61 Supplement: 107-121.

Milić, M. (2010) Važnost individualne osjetljivosti za procjenu rizika od oštećenja genoma pri kroničnoj profesionalnoj izloženosti niskim dozama ionizirajućeg zračenja [The significance of individual genome sensitivity in risk assessment of chronic professional exposure to low doses of ionizing radiation; in Croatian]. [PhD thesis]. Zagreb: Faculty of Science, University of Zagreb.

Mohrenweiser, H.W. & Jones, I.M. (1998) Variation in DNA repair is 1 a factor in cancer susceptibility: a paradigm for the promises and perils of individual and population risk estimation? *Mutat Res* 400: 15–24.

Mohrenweiser, H.W.; Wilson, D.M. & Jones, I.M. (2003) Challenges and complexities in estimating both the functional impact and the disease risk associated with the extensive genetic variation in human DNA repair genes. *Mutat Res* 526: 93–125.

Monsieurs, M.A.; Thierens, H.M.; Vral, A.M.; Van De Wiele, C.; De Ridder, L.I. & Dierckx, R.A. (2000) Adaptive response in patients treated with 131I. *J Nucl Med* 41 (1): 17-22.

Morgan, W.F. (2003) Non-targeted and delayed effects of exposure to ionizing radiation: i. radiation-induced genomic instability and bystander effects *in vitro*. *Radiat Res* 159: 567-580.

Mothersill, C.; Kadhim, M.A.; O' Reilly, S.; Paphworth, D.; Mardsen, S.J.; Seaymoure, C.B. & Wright, E.G. (2000) Dose- and time-response relationships for lethal mutations and chromosomal instability induced by ionizing radiation in an immortalized human keratinocyte cell line. *Int Radiat Biol* 76 (6): 799-806.

Mothersill, C.; Rea, D.; Wright, E.G.; Lorimore, S.A.; Murphy, D.; Seymour, C.B. & O'Malley, K. (2001) Individual variation in the production of a bystander signal following irradiation of primary cultures of normal human urothelium. *Carcinogenesis* 22 (9): 1465-1471.

Muller, W.U.; Bauch, T.; Stuben, G.; Sack, H. & Streffer, C. (2001) Radiation sensitivity of lymphocytes from healthy individuals and cancer patients as measured by the comet assay. *Radiat Environ Biophys* 40: 83–89.

Muller, W.U.; Bauch, T.; Streffer, C. & von Mallek, D. (2002) Does radiotherapy affect the outcome of the comet assay? *Br J Radiol* 75: 608–614.

Naccarati, A.; Soucek, P.; Stetina, R.; Haufroid, V.; Kumar, R.; Vodickova, L.; Trtkova, K.; Dusinska, M.; Hemminki, K. & Vodicka, P. (2006) Genetic polymorphisms and possible gene-gene interactions in metabolic andDNA repair genes: Effects on DNA damage. *Mutat Res* 593: 22–31

Norppa, H. (2004) Cytogenetic biomarkers and genetic polymorphisms. *Toxicol Lett* 149: 309–334.

Nowak, B. & Jankowski, J. (1991) Occupational exposure in operational radiology. *Pol J Occup Med Environ Health* 4: 169–174.

Okayasu, R.; Suetomi, K.; Yu, Y.; Silver, A.; Bedford, J.; Cox, R. & Ullrich, R. (2000) A deficiency in DNA repair and DNA-PKcs expression in the radiosensitive BALB/c mouse. *Cancer Res*. 60: 4342-4345.

Olive, P.L.; Banath, J.P. & Durand, R.E. (1990) Heterogeneity in radiation-induced DNA damage and repair in tumor and normal cells using the "comet" assay. *Radiation Research* 122: 86-94.

Olive, P.L. (1999) DNA damage and repair in individual cells: aplications of the comet assay in radiobiology. *International Journal of Radiation Biology* 75(4): 395-405.

Olivieri, G.; Bodycote, J. & Wolff, S. (1984) Adaptive response of human lymphocytes to low concentrations of radioactive thymidine. *Science* 223: 594–597.

Olivieri, G. & Bosi, A. (1990) Possible causes of variability of the adaptive response in human lymphocytes. In: Obe G, Natarajan A T(ed.) Chromosomal Aberrations, Basic and Applied Aspects. Springer-Verlag, Berlin, 130–140.

Padovani, L.; Appolloni, M.; Anzidei, P.; Tedeschi, B.; Caporossi, D.; Vernole, P. & Mauro, F. (1995) Do human lymphocytes exposed to the fallout of the Chernobyl accident exhibit an adaptive response? I. Challenge with Ionizing Radiation. *Mutat Res* 332 (1-2): 33-38.

Parl, F.F. (2005) Glutathione S-transferase genotypes and cancer 1 risk. *Cancer Lett* 221:123–129.

Plappert, U.; Raddatz, K.; Roth, S. & Fliedner, T.M. (1995) DNA damage detection in man after radiation exposure-the comet assay- its possible application for human monitoring. *Stem Cells* 13(1): 215-222.

Plappert, U.G.; Stocker, B.; Fender, H. & Fliedner, T.M. (1997) Changes in the repair capacity of blood cells as a biomarker for chronic low-dose exposure to ionizing radiation. *Environ Mol Mutagen* 30(2): 153-160.

Price, A. (1993) The repair of ionising radiation- induced damage to DNA. *Cancer Biology* 4: 61-71.

Rajaee-Behbahani, N.; Schmezer, P.; Risch, A.; Rittgen, W; Kayser, K.W.; Dienemann, H.; Schulz, V.; Drings, P., Thiel, S. & Bartsch, H. (2001) Altered DNA repair capacity and bleomycin sensitivity as risk markers for non-small cell lung cancer. *Int J Cancer* 95: 86–91.

Robson, T., Joiner, M.C.; Wilson, G.D.; McCullough, W.; Price, M.E.; Logan, I.; Jones, H.; McKeown, S.R. & Hirst, D.G. (1999) A novel human stress response-related gene with a potential role in induced radioresistance. *Radiat Res* 152 (5): 451-461.

Roos, W.P.; Binder, A. & Bohm, L. (2000) Determination of the initial DNA damage and residual DNA damage remaining after 12 hours of repair in eleven cell lines at low doses of irradiation. *Int J Radiat Biol* 76: 1493-1500.

Rzeszowska-Wolny, J.; Polanska, J.; Pietrowska, M.; Palyvoda, O.; Jaworska, J.; Butkiewicz, D. & Hancock, R. (2005) Influence of polymorphisms in DNA repair genes XPD, XRCC1 and MGMT on DNA damage induced by gamma radiation and its repair in lymphocytes *in vitro*. *Radiat Res* 164: 132–140.

Sankaranarayanan, K.; Duyn, A.; Loos, M.J. & Natarajan, A.T. (1989) Adaptive response of human lymphocytes to low-level radiation from radioisotopes or X-rays. *Mutat Res* 211: 7–12.

Sari-Minodier, I.; Orsiere, T.; Auquier, P.; Martin, F. & Botta, A. (2007) Cytogenetic monitoring by use of the micronucleus assay among hospital workers exposed to low doses of ionizing radiation. *Mutat Res* 629(2): 111-121.

Sasaki, M.S.; Ejima, Y.; Tachibana, A.; Yamada, T.; Ishizaki, K.; Shimizu, T. & Nomura, T. (2002) DNA damage response pathway in radioadaptive response. *Mutat Res* 33 504: 101-118.

Setlow, R.B. (1983) Variations in DNA repair among humans. In: Harris CC, Autrup HN (ed.) Human Carcinogenesis. New York: Academic Press: 231-254.

Seymour, C.B. & Mothersill, C. (2000) Relative contribution of bystander and targeted cell killing to the low-dose region of the radiation dose-response curve. *Radiat Res* 153: 508-511.

Shadley, J.D. & Wiencke, J.K. (1989) Induction of the adaptive response by x-rays is dependent on radiation intensity. *Int J Radiat Biol* 56: 107-118.

Shadley, J.D. (1994) Chromosomal adaptive response in human lymphocytes. *Radiat Res* 138: S9–S12.

Shadley, J.D. & Wolff, S. (1987) Very low doses of X-rays can cause human lymphocytes to become less susceptible to ionizing radiation. *Mutagenesis* 2: 95–96.

Shastry, B.S. (2009) SNPs: impact on gene function and phenotype. *Methods Mol Biol* 578: 3-22.

Singh, N.P.; McCoy, M.T.; Tice, R.R. & Schneider, L.L. (1988) A simple technique for quantitation of low levels of DNA damage in individual cells. *Exp Cell Res* 175:184-191.

Singh, N.P. (2000) Microgels for estimation of DNA strand breaks, DNA protein crosslinks and apoptosis. *Mutat Res* 455: 111-127.

Stecca, C. & Gerber, G.B. (1998) adaptive response to dna-damaging agents: a review of potential mechanisms. *Biochem Pharmacol* 55 (7): 941-951.

Sturgis, E.M.; Castillo, E.J.; Li, L.; Zheng, R.; Eicher, S.A.; Clayman, G.L.; Strom, S.S.; Spitz, M.R. & Wei, Q. (1999) Polymorphisms of DNA repair gene XRCC1 in squamous cell carcinoma of the head and neck. *Carcinogenesis* 20: 2125-2129.

Szumiel, I. (1998) Monitoring and signaling of radiation-induced damage in mammalian cells. *Radiat Res* 150: 92-101.

Tedeschi, B.; Caporossi, D.; Vernole, P.; Padovani, L.; Appolloni, M.; Anzidei, P. & Mauro, F. (1995) Do Human lymphocytes exposed to the fallout of the Chernobyl accident exhibit an adaptive response? II. Challenge with bleomycin. *Mutat Res* 332 (1-2): 299-300.

Tedeschi, B.; Caporossi, D.; Vernole, P.; Padovani, L. & Mauro, F. (1996) Do human lymphocytes exposed to the fallout of the chernobyl accident exhibit an adaptive response? III. Challenge with bleomycin in lymphocytes from children hit by the initial acute dose of ionizing radiation. *Mutat Res* 354 (1): 77-80.

Tice, R.R.;Andrews, P.W.; Hirai, O. & Singh, N.P. (1990) The single cell gel (SCG) assay: an electrophoretic technique for the detection of DN damage in individual cells. In: Witmer, C.M., Snyder, R.R., Hollow, D.J., Kalf, G.F., Kocsis, J.J., Sipes, J.G. (ed.) Biological reactive intermediates, IV Molecular and cellular effects and their impact on human health. New York, Plenum Press, 157-164.

Tice, R.R. (1995) The single cell gel/comet assay: a microgel electrophoretic technique for the detection of DNA damage and repair in individual cells. In: Phillis DH, Venitt S (ed.) *Environmental Mutagenesis*. Bioscientific, Oxford, 315-339.

Touil, N.; Aka, P.V.; Buchet, J.P.; Thierens, H. & Kirsch-Volders, M. (2002) Assessment of genotoxic effects related to chronic low level exposureto ionizing radiation using biomarkers for DNA damage and repair. *Mutagenesis* 17: 223–232.

Trzeciak, A.R.; Barnes, J.; Ejiogu, N.; Foster, K.; Brant, L.J.; Zonderman, A.B. & Evans, M.K. (2008) Age, sex, and race influence single-strand break repair capacity in a human population. *Free Radic Biol Med* 45:1631-1641.

United Nations Scientific Committee on the Effects of Atomic Radiation, Sources and effects of ionizing radiation UNSCEAR 2000 report, vol. 1, http://www.unscear.org. UNSCEAR (United Nations Scientific Committee on theEffects of Atomic Radiation), 2000. Sources and effects of ionizing radiation. Report to the General Assembly.

Valverde, M.; Ostrosky-Wegman, P.; Rojas, E.; Fortoul, T.; Meneses, F.; Ramírez, M.; Díaz-Barriga, F. & Cebrian, M. The application of single cell gel electrophoresis or Comet assay to human monitoring studies. *Salud Publica Mex*. 1999;41 Suppl 2:S109-13.

Vodicka, P.; Kumar, R.; Stetina, R.; Sanyal, S.; Soucek, P.; Haufroid, V.; Dusinska, M.; Kuricova, M.; Zamecnikova, M., Musak, L.; Buchancova, J.; Norppa, H.; Hirvonen, A.; Vodickova, L.; Naccarati, A.; Matousu, Z. & Hemminki, K. (2004) Genetic polymorphismsin DNA repair genes and possible links with DNA repair rates, chromosomal aberrations and single-strand breaks in DNA. *Carcinogenesis* 25: 757-763.

Wang, J.X.; Zhang, L.A.; Li, B.X.; Zhao, Y.C.; Wang, Z.Q.; Zhang, J.Y. & Aoyama, T. (2002) Cancer incidence and risk estimation among medical X-ray workers in China, 1950-1995, *Health Phys* 82: 455–466.

Wang, Z.Q.; Saigusa, S. & Sasaki, M.S. (1991) Adaptive response to chromosome damage in cultured human lymphocytes primed with low doses of X-rays. *Mutat Res* 246: 179-186.

Weiss, J.M.; Goode, E.L.; Ladiges, W.C. & Ulrich, C.M. (2005) Polymorphic variation in hOGG1 and risk of cancer: a review of the functional and epidemiologic literature. *Mol Carcinog* 42: 127–141.

Wiencke, J.K.; Afzal, V; Olivieri, G. & Wolff, S. (1986) Evidence that the (3h) thymidine induced adaptive response of human lymphocytes to subsequent doses of x-rays involves the induction of a chromosomal repair mechanism. *Mutagenesis* 1(5): 375-380.

Winsey, S.L.; Haldar, N.A.; Marsh, H.P.; Bunce, M.; Marshall, S.E.; Harris, A.L.; Wojnarowska, F. & Welsh, K.I. (2000) A variant within theDNA repair gene XRCC3 is associated with the development of melanoma skin cancer. *Cancer Res* 60: 5612-5616.

Wojcik, A.; Sauer, K.; Zolzer, F.; Bauch, T. & Muller, W.U. (1996) Analyses of DNA damage recovery processes in the adaptive response to ionising radiation in human lymphocytes. *Mutagenesis* 11: 291–297.

Wojewodzka, M.; Kruszewski, M.; Iwanenko, T.; Collins, A.R. & Szumiel, I. (1998) Application of the comet assay for monitoring DNA damage inworkers exposed to chronic low-dose irradiation: I. Strand breakage. *Mutat Res* 416:21–35.

Wolff, S.; Wiencke, J.K. & Afzal, V. (1989) Biological Bases of Risk Assessment. In: Baverstock KF and Stather JW (ed.) Low Dose Radiation. Taylor and Francis, London, 439-445.

Wolff, S.; Oliviery, G. & Afzal, V. (1990) Adaptation of human lymphocytes to radiation or chemical mutagens: differences in cytogenetic repair. In: Obe G., Natarajan, A.T. (ed.) Chromosomal Aberrations, Basic and Applied Aspects. Springer-Verlag, Berlin, 140–149.

Wolff, S. (1992) Low-dose exposures and the induction of adaptation. In: Sugahara, T., Sagan, L.A., Aoyama, T. (ed.) Low Dose Irradiation and Biological Defence Mechanisms. Elsevier Science Publishers BV, Amsterdam, 21–28.

Wolff, S. (1996) Aspects of the adaptive response to very low doses of radiation and other agents. *Mutat Res* 358: 135–142.

Yamane, A.; Kohno, T.; Ito, K.; Sunaga, N.; Aoki, K.; Yoshimura, K.; Murakami, H.; Nojima, Y. & Yokota, J. (2004) Differential ability of polymorphic OGG1 proteins to suppress mutagenesis induced by 8-hydroxyguanine in human cell in vivo. *Carcinogenesis* 25: 1689-1694

Yoshinaga, S.; Aoyama, T.; Yoshimoto, Y. & Sugahara, T. (1999) Cancer mortality among radiological technologists in Japan: updated analysis of follow-up data from 1969 to 1993. *J Epidemiol* 9: 61–72.

Youngblom, J.H.; Wiencke, J.K. & Wolff, S. (1989) Inhibition of the adaptive response of human lymphocytes to very low doses of ionizing radiation by the protein synthesis inhibitor cycloheximide. *Mutat Res* 227(4):257-261.

6

New Players in Recognition of Intact and Cleaved AP Sites: Implication in DNA Repair in Mammalian Cells

Svetlana Khodyreva and Olga Lavrik
Institute of Chemical Biology and Fundamental Medicine,
Siberian Branch of the Russian Academy of Sciences,
Russia

1. Introduction

The apurinic/apyrimidinic (AP) sites (called also abasic sites) are common lesion in genomic DNA, arising at a frequency of 10,000 to 50,000 lesions per mammalian cell per day (Lindahl, 1993). Unrepaired AP sites present mutagenic and cytotoxic consequences to the cell (Wilson; & Thompson, 1997). Most of the abasic sites are believed to result directly from spontaneous depurination, or indirectly from deamination of cytosine to uracil, which is then eliminated by uracil glycosylases. AP sites also result from hydrolysis of oxidized or alkylated bases by lesion-specific glycosylases during the early stage of base excision repair (BER) (McCullough et al., 1999). AP sites in isolated DNA are rather stable, but can be converted to single-strand breaks by alkali treatment, heating or nucleophilic attack at the aldehydic C1′ group (Burrows & Muller, 1998). Intact abasic sites are noncoding lesions and *in vivo* can be stable enough to be mutagenic during DNA replication (Loeb & Preston, 1986). To protect genome integrity, eukaryotic organisms have robust enzyme activities, mainly APE1 in mammalian cells (Wilson & Barsky, 2001), that recognize abasic sites and cut the DNA backbone initiating the repair process. The continuous generation and repair of AP sites results in a steady-state levels of AP sites in mammalian cells in the range of approximately 1 site per 10^6 nucleotides (Atamna et al., 2000, Mohsin Ali et al., 2004). The number of AP sites can increase dramatically under stressful conditions such as X-ray or UV light irradiation or oxidative and alkylating agent exposure (Atamna et al., 2000). Considering the ubiquity of these lesions, it is reasonable to assume that wide range of cellular proteins can interact with abasic sites depending on the physiological state and stages of cell cycle.
The chapter is devoted to search of previously unrecognized proteins capable to interact with intact or cleaved AP sites. We mainly focused on proteins that form Schiff base upon this interaction. In most cases, these proteins are able to process AP sites although less efficiently than previously known counterparts. The biological role of these interactions in providing of backup pathways of DNA repair processes is also discussed.

2. Proteins that recognize AP sites

In genomic DNA of higher eukaryotes AP sites irrespectively of their origin are thought to be repaired by base excision repair (Almeida & Sobol, 2007; Hegde et al., 2008).

2.1 Base excision repair (overview)

Base excision repair (BER) is one of the major systems of DNA repair, mostly responsible for removing from DNA of non-bulky base lesions that appear in the genome with high frequency (Almeida & Sobol, 2007; Hegde et al., 2008; Schärer, 2003). The base excision repair pathway essentially removes and replaces nucleotides containing aberrant bases in DNA. Metabolically produced reactive nitrogen and oxygen species can modify the DNA bases due to oxidation, deamination and even alkylation at several positions in the base. BER is usually defined as DNA repair initiated by a lesion-specific DNA glycosylase and completed by either of two sub-pathways: short-patch BER; a mechanism whereby only 1 nucleotide is replaced or long-patch BER; a mechanism whereby 2–13 nucleotides are replaced (Frosina et al., 1996; Klungland & Lindahl, 1997).

The majority of BER is currently thought to occur via the short-patch pathway initiated by either a mono-functional or bi-functional DNA glycosylases. The short-patch BER pathway mediated by a mono-functional glycosylase involves removal of aberrant base by the lesion-specific DNA glycosylases, enzymes that hydrolyze cleavage of *N*-glycosylic bond between base and deoxyribose. This results in apurinic/apyrimidinic (also termed abasic) sites (AP sites), which repair is generally initiated through strand incision at its 5'-side by an AP endonuclease, leaving a nick flanked by a 3'-hydroxyl of an undamaged and a deoxyriboso-5'-phosphate (dRP), to which the damaged base was formerly linked. DNA polymerase then inserts a normal deoxyribonucleotide; however, the ligation step to restore intact DNA is blocked because of the dangling dRP moiety. The situation is resolved by a special enzymatic activity, excising dRP moiety (short-patch), or by continuing DNA synthesis with strand displacement, followed by removal of the displaced strand by flap endonuclease 1 (long-patch BER) (Frosina et al., 1996; Klungland & Lindahl, 1997).

In mammalian cells, the major dRP-removing enzyme is DNA polymerase β (Pol β), a multifunctional enzyme consisting of the 8-kDa amino-terminal domain with deoxyribose phosphate (dRP) lyase activity and the 31-kDa carboxy-terminal domain with nucleotidyl transferase activity (Allinson et al., 2001, Matsumoto & Kim, 1995, Piersen et al., 1996, Podlutsky et al., 2001). Thus, Pol β can mediate both steps in single nucleotide BER: insertion of deoxyribonucleotide and removal of dRP moiety preparing the strand for ligation.

Oxidized bases in DNA are manly produced by reactive oxygen species (ROS). ROS are generated as by-products of metabolic processes, primarily oxidative metabolism in the mitochondria (Dawson et al., 1993), and pathological conditions such as inflammation. ROS are also generated by ionizing radiation and some chemotherapeutic drugs (Almeida & Sobol, 2007; Hegde et al., 2008; Schärer, 2003). Oxidized bases are primarily removed by bi-functional DNA glycosylases that have an additional AP site cleavage activity. In addition to oxidation of DNA bases, ROS attack deoxyribose in DNA to generate strand breaks with nonligatable ends. The 3′ blocking groups include 3′ phosphate, 3′ phosphoglycolaldehyde, or 3′ phosphoglycolate (Breen et al., 1995). The 5′ terminus normally contains phosphate but after ROS reaction the nonligatable ends include 5′ OH and 5′ phosphodeoxyribose derivatives such as 2-deoxyribonolactone (Demple et al., 2002). Repair of single-strand breaks (SSBR) with blocked termini utilizes many of the same proteins as the BER process. The principal difference between SSBR and BER is the initiation step. Further both processes may occur at the single nucleotide level (i.e., short-patch repair) or as a long-patch of repair. BER is initiated via DNA glycosylase activity that results in the removal of a damaged base. SSBR is defined specifically for the repair of single-strand breaks in DNA generated by irradiation or ROS (Fan & Wilson, 2005). AP sites appeared via spontaneous base loss and arising from irradiation are also further processed by the BER machinery.

2.2 Processing of AP sites

AP sites can be incised by three mechanistically different ways represented in Fig.1.

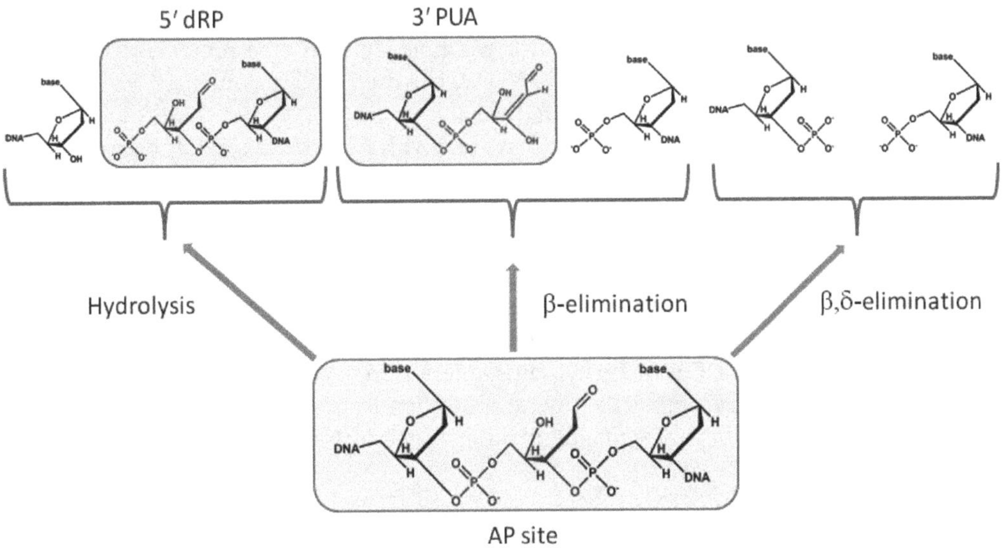

Fig. 1. Structures of intact and cleaved AP sites. DNA structures containing reactive sugar moieties capable of Schiff base formation are marked by grey rectangular boxes.

In mammalian cells, the repair of AP sites is generally initiated through strand incision by APE1, the second enzyme of the canonical BER pathway (Demple et al., 1991). APE1 is thought to process of over 95% of AP sites in mammalian cells (Demple & Harrison, 1994; Wilson & Barsky, 2001). APE1 catalyzes hydrolysis of AP sites by a Mg^{2+}-dependent mechanism, resulting in cleavage of the phosphodiester bond 5′ to the AP site and generation of a single-strand break. This reaction produces a 3′-hydroxyl group and a 5′-dRP group flanking the break. This way of AP site processing fits short-patch pathway of the BER process.

Another way of AP site cleavage by the BER machinery involving the action of bi-functional DNA glycosylases is more complicated and requires the 'end cleaning' of termini prior to the further repair reactions may occur. An intermediate reaction step for these enzymes is the formation of a transient Schiff base between the amino group and the C1′ of deoxyribose for both base excision and subsequent DNA strand cleavage. In solution, AP sites exist predominantly as a mixture of ring-closed α- and β-hemiacetals with a minor amount of ring-opened aldehyde and aldehyde hydrate (<1%) (de los Santos et al., 2004). AP sites can be incised through β-elimination using ε-NH2 of a lysine as the active site nucleophile (David & Williams, 1998; McCullough et al., 1999). Strand incision by β-elimination forms a nick with phospho-α,β-unsaturated aldehyde (PUA) at the 3′ margin and phosphate at the 5′ margin (David & Williams, 1998; McCullough et al., 1999) (Fig. 1). While recently discovered mammalian DNA glycosylases, termed NEIL (Nei-like)-1, -2, catalyze the β,δ-elimination reaction with the N-terminal proline being used as the nucleophile (Hazra et al., 2002; Takao et al., 2002, Das et al., 2006). The β,δ-elimination reaction results in a one nucleotide gap flanked with phosphate groups at the 3′- and 5′ margins. The products of bi-functional DNA glycosylase activity require the trimming of the 3′-ends to produce 3′-end hydroxyl groups that are indispensable for DNA polymerase activity.

Most of mammalian proteins known to form the Schiff base intermediate with the AP site appear to belong to the BER system. On the other hand, an interaction of AP DNA with proteins not formally involved in BER (for example, human ribosomal protein S3 and nucleoside diphosphate kinase - NM23-H2/NDP) has been well documented (Hegde et al., 2004; Postel et al., 2000). These two proteins are able to cleave AP sites. MutY, unlike other monofuctional DNA glycosylases, is able to interact with AP site via a Schiff base formation (Zharkov & Grollman, 1998) without the concomitant cleavage of AP sites. In this particular case formation of the Schiff base intermediate is considered as a mechanism for temporal protection of AP sites (Zharkov & Grollman, 1998).

Since AP sites in DNA appear to be promiscuous in their binding to many cellular factors and they are constantly generated in high frequency in genomic DNA, it may be important to sequester the AP sites immediately upon formation and further process them by the way that is most favorable for DNA integrity. Thus, interaction of cellular proteins with AP sites might be important for their repair/temporal protection from further degradation or might be involved in damage sensing/signaling making search of AP site reactive proteins a very important task.

2.3 Search of new participants of recognition/processing of AP sites

The very promising approach in search for unknown players in AP site recognition is based on a well-known propensity of deoxyribose in AP site, existing in equilibrium between cyclic furanose and acyclic aldehyde forms, to react with amine moieties in its vicinity. The Schiff base intermediate can be reduced by sodium borohydride ($NaBH_4$) or related compounds, forming an irreversible complex between the enzyme and DNA (David & Williams, 1998; Piersen et al., 2000). This reaction is widely used to prove the β-elimination reaction mechanism for the enzymes capable of AP site cleavage (David & Williams, 1998; Piersen et al., 2000), although some proteins (e.g. MutY DNA glycosylase) can form a Schiff base with no further β-elimination (Zharkov & Grollman, 1998). Therefore, upon searching of new players in AP site recognition mediated by the Schiff base formation their ability to cleave AP has to be proved. Along with intact AP site, the product of its cleavage - 3′ PUA and 5′ dRP moieties (Fig. 1, grey rectangular boxes) are also able to form the Schiff base intermediate with primary amino groups of proteins that allows to use these DNA in search and identification of proteins.

2.3.1 Identification of proteins reactive to AP sites

For identification of protein cross-linked to AP DNA in cell extracts immunochemical and/or mass-spectrometry methods can be used. Identification of proteins reactive to AP sites by combination of cross-linking technique and mass-spectrometry is schematically represented in Fig. 2.

In general, search and identification of proteins reactive to AP sites include the following steps: (1) finding of cellular extract proteins forming covalent adducts with AP sites in DNA; (2) the design of AP-DNA probe containing a functional group providing the selective

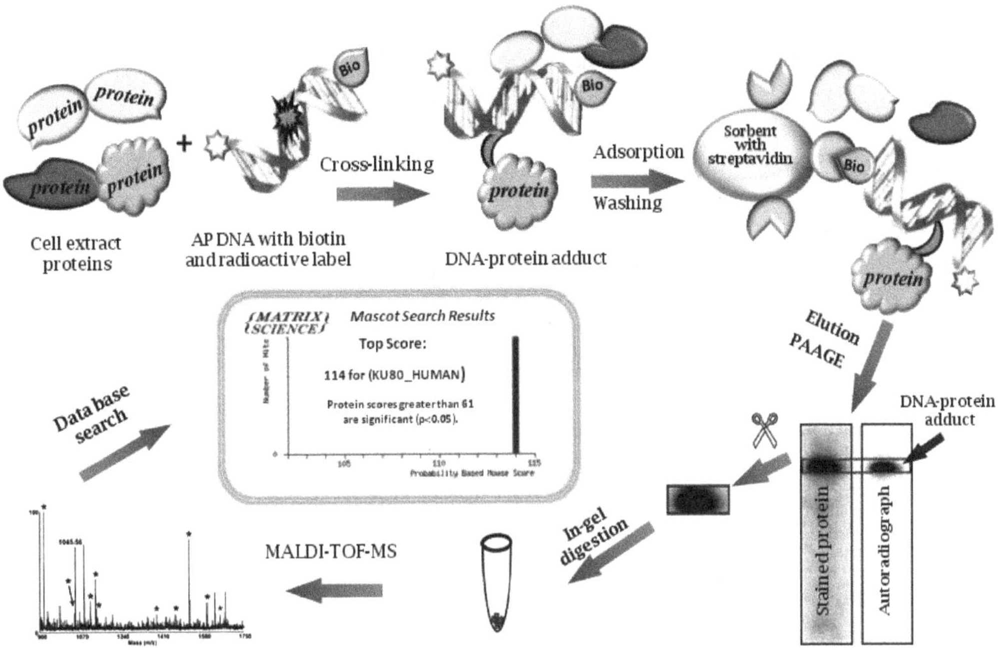

Fig. 2. Workflow of identification of protein cross-linked to DNA containing intact or cleaved AP site.

isolation of cross-linked DNA-protein products; (3) the preparative cross-linking of extract proteins with such DNA; (4) the affinity purification of the resulted products; (5) the identification of the protein in the covalent adduct with DNA using mass-spectrometry methods; (6) the confirmation of the results using purified proteins and/or specific antibodies and the known functions/interactions of the identified protein; and (7) the study of the functional role of the revealed interactions between proteins and AP DNA. A proof-of-principle identification of protein reactive towards AP sites in species from *E. coli* and *S. cerevisiae* was reported in (Rieger et al., 2006).

It should be noted that used protocol includes two steps that increases the selectivity of the method. Affinity purification of cross-linked protein was carried out on commercially available affinity sorbents containing streptavidin, which binds the biotin residue. After adsorption, non-specifically bound proteins were removed by a series of washings. Additional separation of proteins was achieved by electrophoresis under denaturing conditions by the Laemmli method (Laemmli, 1970) followed by staining proteins. The target product was identified by the colocalization in the gel positions of the label in DNA and the stained protein. This approach indicates that only the protein cross-linked to DNA will be subjected to the further analysis. However, one cannot fully exclude the presence of impurity proteins with the same electrophoretic mobility as the target product.

The identification was carried out for a number of proteins forming cross-links with AP sites in extracts of *E. coli* cells at logarithmic and stationary phases of cell growth (Rieger et al., 2006). It should be noted that authors used the previously developed non-enzymatic approach of the creation of AP sites in DNA based on the periodate oxidation of 2,3,5,6-tetrahydroxyhexyl phosphate precursor, which was introduced into an oligonucleotide during the standard phosphoroamidite oligonucleotide synthesis. The periodate oxidation allows one to obtain AP sites in an almost quantitative yield. This method, in the authors' opinion, has several advantages over the more commonly used method that is based on the removal of uracil residues using uracil DNA glycosylase.

The procaryotic proteins AroF, DnaK, MutM, PolA, TnaA, TufA, and UvrA from *E. coli* and eucaryotic ARC1 and Ygl245wp from yeast were identified (Rieger et al., 2006). Protein Ygl245wp with an unknown but essential for cell viability function was prepared in the individual state after its coding sequence was cloned, and the recombinant plasmid was used for the production of the protein in *E. coli* cells followed by its isolation. The obtained protein was shown to bind to AP DNA forming Schiff bases; however, the biological significance of this interaction has not been established. DNA polymerase I, like other DNA polymerases of the A-family, has a weak AP lyase activity and dRP lyase activity (Pinz & Bogenhagen, 2000). However the biological significance of these activities *in vivo* has not been established. The ability of UvrA, the key component of the nucleotide excision repair (NER) in bacteria, to interact with AP sites in the UvrABC complex indicates the possible role of NER as a back-up pathway of AP site repair in bacteria (Showden et al., 1990).

2.3.2 Identification of Ku80 subunit of human Ku antigen as a protein reactive to AP sites

Using the same technique we screened mammalian cell extracts for proteins capable of binding AP site-containing DNA. In HeLa cell extract, a 32-bp DNA duplex with an AP site in the middle of the DNA chain was shown to cross-link predominantly to a protein forming a product with an apparent molecular mass of 95 kDa (Fig. 3) (Ilina et al., 2008).

The subsequent analysis of whole cell extracts of human lung fibroblasts, K-562, and MCF-7 cells revealed the products with the same electrophoretic mobility. The preferential cross-linking of this protein reflected extraordinary specificity in light of the multitude of proteins in the cell. If the AP site in DNA is replaced by its analog (the THF residue) or the treatment with NaBH4 is omitted, DNA–protein cross-linked products are not registered (Fig. 3).

In spite of efficient cross-linking of the above mentioned AP DNA to Ku80 polypeptide (as a part of DNA-PK) no cleavage of AP sites was observed (Ilina et al., 2008). Instead Ku80 formed with AP site a long-living Schiff base intermediate without the concomitant AP site cleavage just as was observed for monofunctional DNA glycosylase MutY and considered as a mechanism for temporal protection of AP sites (Zharkov & Grollman, 1998). AP lyase and 5′-dRP activities are distinctive features of the BER process (Almeida & Sobol, 2007; Hegde et al., 2008). The BER 5′-dRP/AP lyases usually function beyond the DS-breaks. But abasic sites associated with double-strand breaks can be generated by ionizing radiation, by treatment with radiomimetic drugs or as a result of attempted BER of complex damages (Yang et al., 2004). These specifically positioned lesions must be removed prior to or in the course of DS break repair. Ku antigen - DS-end binding protein of NHEJ - has been recently shown to act as a 5′-dRP/AP lyase near double-strand breaks (Roberts et al., 2010).

At DSB ends Ku is approximately tenfold more active than Pol β (Roberts et al., 2010), the most known mammalian 5′-dRP lyase (Matsumoto & Kim, 1995). At the same time, Ku was inefficient as AP lyase at AP sites situated at a distance longer than one helix turn from DS breaks just as was reported in (Ilina et al., 2008). $NaBH_4$-dependent cross-linking of

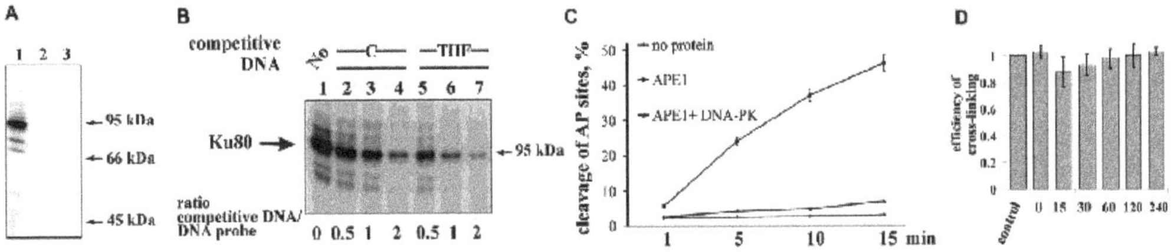

Fig. 3. Interaction of Ku antigen with AP sites (From Ilina et al., 2008). (A) Cross-linking of proteins in HeLa cell extract (lane 1); without borohydride treatment (lane 2); AP DNA probe was replaced by the DNA duplex containing a THF residue (lane 3). (B) Specificity of the Ku80 antigen interaction with AP DNA. Cross-linking of the HeLa cell extract proteins to AP DNA was performed in the absence (lane 1) or presence of competitive DNA at different concentrations (lanes 2-7). The structures of competitive DNAs are shown at the top. Ratio of competitive DNA to DNA probe is shown at the bottom. (C) Influence of DNA-PK on the activity of APE1. (D) Estimation of the stability of Ku complex with AP DNA in HeLa cell extract. AP DNA was preincubated with HeLa cell extract for 15 min at 37°. Then excess of competitive DNA containing a THF residue was added, and the reaction mixture was further incubated at 37° for additional 4 hours. Aliquots at different times were reduced with $NaBH_4$ and analyzed.

appropriate AP lyase substrate and AP lyase activity test in the cell extracts deficient and proficient in Ku antigen unambiguously testify to the role of Ku antigen in processing of AP sites positioned near 5′ termini of DS breaks. Moreover, transfection of Ku deficient or proficient cells with variants of specifically designed substrate DNAs (with natural AP site or its AP lyase-resistant analog or without AP site) followed by PCR amplification of joining products and subsequent restriction analysis of amplicons fully confirmed the necessity of Ku antigen AP lyase activity for removal of near-end AP sites. Altogether the results obtained *in vitro* and *in vivo* testify to use of the 5′-dRP/AP lyase activity of Ku antigen for the excision of near-end abasic sites and explain higher radiosensitivity of mammalian cells deficient in Ku antigen, which is indispensable for classical NHEJ (Schulte-Uentrop et al., 2008). It is worthy of notice, that the same mechanism of AP site cleavage is used by two unrelated DNA repair systems and the suitable positioning of AP sites relative to active site nucleophiles is indispensable for efficient catalysis.

2.3.3 AP site recognition by the 5'-dRP/AP lyase in PARP-1

In further screening for proteins that are reactive to AP sites in addition to a linear DNA duplex with an AP site in the middle of the ^{32}P-5′end-labeled strand, we used circular AP site-containing DNA to exclude interference by Ku80. Circular double-stranded DNA was synthesized, using single-stranded M13 DNA as template, in the presence of dUTP; then, AP sites were generated by uracil DNA glycosylase treatment (Khodyreva et al., 2010a; Khodyreva et al., 2010b). Unlike short duplex DNA with an AP site, that predominantly cross-linked Ku80 in HeLa cell extract (Ilina et al., 2008 and Fig. 4A, lane 5), the use of circular AP site-containing DNA allowed us to detect a novel protein with molecular mass of ~120-kDa that is reactive to AP site (Fig. 4A, lanes 1–4).

To identify the cross-linked protein large-scale cross-linking with the bovine testis nuclear extract (BTNE) and a biotin-containing linear AP DNA was performed. Identification was realized according to the scheme shown in Fig. 2.

Results from the MS analyses were searched against a database, and PARP-1 was identified as the first-rank candidate (Mascot probability score of 248, 38% of coverage).

We tested for and found AP site cross-linking by purified PARP-1 (data not shown). Yet, it was not clear whether the cross-linked complex in the extract resulted from PARP-1's reactivity at the intact AP site or a pre-incised AP site.

We next examined purified PARP-1 cross-linking with a linear DNA containing either an intact AP site or pre-incised AP site; in addition to cross-linking probes, these DNAs are substrates for 5'-dRP and AP lyase enzymatic activity (Fig. 4B).

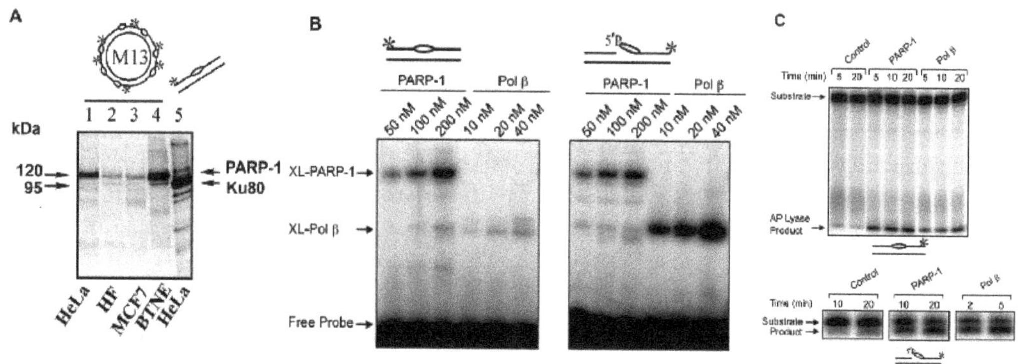

Fig. 4. Interaction of PARP-1 with intact and cleaved AP sites (From Khodyreva et al., 2010b). (A) Cross-linking of mammalian cell extract proteins to circular and linear AP DNA Extracts: whole cell extracts of HeLa, human fibroblasts (HF), MCF-7 and bovine testis nuclear extract (BTNE). (B) Comparison of cross-linking of purified PARP-1 and Pol β with 5'-dRP lyase substrate DNA and AP site-containing DNA. Schematic representations of DNA probes are shown at the top. The * symbol denotes the position of the ^{32}P-label in the DNA. The bubble-like symbol denotes the presence of the AP site in the DNA. (C) 5'-dRP/AP lyase activities of purified PARP-1. The positions of the substrates and products are indicated, and the DNA is illustrated at the bottom.

Cross-linking of PARP-1 was compared with that of Pol β. PARP-1 and Pol β cross-linked to both of these DNA substrates in a concentration-dependent manner. Pol β has a preference for the pre-incised AP site containing-DNA, as compared to the intact AP site. Conversely, PARP-1 does not show a similar preference, yielding similar cross-linking with both probes. The interaction of PARP-1 with the AP site raised the question of the biological relevance of this finding, including whether PARP-1 binds first to the AP site and protects it until repair proteins are recruited. PARP-1 is well known to become activated by binding to DNA strand breaks (Lindahl et al., 1995). Once the AP site became incised by AP endonuclease, PARP-1 became activated and modified by auto-poly(ADP-ribosyl)ation. First, we examined the specificity of PARP-1 interaction with AP site containing-DNA by competition experiments using two types of competitor DNA. A labeled DNA duplex with a 'natural' AP site was used for PARP-1 cross-linking, and the cross-linking was competed either with a control DNA duplex (without an AP site) or a synthetic AP site-containing DNA, tetrahydrofuran (THF), mimicking the AP site. Cross-linking of PARP-1 was reduced with both control and THF-containing DNA. However, the reduction was stronger in the case of

THF-containing DNA than with control DNA. This suggests that PARP-1 has greater affinity for the THF-containing DNA than for the control DNA (data not shown).

The next question regarding PARP-1's interaction with AP sites was whether the enzyme is activated for poly(ADP-ribose) synthesis upon binding to the intact AP site. PARP-1 is well known to become activated by binding to DNA strand breaks (Lindahl et al., 1995), and to avoid the presence of confounding DNA ends, we prepared a double-hairpin DNA for use as probe. First, using this hairpin DNA with internal ^{32}P-label, we confirmed the ability of purified PARP-1 to cross-link to the natural AP site. The results showed that double-hairpin DNA bearing the natural AP site was able to cross-link upon $NaBH_4$ reduction, whereas DNA without the AP site (uracil-DNA) failed to yield cross-linked product (data not shown). As expected, THF-containing DNA failed to cross-link. Next, using similar but unlabeled double-hairpin DNA and ^{32}P-NAD+ as substrate for poly(ADP-ribose) synthesis, we examined the activity of PARP-1. Strong PARP-1 auto-modification was observed only in reaction mixtures containing APE1 (data not shown). PARP-1 auto-modification in reaction mixtures with the natural AP site, but without APE1, was weak; this level, however, was more than the background level (data not shown). Under similar conditions, the THF-containing DNA failed to support poly(ADP-ribose) synthesis, but strong synthesis was observed when APE1 was added. These results indicated that PARP-1 interaction with the intact AP site could result in activation, but this activation involved much less auto-poly(ADP-ribosyl)ation than that observed with APE1-induced strand incision.

Next, to examine PARP-1 auto-modification, purified PARP-1 was first pre-incubated with labeled intact linear AP site-containing DNA. The reaction mixture was then supplemented with NAD^+ to allow poly(ADP-ribose) synthesis. Then, the reaction mixture was treated with $NaHB_4$ and analyzed. The results indicated that poly(ADP-ribose) modified enzyme was cross-linked (data not shown). The mechanism of PARP-1 activation was unclear, but presumably involved single strand break formation within the PARP-1 and DNA complex. In light of this result, we were curious to test PARP-1's capacity to conduct strand incision at the AP site via AP lyase activity. As shown in Fig. 4C, PARP-1 was capable of incising AP site-containing DNA, and the activity was similar to that of Pol β. In light of PARP-1's AP lyase activity, we also tested for 5'dRP lyase activity. PARP-1 conducted 5'-dRP lyase activity against a pre-incised AP site (Fig. 4C), but the activity was much lower than that of Pol β. These results suggested that the endogenous PARP-1 AP lyase activity was sufficient to provide poly(ADP-ribose) synthesis activation at the natural AP site.

Interaction of PARP-1 with AP sites appears to be related with regulation of AP site processing. Such a regulation is particularly important for repair of AP sites included in clustered damage, in which chain breaks, oxidized bases and AP sites are grouped within 1-2 turns of DNA helix and can be situated in both DNA chains. During repair of AP sites within clustered damages additional double strand breaks, which are more cytotoxic, may appear (Yang et al., 2004). PARP-1 influence on hydrolysis of AP sites by APE1 on DNA containing AP site either opposite dAMP or synthetic AP site analogues, was tested (Kutuzov et al., 2011). Along with THF residue, which is most widely used to mimic AP sites, the new AP site analogs were tested (Kutuzov et al., 2011). These analogs were residues of diethylene glycol and decane-1,10-diol. The AP site analogs differ in their sensitivity to the APE1 endonuclease activity. PARP-1 interacts more efficiently with AP sites within clusters that leads to stronger cross-linking with AP sites and more considerable inhibition of APE1 activity as compared with AP DNA containing single AP site.

Thus, by virtue of PARP-1's ability to interact with the intact AP sites (single or within cluster) via Schiff base formation, we demonstrated a new role for PARP-1 in regulation of the BER process. PARP-1's interaction at the AP site could recruit this key enzyme and protect the site until APE1 becomes available to initiate strand incision and BER. Alternatively, PARP-1's 5'-dRP/AP lyase activity could perform strand incision and trigger poly(ADP-ribosyl)ation leading to recruitment of other BER factors.

2.3.4 New function of Neil1 and Neil2 as 5'dRP lyase

According to current view, in mammalian BER the sub-pathway choice is influenced by the rate-limiting step in SN BER, i.e., removal of the 5'-dRP by the dRP lyase activity of Pol β (Horton et al., 2000; Srivastava et al., 1998). For example, if the 5'-dRP cannot be removed efficiently, continued DNA synthesis will emphasize the LP BER sub-pathway (Horton et al., 2000). Yet, both subpathways appear to operate simultaneously to repair most types of DNA lesions *in vitro* (Horton et al., 2000; Prasad et al., 2000). It has been shown previously that the 5'-dRP BER intermediate is the cytotoxic lesion following exposure to methylating agents, and its removal is a pivotal step in BER *in vivo* (Sobol et al., 2000).

Pol β-deficient mouse cells show little dRPase activity (Sobol et al., 2000), but some residual dRP removal by extracts prepared from these cells is still present (Podlutsky et al., 2001). It is possible that while Pol β carries out the bulk of dRP removal from DNA, other activities could be more specifically employed for certain lesions, cell or tissue types, or at certain points of the cell cycle. In *E. coli*, Fpg (formamidopyrimidine-DNA glycosylase) and to a lesser extent endonuclease VIII (Nei) catalyze β-elimination of dRP moiety (Fig. 1). Three mammalian homologues of bacterial Fpg and Nei termed NEIL (Nei-like)-1, -2, and -3 have been identified (Hazra et al., 2002; Hegde et al., 2008). Based on the similarity of their active sites to those of Fpg and Nei, one could expect that they could also display dRPase activity. We have shown that two of these proteins, NEIL1 and NEIL2, are capable of removing dRP lesions from DNA with the efficiency comparable to that of Pol β, and that they can substitute for Pol β dRPase activity in a reconstituted BER assay (Grin et al., 2006).

dRPase activity can be revealed with 3'-labeled nicked abasic oligonucleotide substrates. Such substrates were prepared by end-filling of a 5'-overhanging oligonucleotide duplexes with ^{32}P-labeled dATP and the consecutive treatment of the duplex with uracil DNA glycosylase (Ung) and APE1. The resulting dRP site is unstable in nucleophilic buffers and is degraded during migration through Tris-containing polyacrylamide gels, therefore the products were stabilized by sodium borohydride reduction immediately after the dRPase-catalyzed reaction.

Fig. 5A illustrates that both NEIL1 and NEIL2 possess a dRP-removing activity. The dRPase activities of NEIL1 and NEIL2 demonstrated the enzyme concentration and time dependence expected of an enzyme-catalyzed reaction (Fig. 5B and data not shown). Notably, the activity of NEIL1 in these experiments appeared higher than that of NEIL1 (Fig. 5B). Both NEIL1 and NEIL2 excised with similar efficiency when A, C, or T were placed opposite the lesion, and the excision of dRP opposite G was 1.5–2-fold lower; Pol β removed dRP equally well from all opposite-base contexts. To confirm that dRP removal by NEIL1 and NEIL2 proceeds by β-elimination, as in Pol β and Fpg, we have performed the reaction in the presence of sodium borohydride, which reduces the Schiff base covalent complexes formed between the catalytic amine nucleophile of dRP lyases and C1' of the dRP site during the reaction (Fig. 5C). Such trapped enzyme–DNA complexes are stable enough to be resolved by regular SDS-PAGE. NEIL1 and NEIL2, as well as Fpg and Pol β, formed low-mobility radioactively labeled complexes.

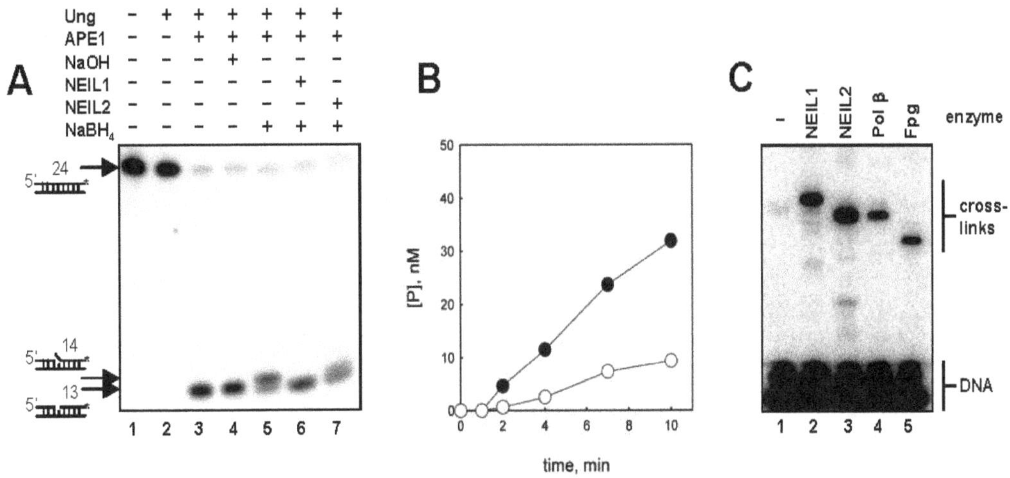

Fig. 5. **dRPase activity of NEIL1 and NEIL2** (From Grin et al., 2006). (A) Cleavage of a dRP moiety by NEIL1 and NEIL2. Lane 1, U-containing oligonucleotide; lane 2, AP-containing oligonucleotide; lanes 3–7, dRP-containing oligonucleotide treated with alkali (lane 4), NEIL1 (lane 6) or NEIL2 (lane 7). In lanes 5–7, the dRP-containing oligonucleotide was stabilized with sodium borohydride to prevent its degradation during electrophoresis. Arrows left to the panels indicate positions of the respective oligonucleotide species after PAGE. (B) Time course of dRP excision by NEIL1 (filled circles) and NEIL2 (open circles). (C) Cross-linking of dRP lyases to a dRP-containing substrate by sodium borohydride: lane 1, no enzyme; lane 2, NEIL1; lane 3, NEIL2; lane 4, Pol β; lane 5, Fpg.

To compare the efficiency of NEIL1 and NEIL2 as dRPases with the same activity of DNA polymerase β, the best-known mammalian dRPase, we have determined steady-state enzyme kinetic constants for all three enzymes. The results of these experiments are summarized in Table 1.

	K_M, μM	k_{cat}, min^{-1}	k_{cat}/K_M, μM^{-1} min^{-1}
NEIL1	0.21±0.03	0.65±0.04	3.1
NEIL2	2.2±0.7	1.6±0.1	0.74
Pol β	1.0±0.1	3.0±0.1	3.0

Table 1. Kinetic parameters of the dRPase reaction catalyzed by NEIL1, NEIL2, and DNA polymerase β.

The kinetic data suggest that NEIL1 is as good a dRPase as Pol β, and they both surpassed NEIL2 in their ability to remove dRP from DNA. K_M of NEIL1 was ~5-fold lower than K_M of Pol β, indicating that NEIL1 might bind dRP-containing substrate more tightly; on the other hand, Pol β processed the substrate ~5-fold faster than did NEIL1, resulting in nearly equal specificity constants for both enzymes. NEIL2 had an intermediate catalytic constant and the poorest binding of all three dRP lyases compared in this experiment.

The experiments with individual enzymes suggest that NEIL1 and NEIL2 possess dRP lyase activities and could substitute for Pol β in removing dRP moiety in the BER process. To analyze the proficiency of NEIL1 and NEIL2 dRPase in a multienzyme BER process, we have reconstituted the base-excision, AP site-incision, gap-filling and dRP-excision stages of BER using mammalian enzymes (UNG, OGG1, APE1, Pol β (wild type and K35A/K68A/K72A mutant deficient in dRP lyase activity) and NEIL1 or NEIL2. Both NEIL1 and NEIL2 could rescue BER of uracil lesions driven by a dRP-deficient Pol β. The proficiency of NEIL1 in the full BER was higher compared with NEIL2, in agreement with the kinetic parameters showing that NEIL2 is the worst of the three dRPases. We have also reconstituted the repair of AP sites pre-formed in DNA by action of *E. coli* UDG. No major difference from the repair of U was observed.

Having established that NEIL1 and NEIL2 could substitute for dRPlyase activity of Pol β in the reconstituted BER system, we then studied whether NEIL proteins could manifest their dRPase activity in some particular systems, e.g. in cell extracts lacking Pol β.

2.3.5 Identification of HMGB1 as cofactor of the BER process

To identify proteins that have dRP lyase activity or influence removal of the dRP from BER intermediates in the absence of Pol β, we used Pol β null mouse embryonic fibroblast (MEF) cell extract for sodium borohydride driven cross-linking of the Schiff base dRP lyase intermediate protein-DNA complex (Prasad et al., 2007). The strong labeling of a single species in the Pol β null cell extracts corresponding to an unknown protein-DNA complex of 37 kDa was observed (Fig. 6A).

The preferential cross-linking of this protein reflected extraordinary specificity in light of the multitude of proteins in the cell. Taking into account the molecular masses of NEIL1 and NEIL2 (43.5 kDa and 38.2 kDa, respectively) the product could not be related to glycosylases. It should be noted that an apparent molecular mass of a covalent adduct protein-nucleic acid estimated by electrophoretic mobility is approximately equal to the sum of molecular masses of protein and attached nucleic acid.

For identification of protein we applied the approach schematically depicted in Fig. 2. The DNA probe contained a ^{32}P-labeled dRP moiety in a single-stranded break and a 3'-biotin tag to facilitate isolation of cross-linked protein-DNA complexes. Eleven of ions observed in MALDI MS spectrum corresponded to peptides of HMGB1. The $(M + H)^+$ ion of m/z 1520.84 was selected automatically during the data dependent acquisition for MS/MS analysis. The values from both the peptide masses and the MS/MS fragment ion masses were used in a database search. The protein was identified as HMGB1 with a Mowse-based score of 102, 32% sequence coverage and a protein score confidence interval of 99.995%. Among the observed ions the ion of m/z 1520.84 corresponds to amino acid residues 113–127 of the mouse HMGB1 and is a 'signature' that distinguishes HMGB1 from the closely related protein, HMGB2 (Bustin & Reeves, 1996). HMGB1 and HMGB2 are nuclear nonhistone DNA-binding proteins that belong to the high-mobility group box family of proteins (Bustin & Reeves, 1996). HMGB1 has an architectural role in the assembly of nucleoprotein complexes and is highly conserved across species (Bustin & Reeves, 1996; Tang et al., 2010 ;Liu et al., 2010; Stros, 2010). HMGB1 binds to DNA in the minor groove without sequence specificity and has the ability to transiently introduce bends or kinks into linear DNA (Liu et al., 2010; Stros, 2010). The intrinsic ability of HMGB1 to alter DNA structures allows it to participate in many biological processes including regulation of chromatin structure, transcription, DNA damage repair and recombination. The importance of HMGB1 in DNA repair was identified in studies that revealed the ability of HMGB1 to bind to a variety of bulky DNA lesions (Liu et al., 2010; Stros, 2010).

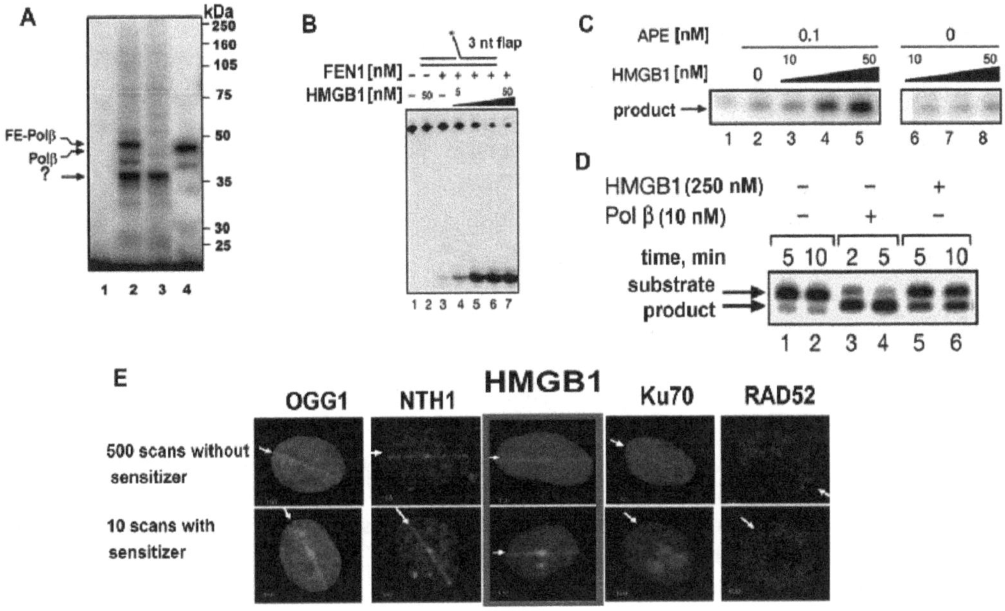

Fig. 6. Identification of HMGB1 as a BER cofactor (from Prasad et al., 2007). (A) Search of extract proteins interacting with the 5'dRP residue in the DNA duplex: lane 2, products of cross-linking between 5' dRP DNA and MEF extract proteins expressing Pol β with flag-epitope (FE), lane 1 control without borohydride treatment. (B) The influence of HMGB1 on FEN1 activity. (C) Influence of HMGB1 on APE1 activity. (D) Comparison of the 5' deoxyribose phosphate lyase activity of HMGB1 and Pol β. (E) Interaction of GFP-HMGB1 in HeLa cells with DNA damage sites induced by scanning laser microirradiation (λ 405 nm) without a sensitizer and in the presence of 8-methoxypsoralen (100 μM). Protein designation: 8-Oxoguanine DNA glycosylase (OGG1); NTH1, DNA glycosylase removing oxidized pyrimidines from DNA; RAD52, protein involved in double-strand break repair, homologous recombination; Ku70, Ku antigen subunit involved in of double-strand break repair, nonhomologous end joining. Arrows show the direction of the scan.

The observed ability of HMGB1 to interact with the BER DNA intermediate poses a question about its role in the process. It was found in the in vitro experiments that HMGB1 isolated from HeLa cells directly interacted with several BER proteins: APE1, Pol β, and FEN1(data not shown) and stimulate the activity of BER enzymes FEN1 and APE1 (Figs. 6B and 6C, respectively). HMGB1 was also revealed to have weak 5' dRP lyase activity (Fig. 6D).

Using HeLa cells expressing HMGB1 in the form of a chimeric protein with green fluorescent protein (GFP-HMGB1), it was found that HMGB1 can be localized in the regions of DNA damage induced by laser microirradiation (Fig. 6E). Irradiation under used conditions generates both single-strand breaks and oxidized bases with high frequency (Lan et al., 2004). Indeed, DNA glycosylases (GFP-OGG1 and GFP-NTH1) efficiently accumulate

in sites of irradiation unlike the proteins recognizing double-strand breaks in DNA (GFP-Ku70 and GFP-RAD52) (Fig. 6E).
Mouse embryonic fibroblasts of the HMGB1+/+ type are more sensitive than HMGB1-/- cells to the combined action of methyl methanesulfonate and methoxyamine, and HMGB1+/+ cells contain a much larger amount of single-strand breaks. The treatment of AP DNA with methoxyamine increases its resistance to APE1 action (Horton et al., 2000).
Another group of researches using two cultivated cell lines of breast cancer found that the increase in the expression level of HMGB1 alters the cells' phenotype by slowing cell growth and increasing the cell sensitivity to ionizing radiation (Jiao et al., 2007).
Interestingly, that in spite of ability of purified NEIL 1/2 to interact with dRP lyase substrate (Grin et al., 2006) we did not reveal abundant products of their cross-linking in the Pol β null MEF extract (Fig. 6 A, lane 2). This interaction appears to be counteracted by effective binding of HMGB1, which is highly abundant in cells.

2.3.6 HMGA as cofactor of the BER process

It is interesting to note that dRP- and AP lyase activities were revealed for another group of chromatin proteins (Summer at al., 2009). Mammalian high mobility group proteins are non-histone chromatin architectural factors encoded by two genes, *HMGA1* and *HMGA2*. Alternative mRNA splicing results in at least four protein isoforms involved in chromatin remodeling and gene transcription (Bustin & Reeves, 1996, Reeves, 2001, Cleynen & van de Ven, 2008). HMGA proteins are characterized by the presence of an acidic C-terminal tail and three DNA binding domains containing short basic repeats, the so called AT-hooks, capable to bind in the minor groove of AT-rich sequences in DNA. In humans, HMGA expression is undetectable or very low in differentiated adult tissues, but high HMGA protein levels are associated with human malignant neoplasias (Berner et al., 1997, Abe et al., 2003, Miyazawa et al., 2004, Meyer et al., 2007). In addition, expression of HMGA1 is functionally linked to chemoresistance of some human carcinomas (Liau & Whang, 2008).
Recombinant human HMGA (HMGA1a, HMGA1b and HMGA2) proteins have been shown to efficiently cleave plasmid DNA containing AP sites (Summer et al., 2009). Further analysis revealed that the proteins could be trapped on AP DNA by $NaCNBH_3$ treatment, the mechanism characteristic of AP lyase activity (David & Williams, 1998; McCullough et al.; 1999, Piersen et al., 2000). To determine the chemical nature of DNA ends generated by the HMGA proteins and the efficiency of AP site cleavage, ^{32}P-labeled double-stranded short DNA duplex containing a single AP site was used as substrate. The analysis revealed that HMGA proteins generated cleavage products, which exhibit the same electrophoretic mobility as those produced by endonuclease III of *E. coli*, an AP lyase catalyzing the β elimination reaction (McCullough et al., 1999; David & Williams, 1998).
To test the possibility that HMGA proteins also possess the related 5'-dRP lyase activity the same DNA duplex bearing label at the 3' end was employed. A 5'-dRP moiety on the labeled strand was produced by endonuclease IV from *E. coli*. To stabilize chemically labile 5'-dRP group and to improve electrophoretic separation of the products, 5'-deoxyribosyl phosphate moiety was adducted with O-benzyl hydroxylamine. The analysis revealed that the HMGA proteins efficiently removed 5'-dRP moiety. Thus, HMGA proteins display the AP/5'-dRP lyase activity characteristic of the BER process.
Having established that the HMGA proteins are lyases, the authors examined the role of this activity in cell context. To this end, cell lines constitutively expressing HMGA2 have been

generated. Then using transgenic and parental cell lines and employing a variety of cell-based assays and biochemical approaches, the authors provided evidence that the AP site/dRP lyase activities indeed had important biological functions. First, it has been demonstrated that HMGA2 could be efficiently trapped on genomic DNA. Parental cells A549, which express HMGA2 below detectable level, were exposed to low pH or physiological pH as control. DNA isolated from treated cells was incubated with recombinant HMGA2 under trapping (+$NaCNBH_3$) or non-trapping (+NaCl) conditions. The subsequent dot-blot analysis revealed that HMGA2 could be only trapped by DNA derived from cells exposed to low pH, conditions leading to generation of AP sites. Moreover, HMGA2 expressed in transgenic cell line A549 (1.6) was efficiently trapped in a covalent complex *in vivo* with genomic AP sites generated when the cells were subjected to low pH. Analysis of cytotoxic effects that might result from depurination in parental and transgenic cells caused by exposure to low pH revealed that all transgenic cell lines were substantially more resistant than parental cells.

In order to unravel the role of HMGA2 in response of cells to genotoxic impact, parental and transgenic cells were exposed to hydroxyurea (Hu) or methyl methanesulphonate (MMS). Hu is able to induce base oxidation and depurination (Sakano et al., 2001). MMS produces genomic AP sites through the action of DNA glycosylases, which remove the alkylated bases (Sedgwik et al., 2006). In the case of both reagents expression of HMGA2 resulted in significant protection against cell death leading to increase in cell survival.

Both AP and dRP lyase activities play central roles in the early steps of BER (Hegde et al., 2008). In order to demonstrate that protection from MMS induced DNA damage observed with transgenic cells involves HMGA2 lyase activities the cells were sequentially exposed to MMS and O-benzyl hydroxylamine (BA). BA alone had no effect on the survival of parental or transgenic cells. However, combined action of MMS and BA sensitized HMGA2-containg cells to MMS treatment. BA (analogously to methoxy amine) reacts with the baseless deoxyribose moieties (in intact or cleaved AP sites) rendering them refractory to mammalian AP endonuclease 1 and AP/dRP lyase activities (Horton et al., 2000).

Direct interaction of HMGA2 with APE1 *in vitro* and *in vivo* (Sgarra et al., 2008, Summer et al., 2009, Sgarra et al., 2010) has been reported. However, the influence of HMGA2 on the AP endonuclease 1 activity is still unknown. HMGA2 protects cells against three different genotoxicants, i.e. Hu, MMS and low pH (Summer et al., 2009), which introduce the DNA damages repaired by the BER machinery. It is noteworthy here, that repair of these lesions involves the common intermediates, AP sites and 5′ dRP moieties, which can be processed by HMGA2. This strongly support the idea developed in (Summer et al., 2009) that intrinsic AP/dRP lyase activities of HMGA2 are responsible for the protective action of this protein. However, one could not exclude that in addition to direct action, HMGA2 influences the BER capacity indirectly by enhancing the activity of APE1 as was observed in the case of HMGB1 (Prasad et al., 2007). Activation of APE1 by protein-protein interaction may be involved both in the stage of AP site hydrolysis and removing the 3′ end PUA group. APE1 is known as the main mammalian protein capable to excise this blocking group producing the 3′ end hydroxyl moiety (Wilson & Barsky, 2001; Pascucci et al., 2002).

2.3.7 Human ALK B homologue (ABH1) is an AP lyase

Methylated bases in DNA generated by endogenous and environmental alkylating agents can be removed by three distinct strategies. While 3-methyladenine (3-alkyladenine) is excised by a specific DNA glycosylase that initiates a base excision repair process, 1-methyladenine, 3-methylcytosine and O6-methylguanine are corrected by direct reversal exploring a different mechanism (for more information see a review Sedgwick et al., 2006). One of the strategies of direct reversal involves the activity of DNA dioxygenases, which release the methyl moiety as formaldehyde (Duncan et al., 2002). Although three human DNA dioxygenases - ABH1–ABH3 - catalyze the same oxidative demethylation reaction they display specificity toward methylated base and nucleic acids (DNA or RNA and single- or double-stranded) (Duncan et al., 2002, Westbye et al., 2008, Ougland et al., 2004; Kurowski et al., 2003). Unexpectedly, ABH1 - the closest AlkB *E. coli* homologue - has been shown to display an AP site cleavage activity (Müller et al., 2010).

Intensive study of discovered activity revealed that the DNA cleavage activity of ABH1 did not require added Fe2+ or 2-oxoglutarate, is not inhibited by EDTA, and is unaffected by mutation of the putative metal-binding residues, indicating that this activity arises from an active site distinct from that used for demethylation.

Enzymes that cleave sugar-phosphate backbone at abasic sites can utilize hydrolysis, β- or β,δ-elimination mechanisms (Fig. 1). First, to assess the cleavage mechanism, the activity of ABH1 was examined with DNA containing THF residue, the AP-site analogue, which could not be cleaved by the β-elimination reaction. No AP site cleavage was observed with ABH1 and EndoIII unlike APE1. Second, the electrophoretic mobility of the products resulting from the activities of ABH1, APE1, EndoIII and EndoVIII were examined. Prior to analysis 5′-[^{32}P]-labeled ds-oligonucleotides containing the AP site were incubated with the corresponding enzymes. In some samples, the products of AP site cleavage were additionally treated with T4 polynucleotide kinase (PNK) to remove possible 3′-terminal phosphate by this phosphatase. It should be noted that authors used proteinase treatment of the reaction mixtures to stop the reaction and degrade the enzymes prior to separation of oligonucleotides by denaturing PAAG electrophoresis (Fig. 7). The products produced by ABH1 migrate slowly (Fig. 7, lane 1) than the product of the β-elimination reaction (Fig. 7, lane 3) and do not contain the 3′ end phosphate group since the mobility of the products was not changed by PNK treatment (Fig. 7, compare lanes 1 and 2). While the products derived from the EndoVIII activity, which explores the β,δ-elimination mechanism resulting in the 3′ phosphate group, migrate slowly after PNK treatment (Fig. 7, compare lanes 5 and 6). The authors proposed that ABH1 cleaves AP sites by β-elimination with ABH1 being bound with the product in tight complex. They attribute the slight decrease in mobility of the products for the ABH1 samples to tight binding of ABH1 fragments with oligonucleotides. The authors demonstrated that both ABH1 and EndoIII in the presence of $NaBH_4$ are able to generate stable products with single-stranded AP-DNA, double-stranded DNA containing one AP site and double-stranded DNA containing two AP sites, but the important control without reducing agent is missed. Taking into account that ABH1 forms stable adducts with AP DNA without reduction, as observed in the activity test (Fig. 7, lanes 1 and 2), it is questionable whether the trapping of ABH1 is the Schiff base dependent.

ABH1 was shown to display specificity in substrate usage with DNA containing two AP sites being the preferable substrate. Further analysis of AP site cleavage activity at different substrate-to-enzyme ratio demonstrated that concentration of product was always sub-stoichiometric to the enzyme concentration that is in agreement with tight binding of ABH1 with the product.

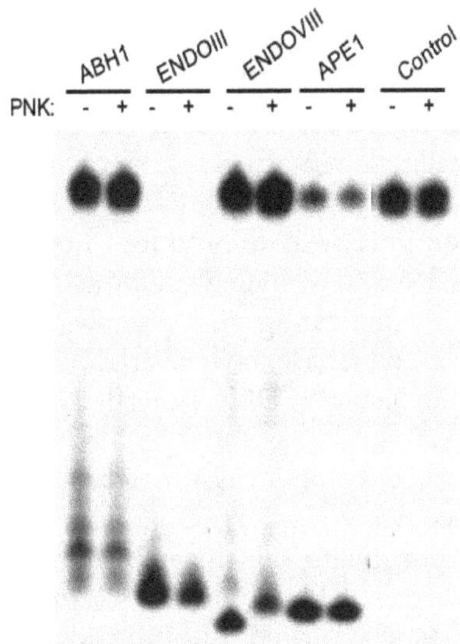

Fig. 7. Comparison of product sizes for ABH1, APE1, ENDOIII, and ENDOVIII, and examination of the effect of phosphatase treatment (from Müller et al., 2010). The uracil containing DNA duplex was cleaved by incubation with ABH1 or the control endonucleases in the presence of UDG for 1 h at 37 °C. Portions of the samples were treated with the phosphatase T4 polynucleotide kinase to remove possible phosphates at the 3′ end of the labeled products. The presence of a 3′-phosphate causes the oligonucleotide to migrate more rapidly than the non-phosphorylated species due to the extra negative charge; removal of the phosphate results in a shift to an apparently larger product, as seen with EndoVIII.

Taking into account ubiquitous expression of APE1 and inefficiency of the ABH1 AP lyase activity, ABH1 hardly play significant role *in vivo* in processing of AP sites. Moreover, the ability of ABH1 to more efficiently cleave opposite AP sites in ds DNA that may result in formation of DS breaks, more toxic for the cells than AP sites, therefore action of ABH1 on clustered AP sites in genomic DNA appears to be dangerous for cells. The authors considered tight binding of ABH1 with the product as a mechanism that protects ends from degradation. On the other hand, tight binding may create hindrances for the repair processes and require special efforts to remove blocking group from the 3′ end. Potentially interesting finding of intrinsic AP lyase activity of ABH1 requires additional studies to draw a conclusion concerning significance of discovered activity *in vivo*.

2.3.8 Tyrosyl-DNA-phosphodiesterase mediates the new APE-independent BER pathway in mammals

As mentioned above AP sites can be cleaved by activity of bifunctional DNA glycosylases with associated AP lyase activities via β- or β,δ-elimination mechanism producing DNA intermediates with 3′ end containing 3′-phosphate or 3′-PUA groups (Fig. 1) that have to be removed prior to DNA synthesis may occur. DNA intermediates with blocked 3′end may also appear from action of ROS and as a result of spontaneous decomposition of AP sites.
The 3' PUA is known to be removed by the only AP-endonuclease, APE1, which possesses 3′ phosphodiesterase activity with α-unsaturated aldehydes, producing a single nucleotide gap flanked by a 3′-hydroxyl group and a 5′ phosphate group (Wilson & Barsky, 2001;

Pascucci et al., 2002). However, APE1 is barely active in removing 3' phosphate generated by mammalian DNA glycosylases NEIL1 and NEIL2. The 3' phosphate is efficiently removed by polynucleotide kinase (PNK) and not APE1 (Wiederhold et al., 2004).

Tyrosyl-DNA phosphodiesterase (Tdp1) was discovered as an enzymatic activity from *Saccharomyces cerevisiae* that specifically hydrolyzes the phosphodiester linkage between the O-4 atom of a tyrosine and a DNA 3′ phosphate (Yang et al., 1996). This type of linkage is typical for the covalent reaction intermediate produced upon Topoisomerase 1 cleavage of one DNA strand. Human Tdp1 can also hydrolyze other 3′-end DNA alterations that are covalently linked to the DNA, indicating that it may function as a general 3′-DNA phosphodiesterase and repair enzyme (Dexheimer et al., 2008). Tdp1 can also remove the tetrahydrofuran moiety from the 3'-end of DNA (Interthal et al., 2005). It is conceivable that Tdp1 acts on the 3′ PUA moiety.

To study an ability of Tdp1 to process the 3′ PUA moiety AP DNA was first incubated with Endo III (Fig. 8A, lane 2) (Lebedeva et al., 2011). Following incubation of this product with Tdp1 results in 15-mer with 3' phosphate, which can be removed by PNKP (Fig. 8A, lane 3). Thus, Tdp1 is able to remove the 3′ PUA that allows to realize the APE1-independent pathway of BER where AP sites are cleaved by bifunctional DNA glycosylases via the β-elimination mechanism.

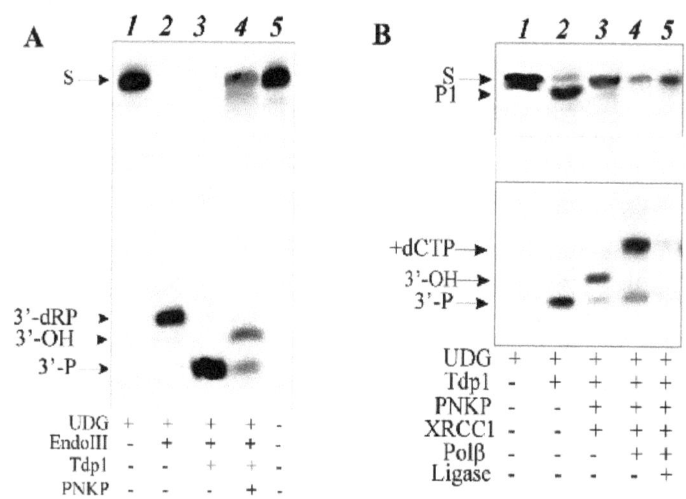

Fig. 8. Tdp1 activity on DNA substrate with 3'-dRP moiety in the single strand break (A) and reconstitution of the AP-DNA substrate repair initiated by Tdp1 (B) (From Lebedeva et al., 2011). **(A)** The 15-mer with 3'-dRP was generated by incubation of AP DNA with EndoIII (lane 2). Following incubation of this product with Tdp1 results in 15-mer with 3'-P (lane 3). Lane 4 shows the 15-mer product with 3'-OH after adding PNKP in the reaction mixture. Lane 1 corresponds to the AP-DNA substrate incubated with UDG. Lane 5 - control. (B) 5'-end labeled AP-DNA substrate was subsequently incubated with the UDG (lane 1), Tdp1 (lane 2), PNKP and XRCC1 (lane 3), Pol β (lane 4), DNA ligase III (lane 5). The components present in different reaction mixtures are indicated.

We tested an ability of Tdp1 to process AP sites (natural or mimicked by THF residue) and found that Tdp1 cleaves both types of AP sites generating the product identical to the product of β,δ-elimination (data not shown). Finally, the repair of AP site was analyzed in a minimal reconstituted BER system consisting of purified proteins (Fig. 8B). The 5′ ^{32}P-labeled 32-mer DNA duplex containing uridine at the position 16 was incubated with the purified recombinant UDG, Tdp1, PNKP, Pol β, DNA ligase III, and XRCC1 to mimic DNA repair system. The reaction mixture containing Tdp1 but lacking PNKP (lane 2) generated a product with a 3′-phosphate, which is identical to that produced by NEIL1. Addition of PNKP resulted in a 15-mer product with the 3′-OH termini (lane 3). XRCC1, a scaffold protein, stimulates the activity of BER proteins, such as DNA polymerase β, PNKP, DNA ligase III (Mani et al., 2004; Caldecott, 2003; Whitehouse et al., 2001).

Lastly, DNA polymerase β replaces the missing DNA segment (lane 4) and DNA ligase reseals the DNA (lane 5). So, the repair of AP site initiated by Tdp1 fully restored the intact DNA and generated the products of the expected lengths at each intermediate stage. In summary, human Tdp1 protein can initiate APE1-independent repair of AP sites and 3′ PUA termini that expands the ability of the BER process.

2.3.9 XRCC1 interactions with base excision repair DNA intermediates

XRCC1 is known to play a crucial role in the coordination of two overlapping repair pathways, SSBR and BER (Caldecott, 2003). Although the main role of XRCC1 during BER has been attributed to its participation in the post-incision steps (Wong et al., 2005), which are shared with SSBR, the physical and functional interactions with proteins involved in the initiation of modified bases or abasic sites repair (Marsin et al., 2003, Campalans et al., 2005, Vidal et al., 2001, Wiederhold et al., 2004) suggest that XRCC1 presence at the early steps of BER could be important for assuring a correct repair process. One possible role of XRCC1 could be to optimize the passage of DNA substrates from one enzyme to the next one in the pathway by holding the proteins together through its different interacting domains (Caldecott, 2003).

Investigating the interactions of with different BER DNA intermediates generated either by DNA glycosylase hOGG1 or AP endonuclease APE1 we have found that XRCC1 is able to interact with AP sites via formation of the Schiff base intermediate (Nazarkina et al., 2007). Because hOGG1 possesses both, DNA glycosylase and AP lyase activities, either of two DNA intermediates can be produced: DNA duplex containing an intact AP site or a nick with a 3′ PUA moiety (See Fig. 1). By competition experiments using the THF-containing or regular DNA duplex it was demonstrated that XRCC1 binds DNA with an AP site, or its synthetic analogue, with considerably higher affinity than regular DNA duplex.

XRCC1 is known to bind DNA with single-strand breaks with higher affinity that regular DNA duplex (Mani et al., 2004). We then investigated the relative affinities of XRCC1 to different DNA structures that could be BER intermediates in the repair of single or double DNA lesions. The efficiency of cross-linking is maximal with an incised AP site 3′ PUA (Fig. 9A, lane 3). Interestingly, the presence of a strand interruption on the complementary oligonucleotide strongly stimulated the cross-linking of XRCC1 to the AP site. These results suggest that XRCC1 could be important to hold the DNA together during the repair of clustered DNA damage. XRCC1 is also able to cross-link to a 5′ dRP residue downstream of a nick (Fig. 9A, lane 6). Comparative analysis of the patterns of protein cross-linking to AP DNA in cell extracts deficient (EM9) and proficient in XRCC1 (EM9-X) (Fig. 9B, lanes 3-6) revealed the product that can be related with XRCC1 (lane 6). Interestingly, that the band is observed with DNA containing interruption opposite AP site (Fig. 9B, lanes 4 and 6).

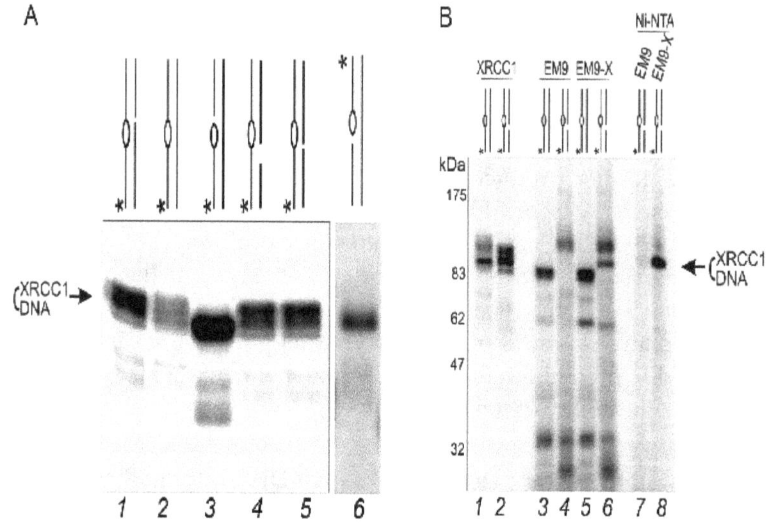

Fig. 9. Interactions of XRCC1 with BER DNA intermediates (From Nazarkina et al., 2007). (A) Cross-linking of XRCC1 to different 5′-^{32}P-labeled AP DNA. DNA containing intact AP sites (lanes 1, 2, 4, and 5) and cleaved AP site (3′ PUA) (lane 3) were 5′ end labeled, while DNA containing hydrolyzed AP site (5′ dRP) (lane 6) was 3′ end labeled. (B) Cross-linking of XRCC1 with AP DNA in CHO cell extracts deficient in XRCC1 (EM9) or EM9 expressing His-tagged human XRCC1 (EM9-9). Position of radioactive label in DNA is designated by the asterisk.

To confirm that this product corresponds to the XRCC1 containing conjugate, after trapping with $NaBH_4$, His-tagged XRCC1 was recovered by pull-down using a Ni-NTA resin. After this purification step, the product was recovered from the EM9-X extract (lane 8) but not the EM9 one (lane 7).

Taken together, these results demonstrate XRCC1 ability to interact with intact and cleaved AP sites, including cell extracts, e.g. in the presence of cellular proteins that can interfere with XRCC1 binding to AP DNA.

Thus, using the Schiff-base-mediated cross-linking, we show that XRCC1 displays a specific affinity for AP containing substrates. Although at this time we cannot evaluate the in vivo relevance of covalent complexes between XRCC1 and DNA, considering the Schiff base reversibility, it is tempting to speculate that its formation during BER of AP sites could be a physiological response to situations where a reactive intermediate needs to be protected until the next enzyme recruited by XRCC1 is able to process it.

3. Conclusion

Combination of affinity based cross-linking of proteins with specific DNA probes containing intact or cleaved AP sites and MS analysis allowed to identify new players in recognition/processing of these ubiquitous lesions. Some identified proteins are known as regulatory proteins of specific DNA repair processes, not necessarily involved in repair of AP sites, but all these proteins are related to cell radiosensitivity. Two of them—XRCC1 and PARP1—belong to the base excision repair system, but have been previously considered as participants of later stages of the BER process. By virtue of its interaction with AP sites,

PARP1 and XRCC1 can regulate initial stage of BER persisting at AP sites until APE1 could come and initiate AP sites cleavage. The PARP1 activation upon interaction with AP sites and resultant automodification appear to facilitate the BER factor recruitment to stimulate the repair process. In the absence or deficiency of APE1, PARP1 can provide temporal protection of AP sites. Ku antigen can temporarily protect AP sites situated within 1-2 turns of DNA helix from double-strand breaks or displays AP/dRP lyase activity near double-strand ends. The last activity has no analogues and is indispensable for proper repair of DS breaks with particular blocking groups at the ends, which can result from action of ionizing radiation.

In other case of revealed AP/dRP lyase activities, they appear to function under particular physiologic or stressful conditions modulating the capacity of the BER system or providing the appropriate functions of the repair machinery when some participants are missed or inactive. Interestingly, that structural chromatin proteins -HMGB1 and HMGA - were found to interact with AP sites displaying an enzymatic activity. Although being a relative weak, this activity may be biologically significant due to high abundance of these proteins.

4. Acknowledgments

This work was supported in part by the Russian Foundation for Basic Research (Project No 10-04-01083) and Program of the Russian Academy of Sciences "Molecular and Cellular Biology".

5. References

Abe, N.; Watanabe, T.; Suzuki, Y.; Matsumoto, N.; Masaki, T.; Mori, T.; Sugiyama, M.; Chiappetta, G.; Fusco, A.; & Atomi, Y. (2003). An increased high-mobility group A2 expression level is associated with malignant phenotype in pancreatic exocrine tissue. *Br J Cancer* 89, 2104.

Allinson, S.L.; Dianova, I.I.; & Dianov, G.L. (2001). DNA polymerase β is the major dRP lyase involved in repair of oxidative base lesions in DNA by mammalian cell extracts. *EMBO J* 20, 6919.

Almeida, K.H. & Sobol, R.W. (2007). A unified view of base excision repair: lesion-dependent protein complexes regulated by post-translational modification. *DNA Repair* 6, 695.

Atamna, H.; Cheung, I.; & Ames, B.N. (2000). A method for detecting abasic sites in living cells: age-dependent changes in base excision repair. *Proc Natl Acad Sci USA* 97, 686.

Berner, J.M.; Meza-Zepeda, L.A.; Kools, P.F.; Forus, A.; Schoenmakers, E.F.; Van de Ven, W.J.; Fodstad, O.; & Myklebost, O. (1997). HMGIC, the gene for an architectural transcription factor, is amplified and rearranged in a subset of human sarcomas. *Oncogene* 14, 2935.

Breen, A.P.; & Murphy, J.A. (1995). Reactions of oxyl radicals with DNA. *Free Rad Biol Med* 18, 1033.

Burrows, C.J.; & Muller, J.G. (1998). Oxidative nucleobase modifications leading to strand scission. *Chem Rev* 98, 1109.

Bustin, M. & Reeves, R. (1996) High-mobility-group chromosomal proteins: architectural components that facilitate chromatin function. *Prog Nucleic Acid Res Mol Biol* 54, 35.

Caldecott, K.W. (2003). XRCC1 and DNA strand break repair. *DNA Repair* 2, 955.

Campalans, A.; Marsin, S.; Nakabeppu, Y.; O'connor, T.R; Boiteux, S.; & Radicella, J.P. (2005). XRCC1 interactions with multiple DNA glycosylases: a model for its recruitment to base excision repair. *DNA Repair* 4, 826.

Cleynen, I.; & van de Ven, W.J. (2008). The HMGA proteins: a myriad of functions *Int J Oncol* 32, 289.

Das, A; Wiederhold, L.; Leppard, J.B, Kedar, P.; Prasad, R.; Wang, X.; Boldogh, I.; Karimi-Busheri, F.; Weinfeld, M.; Tomkinson, A.E.; Wilson, S.H., Mitra, S.; & Hazra, T.K. (2006). NEIL2-initiated, APE-independent repair of oxidized bases in DNA: Evidence for a repair complex in human cells *DNA Repair* 5, 1439.

David, S.S. & Williams, S.D. (1998). Chemistry of glycosylases and endonucleases involved in base-excision repair. *Chem Rev* 98, 1221.

Dawson, T.L.; Gores, G.J.; Nieminen, A.L.; Herman, B.; & Lemasters, J.J. (1993). Mitochondria as a source of reactive oxygen species during reductive stress in rat hepatocytes. *Am J Physiol* 264, C961.

de Los Santos, C.; El-Khateeb, M.; Rege, P.; Tian, K.; & Johnson, F. (2004). Impact of the C1' configuration of abasic sites on DNA duplex structure. *Biochemistry* 43, 15349.

Demple, B & Harrison, L. (1994). Repair of oxidative damage to DNA: enzymology and biology. *Annu Rev Biochem* 63, 915.

Demple, B. & DeMott, M.S. (2002). Dynamics and diversions in base excision DNA repair of oxidized abasic lesions. *Oncogene* 21, 8926.

Demple, B; Herman, T; & Chen, D.S. (1991). Cloning and expression of APE, the cDNA encoding the major human apurinic endonuclease: definition of a family of DNA repair enzymes. *Proc Natl Acad Sci U S A* 88, 11450.

Dexheimer, T.S., Antony, S., Marchand, C. & Pommier, Y. (2008). Tyrosyl-DNA phosphodiesterase as a target for anticancer therapy.phosphodiesterase as a target for anticancer therapy. *Anticancer Agents Med Chem* 8, 381.

Downs, J.A.; & Jackson, S.P. (2004) A means to a DNA end: the many roles of Ku. Nat Rev *Mol Cell Biol* 5, 367.

Duncan, T.; Trewick, S.C.; Koivisto, P.; Bates, P.A.; Lindahl, T.; & Sedgwick, B. (2002). Reversal of DNA alkylation damage by two human dioxygenases. *Proc Natl Acad Sci USA* 99, 16660.

Fan, J.; & Wilson, D.M. 3rd. (2005). Protein-protein interactions and posttranslational modifications in mammalian base excision repair, *Free Radic Biol Med* 38, 1121. Frosina, G.; Fortini, P.; Rossi, O.; Carrozzino, F.; Raspaglio, G.; Cox, L.S.; Lane, D.P.; Abbondandolo, A.; & Dogliotti, E. (1996). Two pathways for base excision repair in mammalian cells. *J Biol Chem* 271, 9573.

Grin, I.R.; Khodyreva, S.N.; Nevinsky, G.A.; & Zharkov, D.O. (2006). Deoxyribophosphate lyase activity of mammalian endonuclease VIII-like proteins. *FEBS Lett* 580, 4916.

Gullo, C.; Au, M.; Feng, G.; & Teoh, G. (2006) The biology of Ku and its potential oncogenic role in cancer. *Biochim Biophys Acta* 1765 223-234

Hazra, T.K.; Izumi, T.; Boldogh, I.; Imhoff, B.; Kow, Y.W.; Jaruga, P.; Dizdaroglu, M.; & Mitra, S. (2002). Identification and characterization of a human DNA glycosylase for repair of modified bases in oxidatively damaged DNA. *Proc Natl Acad Sci USA* 99, 3523.

Hegde, M.L.; Hazra, T.K.; & Mitra, S. (2008). Early steps in the DNA base excision/single-strand interruption repair pathway in mammalian cells. *Cell Research* 18, 27.

Hegde, V.; Wang, M.; & Deutsch, W.A. (2004). Human ribosomal protein S3 interacts with DNA base excision repair proteins hAPE/Ref-1 and hOGG1. *Biochemistry* 43, 14211.

Horton, J.K.; Prasad, R.; Hou, E.; & Wilson, S.H. (2000). Protection against methylation-induced cytotoxicity by DNA polymerase β-dependent long patch base excision repair. *J Biol Chem* 275, 2211.

Ilina, E.S.; Lavrik, O.I.; & Khodyreva, S.N. (2008). Ku antigen interacts with abasic sites. *Biochim Biophys Acta* 1784, 1777-1785.

Interthal, H.; Chen, H.J. & Champoux, J.J. (2005). Human Tdp1 cleaves a broad spectrum of substrates, including phosphoamide linkages. *J Biol Chem* 280, 36518.

Jiao Y., Wang, H.C., and Fan, S.J., Growth suppression and radiosensitivity increase by HMGB1 in breast cancer. *Acta Pharmacol. Sin.*, 2007, vol. 28, pp. 1957–1967.

Khodyreva, S.N.; Ilina, E.S.; Sukhanova, M.V.; Kutuzov, M.M. & Lavrik, O.I. (2010a). Poly(ADP-ribose) polymerase 1 interaction with apurinic/apyrimidinic sites. *Dokl Biochem Biophys* 431, 69.

Khodyreva, S.N.; Prasad, R.; Ilina, E.S.; Sukhanova, M.V.; Kutuzov, M.M.; Liu, Y.; Hou, E.W.; Wilson, S.H.; & Lavrik, O.I. (2010b). Apurinic/apyrimidinic (AP) site recognition by the 5′-dRP/AP lyase in poly(ADP-ribose) polymerase-1 (PARP-1) *Proc Natl Acad Sci USA* 107, 22090.

Klungland, A & Lindahl, T. (1997). Second pathway for completion of human DNA base excision-repair: reconstitution with purified proteins and requirement for DNase IV (FEN1). *EMBO J* 16, 3341.

Kurowski, M.A.; Bhagwat, A.S.; Papaj, G.; & Bujnicki, J.M. (2003). Phylogenomic identification of five new human homologs of the DNA repair enzyme AlkB. *BMC Genomics* 4, 48.

Kutuzov, M.M.; Ilina, E.S.; Sukhanova, M.V.; Pyshnaya, I.A.; Pyshnyi, D.V.; Lavrik, O.I.; & Khodyreva, S.N. (2011). Interaction of poly(ADP-ribose) polymerase 1 with apurinic/apyrimidinic sites within clustered DNA damage. *Biochemistry (Moscow)* 76, 147.

Laemmli, U.K. (1970). Cleavage of structural proteins during the assembly of the head of bacteriophage T4. *Nature* 277, 680.

Lan, L.; Nakajima, S.; Oohata, Y.; Takao, M.; Okano, S.; Masutani, M.; Wilson, S.H.; & Yasui, A. (2004). In situ analysis of repair processes for oxidative DNA damage in mammalian cells. *Proc Natl Acad Sci USA* 101, 13738.

Lebedeva, N.A.; Rechkunova, N.I.; and Lavrik, O.I. (2011). AP-site cleavage activity of tyrosyl-DNA phosphodiesterase 1. *FEBS Lett* 585, 683.

Liau, S.S. & Whang, E. (2008). HMGA1 is a molecular determinant of chemoresistance to gemcitabine in pancreatic adenocarcinoma. *Clin Cancer Res* 14, 1470.

Lindahl, T. (1993). Instability and decay of the primary structure of DNA. *Nature* 362, 709.

Lindahl, T.; Satoh, M.S.; Poirier, G.G.; & Klungland, A. (1995). Post-translational modification of poly(ADP-ribose) polymerase induced by DNA strand breaks. *Trends Biochem Sci* 20, 405.

Liu, Y.; Prasad, R.; & Wilson, S.H. (2010). HMGB1: roles in base excision repair and related function. *Biochim Biophys Acta* 1799, 119.

Loeb, L.A. & Preston, B.D. (1986). Mutagenesis by apurinic/apyrimidinic sites. *Annu Rev Genet* 20, 201.

Mani, R.S.; Karimi-Busheri, F.; Fanta, M.; Caldecott, K.W.; Cass, M.; & Weinfeld, C.E. (2004) Biophysical characterization of human XRCC1 and its binding to damaged and undamaged DNA. *Biochemistry* 43, 16505.

Marsin, S. Vidal, A.E.; Sossou, M.; Menissier-de Murcia, J.; Le Page, F.; Boiteux, S.; de Murcia, G.; & Radicella, J.P., (2003). Role of XRCC1 in the coordination and stimulation of oxidative DNA damage repair initiated by the DNA glycosylase hOGG1. *J Biol Chem* 278, 44068.

Matsumoto, Y. & Kim, K. (1995). Excision of deoxyribose phosphate residues by DNA polymerase β during DNA repair. *Science* 269, 699.

McCullough, A.K.; Dodson, M.L.; & Lloyd, R.S. (1999). Initiation of base excision repair: glycosylase mechanisms and structures. *Annu Rev Biochem* 68, 255.

Meyer, B.; Loeschke, S.; Schultze, A.; Weigel, T.; Sandkamp, M.; Goldmann, T.; Vollmer, E.; & Bullerdiek, J. (2007). HMGA2 overexpression in non-small cell lung cancer. *Mol Carcinog* 46, 503.

Miyazawa, J.; Mitoro, A.; Kawashiri, S.; Chada, K.K.; & Imai, K. (2004). Expression of mesenchyme-specific gene HMGA2 in squamous cell carcinomas of the oral cavity. *Cancer Res* 64, 2024.

Mohsin Ali, M.; Kurisu, S.; Yoshioka, Y.; Terato, H.; Ohyama, Y.; Kubo, K.; & Ide, H. (2004). Detection of endonuclease III- and 8-oxoguanine glycosylase-sensitive base modifications in gamma-irradiated DNA and cells by the aldehyde reactive probe (ARP) assay. *J Radiation Res* 45, 229.

Müller, T.A.; Meek, K.; & Hausinger, R.P. (2010). Human AlkB homologue 1 (ABH1) exhibits DNA lyase activity at abasic sites. *DNA Repair* 9, 58.

Nazarkina, Z.K.; Khodyreva, S.N.; Marsin, S.; Lavrik, O.I.; & Radicella, J.P. (2007). XRCC1 interactions with base excision repair DNA intermediates. *DNA Repair* 6, 254.

Ougland, R.; Zhang, C.M.; Liiv, A.; Johansen, R.F.; Seeberg, E.; Hou, Y.M.; Remme, J.; & Falnes, P.Ø. (2004). AlkB restores the biological function of mRNA and tRNA inactivated by chemical methylation. *Molec Cell* 16, 107.

Pascucci, B.; Maga, G.; Hübscher, U.; Bjoras, M.; Seeberg, E.; Hickson, I.D.; Villani, G.; Giordano, C.; Cellai, L.; & Dogliotti, E. (2002). Reconstitution of the base excision repair pathway for 7,8-dihydro-8-oxoguanine with purified human proteins. *Nucleic Acids Res* 30, 2124.

Piersen, C.E.; McCullough, A.K.; & Lloyd, R.S. (2000). AP lyases and dRPases: commonality of mechanism. *Mutat Res* 459, 43.

Piersen, C.E.; Prasad, R.; Wilson, S.H.; & Lloyd, R.S. (1996). Evidence for an imino intermediate in the DNA polymerase β deoxyribose phosphate excision reaction. *J Biol Chem* 271, 17811.

Pinz, K.G., & Bogenhagen, D. (2000). Characterization of a catalytically slow AP lyase activity in DNA polymerase γ and other family A DNA polymerases. *J Biol Chem* 275, 12509.

Podlutsky, A.J.; Dianova, I.I.; Wilson, S.H.; Bohr, V.A.; & Dianov, G.L. (2001). DNA synthesis and dRPase activities of polymerase β are both essential for single-nucleotide patch base excision repair in mammalian cell extracts. *Biochemistry* 40, 809.

Postel, E.H.; Abramczyk, B.M.; Levit, M.N.; & Kyin, S. (2000). Catalysis of DNA cleavage and nucleoside triphosphate synthesis by NM23-H2/NDP kinase share an active site that implies a DNA repair function. *Proc Natl Acad Sci USA* 97, 14194.

Prasad, R.; Liu, Y.; Deterding, L.J.; Poltoratsky, V.P.; Kedar, P.S.; Horton, J.K.; Kanno, S.; Asagoshi, K.; Hou, E.W.; Khodyreva, S.N.; Lavrik, O.I.; Tomer, K.B.; Yasui, A.; & Wilson, S.H. (2007). HMGB1 is a cofactor in mammalian base excision repair. *Mol Cell* 27, 829.

Reeves, R. (2001). Molecular biology of HMGA proteins: hubs of nuclear function. *Gene* 277, 63.

Rieger, R.A.; Zaika, V.; Xie, W.; Johnson, F.; Grollman, A.P.; Iden, C.R.; & Zharkov, D.O. (2006). Proteomic approach to identification of proteins reactive for abasic sites in DNA. *Mol Cell Proteomics* 5, 858.

Roberts, S.A.; Strande, N.; Burkhalter, M.D.; Strom, C.; Havener, J.M.; Hasty, P.; & Ramsden, D.A. (2010). Ku is a 5'-dRP/AP lyase that excises nucleotide damage near broken ends. *Nature* 464, 1214.

Sakano, K.; Oikawa, S.; Hasegawa, K.; & Kawanishi, S. (2001). Hydroxyurea induces site-specific DNA damage via formation of hydrogen peroxide and nitric oxide. *Jpn J Cancer Res* 92, 1166.

Schärer, O.D. (2003). Chemistry and biology of DNA repair. *Angew Chem Int Ed* 42, 2946.

Schulte-Uentrop, L.; El-Awady, R.A.; Schliecker, L.; Willers, H.; & Dahm-Daphi, J. (2008) Distinct roles of XRCC4 and Ku80 in non-homologous end-joining of endonuclease- and ionizing radiation-induced DNA double-strand breaks. *Nucleic Acids Res.* 36, 2561.

Sedgwick, B.; Bates, P.A.; Paik, J.; Jacobs, S.C.; & Lindahl, T. (2006). Repair of alkylated DNA: recent advances. *DNA repair* 6, 429.

Sgarra, R.; Furlan, C.; Zammitti, S.; Lo Sardo, A.; Maurizio, E.; Di Bernardo, J.; Giancotti, V.; & Manfioletti, G. (2008). Interaction proteomics of the HMGA chromatin architectural factors. *Proteomics* 8, 4721.

Sgarra, R.; Zammitti, S; Lo Sardo, A.; Maurizio, E.; Arnoldo, L., Pegoraro, S.; Giancotti, V.; & Manfioletti, G. (2010). HMGA molecular network: From transcriptional regulation to chromatin remodeling. *Biochim Biophys Acta* 1799, 37.

Snowden, A.; Kow, Y.W.; & Van Houten, B. (1990). Damage repertoire of the *Escherichia coli* UvrABC nuclease complex includes abasic sites, base-damage analogues, and lesions containing adjacent 5' or 3' nicks. *Biochemistry* 29, 7251.

Sobol, R.W.; Prasad, R.; Evenski, A.; Baker, A.; Yang, X.-P.; Horton, J.K.; & Wilson, S.H. (2000). The lyase activity of the DNA repair protein β-polymerase protects from DNA-damage-induced cytotoxicity. *Nature* 405, 807.

Srivastava, D.K.; Vande Berg, B.J.; Prasad, R.; Molina, J.T.; Beard, W.A.; Tomkinson, A.E.; & Wilson, S.H. (1998). Mammalian abasic site base excision repair. Identification of the reaction sequence and rate-determining steps. *J Biol Chem* 273, 21203.

Stros, M. (2010) HMGB proteins: interactions with DNA and chromatin. *Biochim Biophys Acta* 1799, 101.

Summer, H.; Li, O.; Bao, Q.; Zhan, L.; Peter, S.; Sathiyanathan, P.; Henderson, D.; Klonisch, T.; Goodman, S.D.; & Droge, P. (2009). HMGA2 exhibits dRP/AP site cleavage activity and protects cancer cells from DNA-damage-induced cytotoxicity during chemotherapy. *Nucleic Acids Res* 37, 4371.

Takao, M.; Kanno, S.; Kobayashi, K.; Zhang, Q.M.; Yonei, S.; van der Horst, G.T.; & and Yasui, A. (2002). A back-up glycosylase in Nth1 knock-out mice is a functional Nei (endonuclease VIII) homologue. *J Biol Chem* 277, 42205.

Tang, D.; Kang, R.; Zeh, H.J. 3rd; & Lotze, M.T. (2010). High-mobility group box 1 and cancer. *Biochim Biophys Acta* 1799, 131.

Vidal, A.E.; Boiteux, S.; Hickson, I.D.;& Radicella, J.P. (2001). XRCC1 coordinates the initial and late stages of DNA abasic site repair through protein–protein interactions, *EMBO J* 20, 6530.

Westbye, M.P.; Feyzi, E.; Aas, P.A.; Vagbo, C.B.; Talstad, V.A.; Kavli, B.; Hagen, L.; Sundheim, O.; Akbari, M.; Liabakk, N.B.; Slupphaug, G.; Otterlei, M.; & Krokan, H.E. (2008). Human AlkB homolog 1 is a mitochondrial protein that demethylates 3-methylcytosine in DNA and RNA. *J Biol Chem* 283, 25046.

Whitehouse, C.J.; Taylor, R.M.; Thistlethwaite, A.; Zhang, H.; Karimi-Busheri, F.; Lasko, D.D.; Weinfeld, M.; & Caldecott, K.W. (2001). XRCC1 stimulates human polynucleotide kinase activity at damaged DNA termini and accelerates DNA single-strand break repair. *Cell* 104, 107.

Wiederhold, L.; Leppard, J.B.; Kedar, P.; Karimi-Busheri, F.; Rasouli-Nia, A.; Weinfeld, M. ; Tomkinson, A.E.; Izumi, T.; Prasad, R.; Wilson, S.H.; Mitra, S. & Hazra, T.K. (2004). AP endonuclease-independent DNA base excision repair in human cells. *Mol Cell* 15, 209.

Wilson 3rd, D.M. & Barsky, D. (2001). The major human abasic endonuclease: formation, consequences and repair of abasic lesions in DNA. *Mutat Res* 485, 283.

Wilson, D.M. 3rd & Thompson, L.H. (1997). Life without DNA repair. *Proc Natl Acad Sci USA* 94, 12754.

Wong, H.; Kim, D.; Hogue, B.A.; McNeill, D.R.; & Wilson, D.M. III. (2005). DNA damage levels and biochemical repair capacities associated with XRCC1 deficiency, *Biochemistry* 44, 14335.

Yang, N.; Galick, H.; & Wallace, S.S. (2004). Attempted base excision repair of ionizing radiation damage in human lymphoblastoid cells produces lethal and mutagenic double-strand breaks. *DNA Repair* 3, 1323.

Yang, S.W.; Burgin, A.B. Jr.; Huizenga, B.N.; Robertson, C.A.; Yao, K.C.; & Nash, H.A. (1996). A eukaryotic enzyme that can disjoin dead-end covalent complexes between DNA and type I topoisomerases. *Proc Natl Acad Sci USA* 93, 11534.

Zharkov, D.O. & Grollman, A.P. (1998). MutY DNA glycosylase: base release and intermediate complex formation. *Biochemistry* 37, 12384.

7

DNA Radiosensitization: The Search for Repair Refractive Lesions Including Double Strand Breaks and Interstrand Crosslinks

Tsvetan G. Gantchev[1,2], Marie-Eve Dextraze[1] and Darel J. Hunting[1]
[1]*Department of Nuclear Medicine & Radiobiology, Faculté de medicine, Université de Sherbrooke, Sherbrooke, Québec,*
[2]*Department of Gene Regulations, Institute of Molecular Biology, Bulgarian Academy of Sciences, Sofia,*
[1]*Canada*
[2]*Bulgaria*

1. Introduction

More than half of all cancer patients receive radiotherapy (RT) as part of their treatment regimens. The cytotoxicity of ionizing radiation is mainly mediated by the ensuing DNA damage. Double-stranded DNA breaks (DSB) are generally accepted to be the most important lesions for the induction of cell death by ionizing radiation because they are much more difficult to repair than single strand breaks, although their radiation yield is very low, at two orders of magnitude less than that of single strand breaks (SSB) (Hempel & Mildenberger, 1987). The role of other DNA lesions such as base damage and interstrand crosslinks in cell killing has not been yet fully elucidated. Gamma-radiation inflicts DNA damage *via* two separated processes: i) direct interaction with DNA and; ii) indirect damage produced by secondary radicals ($^{\bullet}OH$, $^{\bullet}H$ and e^{-}_{aq}) generated after water radiolysis (Michaels & Hunt, 1978). Among the H_2O derived radicals, hydroxyl radicals ($^{\bullet}OH$) are the species primarily responsible for strand break formation and DNA base damage (> 35%). Hydrated electrons, e^{-}_{aq}, which are generated at a yield comparable to the $^{\bullet}OH$ (G-values of ~ 2.8×10^{-7} mol.J^{-1}), participate in only ~ 8% of the total damage and the exact nature of DNA damage formed *in vivo* by e^{-}_{aq} is obscure (Nabben *et al.*, 1982). In vertebrate cells, the majority of RT-induced DSB are repaired by non-homologous end joining (NHEJ) with some contribution from homologous recombination repair (HRR) during the late S and G2 phases of the cell cycle (Jackson, 2002; Takata *et al.*, 1998). The repair of other DNA damages, such as interstrand crosslinks (ICL) is more complicated and less understood (Wang, 2007; Moldovan & D'Andrea, 2009). ICLs can be recognized by the nucleotide excision repair (NER) system and it is accepted that ICL repair involves nucleolytic cleavage at or near the site of ICL to produce a suitable substrate that can subsequently be repaired by homologous recombination (HR) (D'Andrea & Grompe, 2003; Moldovan & D'Andrea, 2009a, Liu *et al.*, 2010).

An approach to improve the effectiveness of RT is either to enhance the formation of lethal DNA lesions, or to use inhibitors of DNA repair pathways (or both) and thus to render tumor cells more sensitive to ionizing radiation. A novel strategy to inhibit radiation-induced double strand break repair was recently promoted by using short modified DNA molecules that mimic double strand breaks (Dbaits) and artificially activate the DNA-PK pathway (Quanz *et al.*, 2009). Likewise, using siRNA screening of genes involved in DNA damage repair, Higgins *et al.* (2010) identified POLQ (DNA polymerase θ) as a potential tumor-specific target whose knockdown led to tumor cell-specific radiosensitization. However, with the exception of oxygen-enhancing or mimetic agents and platinum derivatives such as cis-platinum, which amplify DNA damage, the only direct DNA radiosensitizing agents known to date are halogenated uracils, such as 5-bromodeoxyuridine (BrdU). BrdU administration to cultured cells, animals and humans leads to replacement of isosteric thymine by 5-bromouracil during replication and excision repair of DNA. The basic pathway of BrdU radiolysis and DNA strand break formation in solution was described many years ago (Zimbrick *et al.*, 1969a,b). It involves dissociative e^-_{aq} attachment to BrdU, followed by the formation of a 5-uracil-yl σ-radical (•U) and a bromine ion (Br^-, Fig. 1). The reaction is very efficient in air-free solutions, with $k(e^-_{aq}+ BrU) = 2.6x10^{10}\ M^{-1}s^{-1}$ and $G(U) = 2.4x10^{-7}$ mol.J^{-1}, but interactions with •OH may intervene and can lead to somewhat different products. BrdU is also an efficient UV-light absorbing phtotosensitizer; the homolytic Br−C bond cleavage, however, results in two

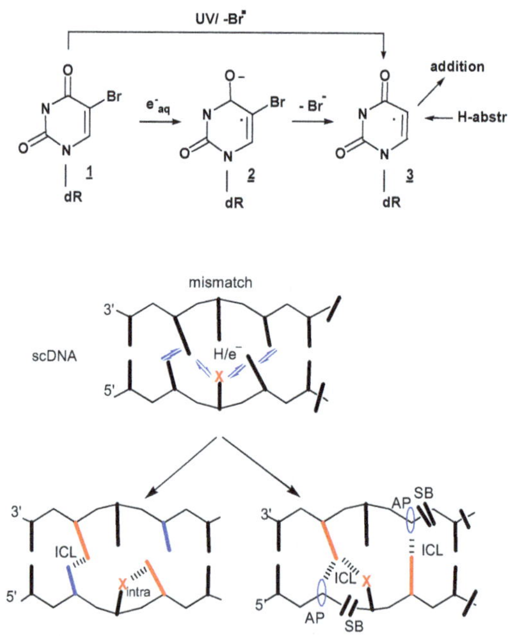

Fig. 1. Primary reaction mechanism of 5-BrdU sensitization and subsequent damages in wobble scDNA. The dynamic structure of scDNA facilitates electron (hydrogen atom) transfer (ET) between the two strands. The ET direction depends on the BrdU local sequence context (e.g. purine *vs.* pyrimidine environment). In the scheme the 5-uracil-yl radical (3) and its products are denoted by X. Modified bases (reduced or oxidized; red and blue), uracil and/or 2′-deoxyribose may further interact between and/or with undamaged bases and oxygen to form various products, including AP-sites, intra- and inter-strand crosslinks (ICL) and strand breaks (SB).

radical species (•U and •Br). It is generally assumed that •U abstracts an H-atom from 2′-deoxyribose to form a strand break or accepts an electron from a neighboring base (inter-base chain e^- transfer (ET), generating an oxidized base), which eventually terminates with the formation of a guanine cation radical, $G^{+\bullet}$ (Nese *et al.*, 1992). •U-radical addition reactions may result in DNA crosslinks (Fig. 1), but this was only recently shown experimentally (Zeng & Wang, 2007). New findings show that electron capture and migration along BrdU-substituted DNA might be contra-thermodynamically selective and, thus far more complicated (Yoshioka *et al.*, 1999; Aflatooni *et al.*, 1998). In cells, radiosensitization by BrdU (typically at ~20-30% thymine replacement) gives about 2-3 fold radiotoxicity enhancement and in most cell types parallels similar increase in the DSB yield, and/or the decreased rate of their repair (Sawada & Okada, 1972). Further characteristics of BrdU-mediated DSB and other DNA damages *in vivo* (*e.g.* DNA crosslinks) are scarcely available.

2. DNA-structure/conformation dependent BrdU-sensitized formation of strand breaks

A crucial difference between the radiosensitization of single and double stranded DNA by BrdU was not known until our work with purified *semi*-complementary (mismatched) DNA showing the single stranded specificity of BrdU-induced DNA damage (Cecchini *et al.*, 2004). In parallel experiments, using BrdU-substituted (or not) single-stranded (ssDNA), double-stranded (dsDNA) and mismatched (wobble) semi-complementary (scDNA) DNA we have found that BrdU efficiently sensitizes single stranded BrdU-substituted (brominated) oligonucleotides, but not when these are hybridized to completely complementary oligonucleotides to form normal dsDNA duplexes. We estimate that BrdU radiosensitization efficiency in dsDNA drops up to 20-fold compared to that in ssDNA. Comparative measurements of radiolytic loss of the bromine atom in ssDNA *vs.* dsDNA likewise indicate that this process is greatly suppressed in dsDNA (Cecchini *et al.*, 2004, 2005a). In mismatched, scDNA duplexes, strand brakes are formed in loci encompassing nucleotides surrounding BrdU. However, high efficiency single strand break formation takes place on the brominated strand, or on the opposite, non-brominated strand but have not been detected on both, suggesting that they are mutually exclusive events (Hunting *et al.*, unpublished; Cecchini *et al.*, 2005b). Experiments performed with scDNA bearing variable number of mismatches (from one to five) and containing a single BrdU substitution gave qualitatively similar results. The radiation dose-response for strand break formation was linear for both the brominated and the opposite, non-brominated strand within the single-stranded regions of a standard model scDNA containing a bulge formed by up to five mismatched bases (Dextraze *et al.*, 2007). Interestingly, UVB-irradiation of BrdU-substituted DNA also demonstrated DNA-structure specificity, but in this situation BrdU greatly enhances breakage of only the brominated strand in dsDNA, or either the brominated or the non-brominated strand in the case of scDNA (Cecchini *et al.*, 2005b; Chen *et al.*, 2000). The different effects initiated by radiolysis and photolysis, especially with BrdU-dsDNA, underline the role of DNA structure-conformation properties in solution as a prerequisite for the initial electron-capture by BrdU and/or the propagation of an excess-electron along the polymer after gamma-irradiation.

The importance of DNA structure during sensitization by BrdU is further demonstrated by comparison of the damages induced in A- and B-form DNA. Using brominated 25-mer oligonucleotides hybridized to complementary or semi-complementary ones with five mismatched bases: AAT(orBU)AA, we have shown that strand breaks are specific for B-DNA, whereas A-DNA only undergoes formation of alkali-labile DNA lesions (Dextraze *et al.*, 2007). Piperidine-sensitive lesions are observed exclusively at the site of BrdU substitution. Generally, the cleavage reaction is a confluence of at least three factors: e^{-}_{aq} capture, forward electron transfer and charge recombination. The strand break positions migrate along the DNA strand, however, there is a clear preference for the dA 5′-flanking BrdU. Similarly, 5′-dABrdU-sequence preference has been observed in UV-induced BrdU DNA cleavage (Chen *et al.*, 2000). This is to be expected since in B-DNA the 5′ proximal 2′-deoxyribose would be the ultimate H-atom donor to the uracil-5-yl radical, whereas in A-DNA conformational (spatial) restrictions render the same 5′dA 2′-deoxyribose a less-accessible H-donor. Therefore, in A-DNA the uracil-5-yl radical is more likely to abstract H-atoms from other donors (bases), thus oxidizing proximal to the BrdU-site bases which results in alkali-labile site formation.

Sequence-preferential strand break formation was examined in a series of 25-mer scDNA encompassing a central 1- or 5-mer mismatched site with BrdU incorporated (brominated strand) in a purine 5′d(AABrdUAA), 5′d(GGBrdUGG), or a pyrimidine 5′d(ATBrdUTA) environment, and the semi-complimentary (non-brominated) strand contained any of the sequences: 5′d(AATAA), 5′d(CCCCC), 5′d(GGGGG), or 5′d(ATTTA) (twelve permutations in total) (Dextraze *et al.*, 2007; 2009). While there was no significant change between the strand-break yields in ssDNA and typically there were no changes in strand breaks produced on each strand (*i.e.*, brominated *vs.* nonbrominated), two wobble sequence permutations derived from the above pattern: d(GGBrdUGG)^d(GGGGG) and d(ATBrdUTA)^d(ATTTA) produced more breaks on the brominated strand, whereas the generation of breaks was enhanced in the non-brominated strand in the combinations: d(GGBrdUGG)^d(AATAA), d(GGBrdUGG)^d(ATTTA), and d(AABrdUAA)^d(GGGGG). Similarly irradiation of the same scDNA, gave different patterns of interstrand crosslinks (see below).

3. BrdU sensitized formation of interstrand crosslinks (ICL) in mismatched (wobble) DNA duplexes

In addition to increasing strand break generation by ionizing radiation, the presence of bromouracil induces formation of DNA interstrand crosslinks (ICL). This process occurs in single stranded regions within double stranded DNA (*i.e.*, in scDNA) and requires the presence of B-DNA (Dextraze *et al.*, 2007; 2009). Although anticipated, the generation of ICL during radiosensitization with BrdU has not been demonstrated experimentally prior to our work (Cecchini *et al.*, 2005a). Formation of intra-strand crosslinks has been reported in UVB-irradiated BrdU-substituted synthetic DNA (Zeng & Wang, 2006) and in cells (Zeng & Wang, 2007). However, the generation of DNA ICLs by ionizing radiation has been largely ignored in favor to studies on double-strand breaks and their repair. At least part of the problem is technical; it is difficult to detect and quantify ICLs when the same agent forms both strand breaks and ICL, because the analysis of ICL generally involves a denaturing step. Apart from multiple damage events that may cause the disappearance of ICL-products due to DNA backbone cleavage at nucleotides located between the ICL-site and the radiolabel, another factor that obstructs DNA-ICL detection is that ICLs may decompose under prolonged irradiation, especially in the presence of O_2 (Ding & Greenberg, 2007).

Therefore, ICL detection and quantitation implies careful selection of the irradiation conditions. In our experience, the presence of a mild •OH-radical scavenger (20 mM EDTA) sufficiently protects against ICL destruction, and even enhances ICL yields up to 1 kGy irradiation dose. A typical ICL- migration pattern observed in agarose denaturing gel electrophoresis of ^{32}P-labeled scDNA samples containing different mismatched regions and subjected to γ-irradiated (750 Gy) is shown in Fig. 2. The figure exemplifies the fact that, depending on the mismatched-sequence context of the incorporated BrdU, ICL-DNA segments are formed, which differ in their length, structure and yield. Comparative analyses of ICL yields and various electrophoretic-band patterns depending on DNA structure are presented in (Dextraze *et al.*, 2009). Although, no ICL chemical structure identification has been done yet, quantitative data show that d(AABrdUAA)^d(GGGGG) and d(GGBrdUGG)^d(CCCCC) bulge patches are the least prone to crosslink formation in DNA wobbles, while efficient crosslinking takes place in T-enriched bulge structures, *e.g.* d(GGBrdUGG)^d(ATTTA) and d(ATBrdUTA)^d(ATTTA). The calculated total ICL radiation yield (G) in the later sequences (*i.e.* including all ICL bands) is in the range of (1-4) $x10^{-8}$ mol.J^{-1}. Taking into account that $G(e^{-}_{aq}) = 2.75x10^{-7}$ mol J^{-1} it follows that the formation of interstrand crosslinks in BrdU-scDNA is an event that occurs at least once with every ten solvated electrons produced. Ding and Greenberg (2007) reported γ-radiolysis production of ICL in unsubstituted dsDNA and identified the structure as T[5m-6n]A (Fig. 6B). Under their irradiation conditions the estimated G-value of the single ICL is ~ (3-4) $x10^{-4}$ nmol.J^{-1}. These data underline that BrdU-sensitized ICL formation in mismatched scDNA duplex is much more efficient (> 10^4 - fold) than in normal dsDNA.

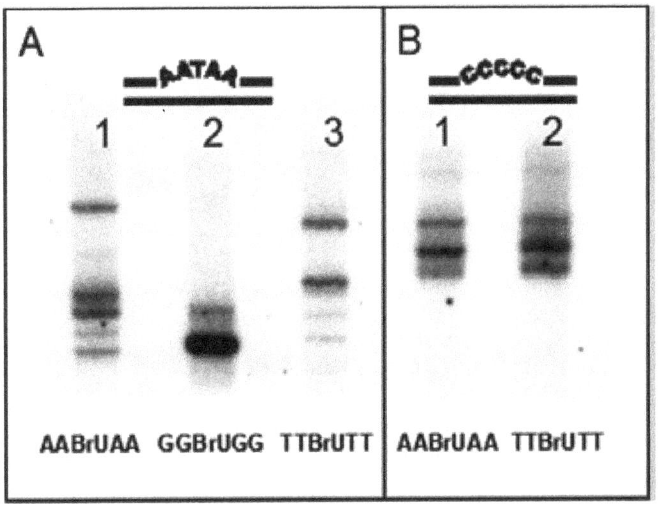

Fig. 2. Sequence-dependent BrdU-radiosensitized formation of ICL in wobble scDNA, as seen by the different electrophoretic mobility of the ICL bands. The central quintet sequence of the brominated strand is shown at the bottom; the opposite strand comprises $d(A_2TA_2)$ or $d(C)_5$ as shown on the top; there is a 5-b.p. central mismatch in all samples, except for lane-3 (panel A) where a single BU^T mismatch is present. The figure exemplifies the role of mismatched sequence (length and composition) on the ICL nature and yields; the individual chemical structures, however have not been yet determined. For a tentative ICL assignment, see Dextraze M.-E., *et al.*, (2009); for recently identified ICL structures, see Fig. 6.

4. Peptide nucleic acids (PNA) as sequence targeted radiosensitizers

In searching for new RT approaches to inflict heavy DNA damage (specific, repair-refractive and lethal) we developed the concept of cell radiosensitization by non-covalently bound DNA radiosensitizers. Our original idea was to use *semi*-complementary BrdU-substituted oligonucleotide vectors which would hybridize to specific genomic sequences and create a mismatch at the site of the bromouracil. In theory, the sequences of the BUdR-loaded oligonucleotide vectors could be designed to efficiently form crosslinks with the target DNA upon radiation, since, as discussed above, the crosslinking efficiency is dependent on the target sequence. However, the use of oligonucleotides as vectors to bring BrUdR close to cellular DNA has many pitfalls (similarly to the antisense RNA applications) and instead we focused on peptide nucleic acids (PNA) as vectors, because PNAs are resistant to degradation and are able to invade DNA duplexes under physiological conditions. To our surprise, PNA were found to efficiently form crosslinks with DNA under ionizing radiation even without bearing halogenated bases.

PNA: R_1-ATG-CCG-ATC-GTA-R_2

DNA: 3'-TAC-GGC-TAG-CAT-5'

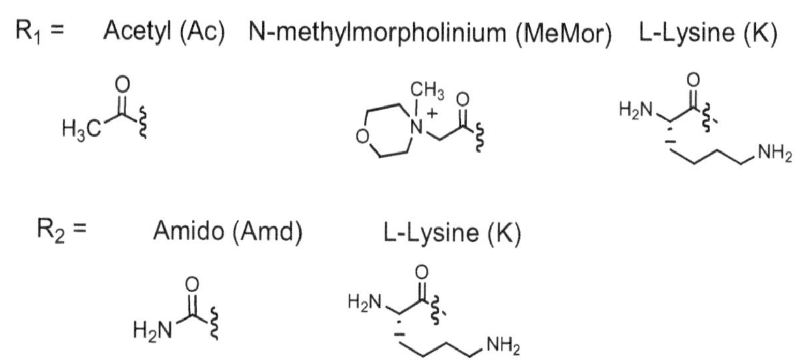

Fig. 3. The 12-mer PNA-DNA heteroduplex sequence (top) used in γ-radiation experiments to induce ICL and the variable N- and C-capping groups (R_1 and R_2) on PNA.

PNAs are nucleic acid analogues with an uncharged peptide-like backbone (Nielsen, 1995; Porcheddu & Giacomelli, 2005; Pellestor *et al.*, 2008). PNAs bind strongly to complimentary DNA and RNA sequences. Originally designed as ligands for the recognition of double stranded DNA (Egholm *et al.*, 1993; Demidov *et al.*, 1995) their unique physicochemical properties allow them to recognize and invade complimentary sequences in specific genes and to interfere with the transcription of that particular gene (antigene strategy) (Nielsen *et al.*, 1994; Ray & Norden, 2000; Pooga *et al.*, 2001; Cutrona, *et al.*, 2000; Doyle *et al.*, 2001; Romanelli *et al.*, 2001; Kaihatsu *et al.*, 2004). The introduction of a bulky charged amino acid (*e.g.* lysine, Fig. 3) improves binding specificity, solubility and cell uptake (Menchise *et al.*, 2003). PNAs have several advantages over oligo-deoxyribonucleotides including: greater chemical and biochemical stability (PNAs are not substrates for proteases, peptidases and nucleases), greater affinity towards targets (lack of electrostatic repulsion between hybridizing strands, Fig. 4), and more sequence-specific binding.

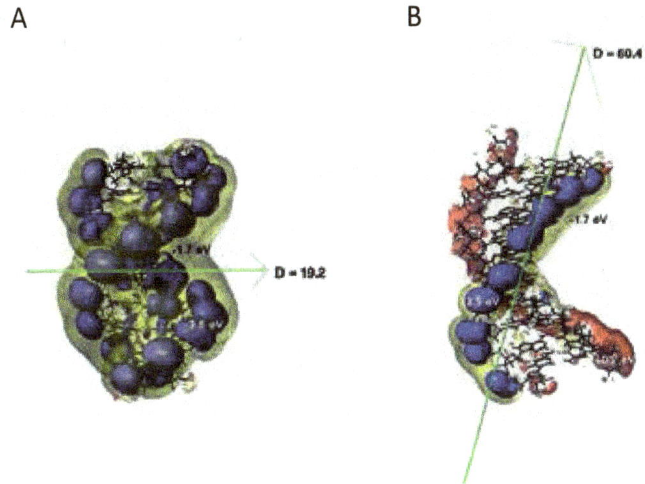

Fig. 4. Electrostatic potentials surrounding 10-mer 3D-models of $(DNA)_2$ and DNA-PNA duplexes, calculated using Sybyl modeling interface and dielectric constant, D = 4. Color-codes as indicated: electronegative potentials -3.5 eV, -1.7 eV (dark blue and yellow) and electropositive +0.2 eV (red). (A) Symmetric electronegative potential surfaces along the two strands of the DNA duplex expand over all backbone atoms (blue) and the two grooves (yellow). (B) Asymmetric isopotential surfaces around PNA-DNA duplex. The electropositive/neutral PNA backbone region (red) extends over the minor and major groove atoms (0 - 0.2 eV at distances ~ 0.1 Å), but the DNA backbone atoms remain enveloped by a negative surface (-3.5 eV). The resultant dipole momenta (green vectors) are 19.2 D and 60.4 D for the DNA-DNA and PNA-DNA duplexes, respectively. In the latter case it is oriented diagonally from PNA to DNA strand and can be a driving force for $e^{-}aq$ interaction with accessible PNA backbone and groove atoms.

We have studied hybridization of DNA oligonucleotides with PNA, where PNA bear (or not) N- or C-terminal amino groups ($-NH_2$, lysine, or methylmorpholinium) (Fig. 3, Gantchev *et al.*, 2009). After γ-irradiation (typically 750 Gy) of PNA-DNA heteroduplexes, those with PNA containing free amino group ends formed ICLs (Fig. 5). The multiple bands in each lane represent different crosslinked products and match the number of available amino groups in each heteroduplex. The ICL-formation efficiency is high, G = (5-8) $\times 10^{-8}$ mol.J^{-1}. This G-value even exceeds the ICL yields observed after irradiation BrdU-substituted wobble DNA under identical conditions. Using selective scavengers it was shown that ICL formation in PNA-DNA heteroduplexes strongly depends on the availability of solvated electrons (e^{-}_{aq}), but proceeds only with a concomitant presence of •OH radicals (Gantchev *et al.*, 2009). Thus, it appears that PNA-DNA ICLs arise in a concerted free radical mechanisms resembling those involved in DNA multiply damaged sites (MDS). By hybridizing 12-mer PNAs with shorter (11-mer), or longer (up to 16-mer) complementary oligo-deoxyribonucleotides thus creating unpaired (single-stranded) regions (deletions and overhangs) at one, or both duplex ends we compared sequence effects on the cross-linking reaction (*e.g.* dT vs. dA termini), the susceptibility of duplex ends to radiation damage, *etc.* The 3′- and 5′- DNA terminal dT nucleotides proved to be of most importance for the efficient ICL formation. Since hydrolysis of N-glycosidic bonds in γ-

damaged nucleotides and/or direct 2′-deoxiribose oxidation yields AP (apurinic/apyrimidinic) abasic sites as a common DNA lesion; we also assessed the role of AP-sites in the PNA-DNA ICL formation using synthetic AP-containing oligo-deoxyribonucletides. We found that presence of AP-sites at different positions of the DNA strand (3′- or 5′-end, and/or penultimate to the ends) results in ICL formation without radiation, but instead required addition of a strong reductant, *e.g.* $NaCNBH_3$. The electrophoretic gel-mobility of thus formed ICL bands resembled that of γ-radiation generated ones. Therefore, we concluded that AP-sites on the DNA strand are the likely partners of the free NH_2, or α- and ε-amino groups of Lys at the PNA ends in the formation of DNA-PNA crosslinks *via* a Schiff-base reaction, followed by imine reduction.

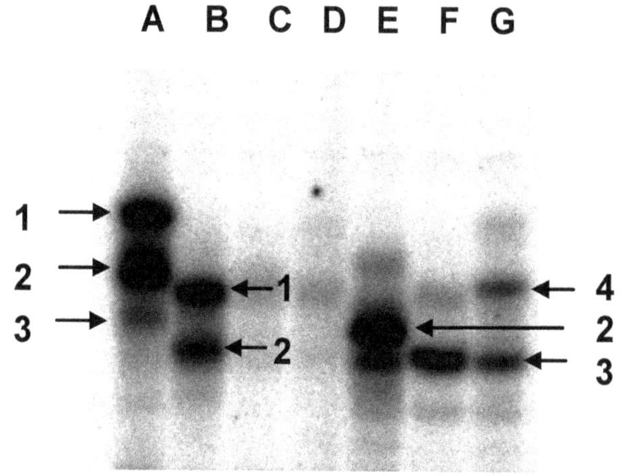

Fig. 5. Electrophoretic migration of bands representing the covalent PNA-DNA dimers (ICL). Aqueous solutions of ^{32}P-DNA hybridized with various PNA were γ-irradiated (750 Gy) under N_2 - atmosphere and in the presence of 25 mM EDTA. Samples differ only by the type of capping groups on PNA ends (R_1 and R_2, Fig. 3). Lanes from left to right: (A) NH_2-K-PNA; (B) NH_2-PNA; (C) Ac-PNA; (D) MeMor-K-PNA; (E) NH_2-PNA-K; (F) Ac-PNA-K; and (G) MeMor-PNA-K; (1- 4): different crosslinked products involving the different amino groups. No ICL are formed with Ac-PNA (C) and MeMor-K-PNA (D). Adapted from Gantchev *et al.*, (2009).

5. Mechanistic and structural aspects of the ICL formation in DNA duplexes and DNA-PNA heteroduplexes

In comparison to inter-strand crosslinks (ICLs), the intra-strand DNA crosslinks have been better studied, mostly as part of locally multiply damage sites (MDS, clustered/tandem DNA lesions). Recently, Wang and co-workers (Lin *et al.*, 2010) found that the exposure of BrdU-substituted telomer G-quadruplex DNA to UVA light results in the formation of G[8-5]U intra-strand crosslink (Fig. 6A). This finding presents evidence that free radical reactions, involving 5-uracil-yl-radical (•U) can also be a source of ICL, albeit not in completely dsDNA duplexes. Thus, Ding & Greenberg (2010) reported radiolytic formation of ICL in anaerobic solutions by BrdU-mimetic iodo-aryl nucleotides incorporated into synthetic dsDNA duplex. Similarly to BrdU-dsDNA irradiation, in these model systems stand breaks and alkali-labile lesions were also induced at the halogenated site and at the flanking nucleotides. The conclusions from this study highlight the importance of the local DNA structure (wobble *vs.* normal duplex) in terms of Watson-Crick pairing restrictions that likely prevent the 5-uracil-yl σ-radical (in contrast to the aryl radical) interaction with the opposite strand bases to produce ICL. The chemical structures of several DNA inter-strand crosslinks have been reported only recently. Several groups have focused on the identification of ICL structures synthesized in model systems using light- and/or oxidation-sensitive precursors (Hong *et al.*, 2006; Weng *et al.*, 2007; Peng *et al.*, 2008; Kim & Hong, 2008; Op de Beeck & Madder, 2011). A few structures have been definitively identified in natural conditions and, to our knowledge, only one in cellular DNA (Regulus *et al.*, 2007) (Fig. 6C). However, the authors in Regulus *et al.*, (2007) failed to present evidence that this crosslink is exclusively an inter-strand crosslink in cells. Mechanistically, the sole ICL-structure that is exclusively generated with the participation of a primary radiation-induced 5-(2′-deoxyuridinyl) methyl free radical, a product of •OH-induced hydrogen-atom abstraction from thymine, is the T[5m-6n]A crosslink (Ding & Greenberg, 2007; Ding *et al.*, 2008) (Fig. 6B).

A common pathway for ICL formation in dsDNA is the condensation reaction between aldehydes (*e.g.* in abasic DNA sites) and exocyclic amines of opposite bases. Under γ-radiation abasic (AP-apurinic/apyrimidinic) sites are generated either *via* direct H-atom abstraction by •OH radicals from 2′-deoxyribose or after oxidative base damage followed by N-glycosidic bond-cleavage. Oxidation of each of the five positions in 2′-deoxyribose in DNA is possible, but under γ-radiation the best known reactions involve H-atom abstraction at C1′-, C2′- and C4′-positions. The 4′-keto abasic site formed after C4′-oxidation (C4′-AP) is generally known as the "native" abasic site (Chen & Stubbe 2004). Subsequent interactions of sugar radicals with oxygen and/or elimination reactions give a variety of closed-cycle/open-chain aldehydic products, accompanied (or not) by DNA strand-cleavage (Dedon, 2008). One of the first reported, and structurally identified DNA-ICL generated by γ-radiation and/or selective 4′-position 2′-deoxyribose oxidation by bleomycin in model systems and in cells (Fig. 6C; Regulus *et al.*, 2007; Cadet *et al.*, 2010) is produced *via* electrophilic interaction between 2′-deoxypentos-4-ulose abasic site (opened C4′-AP) and N4-dC. Formation of this ICL is accompanied by a DNA strand break. In a series of works, Greenberg and collaborators studied the ICL formation with participation of oxidized native C4′-AP (Sczepanski *et al.*, 2008, 2009a) and 5′-(2-phosphoryl-1,4-dioxobutane, DOB) (Guan & Greenberg, 2009) sites. DOB is produced concomitantly with a single-strand break byDNA-damaging agents capable of abstracting an H-atom from the C5′-position. When oxidized C4′-AP was opposed by dA, a single crosslink formation occurred exclusively with an adjacent dA on the 5′-side. The crosslink formation was attributed to condensation of C4′-AP with the N6-amino group of dA and less favorably with N4-amino group of dC, but not with dG or dT. Interestingly, C4′-AP produced ICLs in which both strands are either intact or ICLs, where the C4-AP containing strand was cleaved (3′ to the AP-site), while DOB-ICLs were always accompanied by an adjacent to the AP-site single-strand break, and thus constituting a clustered type (MDS) lesion.

In contrast, following γ-radiation of BrdU-substituted wobble-DNA (scDNA) duplexes multiple crosslinked products were generated which impedes their chemical identification (Cecchini et al., 2005a; Dextraze et al., 2009). However, in DNA-PNA heteroduplexes, because the amino-groups attached to PNA are exogenous and could be omitted/varied,

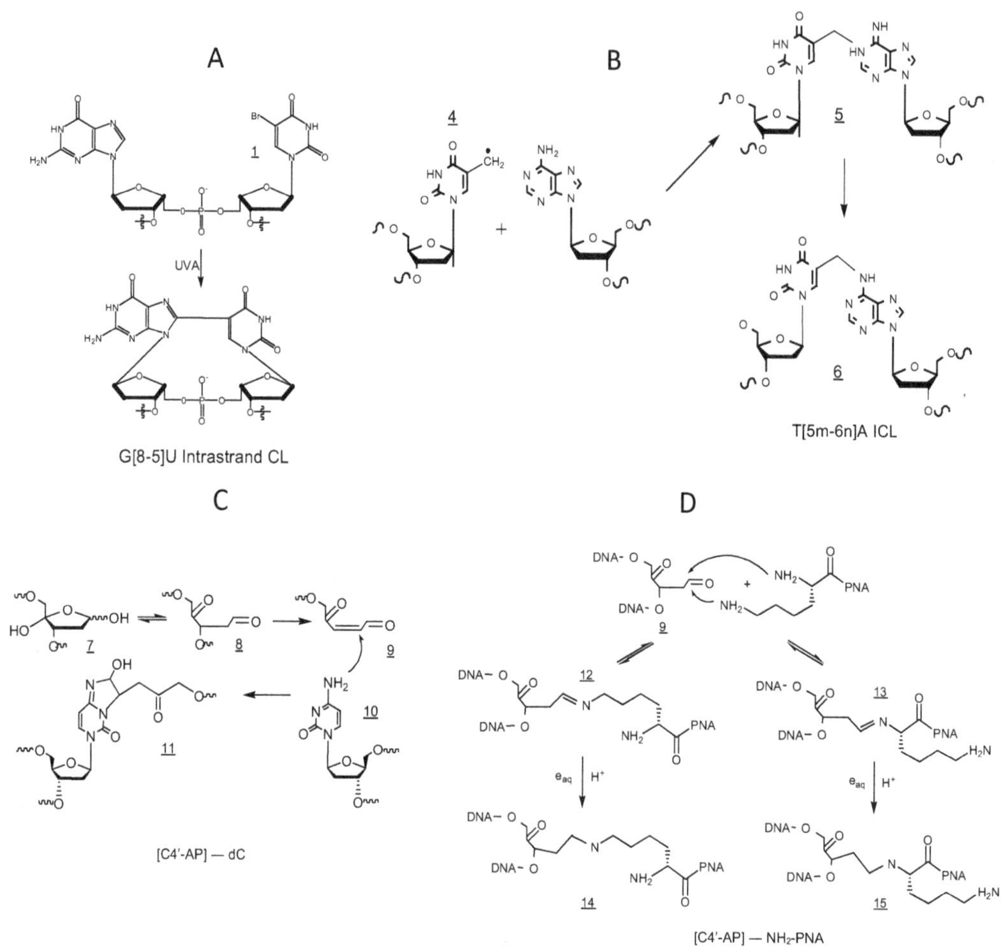

Fig. 6. Chemical structures of known intra- and interstrand crosslinks as generated in model DNA systems, UV and ionizing radiation: (A) The structure of G[8-5]U intrastrand crosslink; the only known crosslink formed *via* direct addition to •U-radical (3). This pathway was not found for ICL formation in normal dsDNA, probably due to steric restrictions, however interstrand crosslinks generated with the participation of 5-uracil-yl radical are possible in wobble scDNA (Fig. 1); (B) The formation of T[5m-6n]A ICL initiated by •OH radical H-abstraction from 5-CH_3dT (4); the intermediate product is addition to N1 (5), which is further rearranged to the final product (6), (Ding *et al.*, 2008); (C) The ICL (11) formed *via* condensation reaction of exocyclic NH_2-group of dC with β-elimination product (9) of an oxidized C4′-AP abasic site (7 and 8). This ICL is associated with a SSB formation, (Regulus *et al.*, 2007) and; (D) Reaction of C4′-AP native abasic site (9) with L-Lys-capped PNA resulting in the formation of PNA-DNA interstrand crosslinks *via* Schiff base (12 and 13). Two free NH_2-groups are equally reactive which can produce two ICLs of different structure (14 and 15). The abasic sites are formed by γ-radiation oxidation of DNA (*e.g.* by •OH radicals). The concomitant solvated electrons, e_{aq}^- are the essential reducing species required to convert Schiff bases in irreversible ICLs, (Gantchev *et al.*, 2009).

together with the synthetically positioned AP-sites on DNA the participation of these two entities in the ICL formation was positively identified (Gantchev *et al.*, 2009). Our data are consistent with a mechanism of ICL formation that involves formation of Schiff bases between PNA-amino functional groups and radiation-damage induced AP-sites on DNA. This type of covalent bonding is widely accepted to take place in the formation of covalent links between NH_2-peptide (protein) groups and damaged (aldehydic) DNA sites, albeit in the presence of an exogenous reducing agent (Mazumder *et al.*, 1996). The new finding is that apart from the prerequisite •OH-mediated, or direct γ-damage of DNA (formation of AP-sites), γ-radiation also provides reducing equivalents to transform the initially formed Schiff base linkage into a more stable reduced bond (amine), *i.e.* to produce irreversible ICL (Fig. 6D). This presents a typical case of radiation-induced MDS, where the synergism of the interactions of •OH, e^-_{aq}, and possibly even •H radicals on PNA-DNA results in ICL. The 3D-modeling (Gantchev *et al.*, 2009) confirms experimental data that open-chain C4′-AP at several DNA-strand end, or penultimate positions are structurally allowed to form covalent bonds with the ε- and α-amino groups of opposite Lys residues, or PNA NH_2-terminal groups and in all cases although, intra-helical ICLs are solvent accessible (*e.g.* the transient Schiff bases are available for interaction with e^-_{aq}). Importantly, if dsDNA duplexes are compared, the e^-_{aq} and solvent accessibility holds for the open structures in BrdU-DNA bubbles in scDNA, only (see below).

Solvated electrons (e^-_{aq}) are indispensible species for the formation of both strand breaks and interstrand crosslinks sensitized by BrdU in scDNA and crosslinks in DNA-PNA heteroduplexes. The e^-_{aq} interaction rate with oxygen, $k(e^-_{aq} + O_2) = 2x10^{10}\ M^{-1}s^{-1}$ is high, therefore hypoxic experimental conditions are important. The radiosensitization properties of BrdU are based on its ability to undergo dissociative electron transfer (ET) which is initiated by electron capture either from solution, or following excess ET from surrounding DNA bases (Fig. 1). The classical reducibility (electron affinity, EA) trend of nucleobases is BrU>U~T>C>A>G (Aflatooni *et al.*, 1998; Richardson *et al.*, 2004), with BrU being only ~ 40 mV easier to reduce than thymidine (Gaballah *et al.*, 2005). Using the approach described by Michaels & Hunt (1978) and quantitation of BrdU-mediated damage in mismatched duplexes, we calculated a value for $k(e^-_{aq}$ + BrdU-scDNA) of $\sim 2x10^{10}\ M^{-1}s^{-1}$. This value is particularly interesting in that the rate constant for BrdU interaction with e^-_{aq} in mismatched, scDNA (single-stranded regions of the duplex) is practically the same as for the free base BrU in solution (Zimbrick *et al.*, 1969a) (*i.e.* essentially diffusion controlled) and, about two orders of magnitude higher than in normal dsDNA. Based on our results from the irradiation of solutions containing PNA-DNA hybrids, we calculated a rate constant for the formation of PNA-DNA crosslinks, assuming only interactions with hydrated electrons, equal to: $k(e^-_{aq}$ + PNA) ~ $5x10^9\ M^{-1}s^{-1}$, which is also high. While high rate interaction of e^-_{aq} with PNA-DNA hetereoduplexes can be attributed to the lack of electrostatic repulsion (see Fig. 4 and legend), the increased rate of interaction with wobble scDNA is less obvious. We hypothesized that e^-_{aq} may have a restricted access to BrdU when incorporated in a normal DNA duplex, although the Br-atom is partially solvent-exposed in the major groove. To address this issue we applied molecular modeling and nanosecond scale molecular dynamics (MD) simulations, where the excess electron in solution was modeled as a localized $e^-(H_2O)_6$ anionic cluster (Gantchev & Hunting, 2008, 2009). We compared the dynamics and interactions of e^-_{aq} with dsDNA containing a normal BrdU•dA pair in the center of the duplex (dsDNA) with that of a wobble DNA containing a single mismatched

BrdU^dT pair (scDNA), *i.e.* replacing dA with dT. Rather unexpectedly we found that the occupancy of the close-to-DNA space for scDNA and dsDNA at cut-off distance <5 Å was 0.7% vs. 1.6%, respectively (from a total of 4,000 MD configurations). However, the electron interacted with a larger number of individual bases in scDNA. For instance, in dsDNA, the electron moved closely toward only four nucleobases, all from the non-brominated DNA strand, while in scDNA eleven nucleobases from both strands were found to come within reach of e_{aq}^-. The different clustering of the electron (occupation of close to DNA sites) in both duplexes is presented graphically in Fig. 7 (see legend for details). Notably, BrU incorporated in the central (sixth) position of both DNA duplexes, was approached by e_{aq}^- several times in scDNA only. Likewise only in scDNA, the e_{aq}^- preferentially occupied close sites and formed contacts with the two most perturbed thymidines (dT5 and dT7) flanking BrdU. At present, there is no explanation for the disparity of e_{aq}^- interactions with dsDNA *vs.* scDNA, other than the different dynamic structure of the isosteric DNA sequences under study, including the dynamics of structured water and Debay-Hückel layers (Gantchev & Hunting, 2008, 2009). The exposure of wobble-pair pyrimidine carbonyl groups into the DNA grooves results in excess solvation of the mismatched pairs (Sherer & Cramer, 2004).

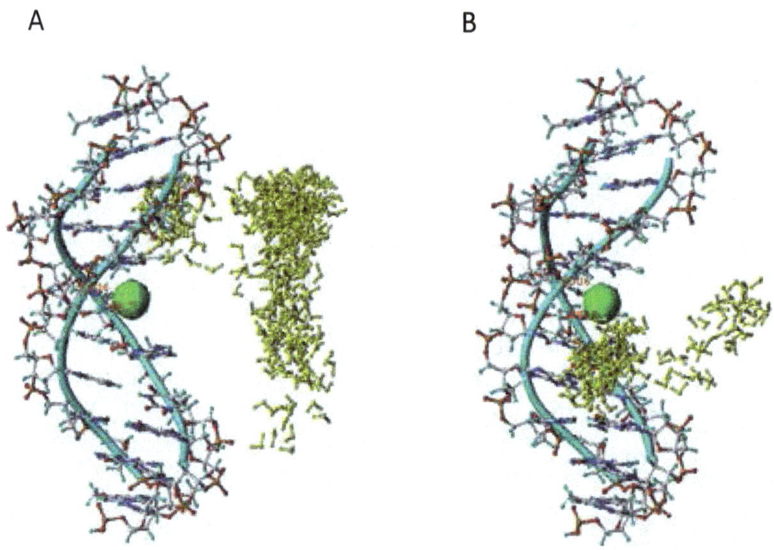

Fig. 7. Superimposed snapshots from ns MD of regular (left) and mismatched (right) 11-mer DNA containing a Watson-Crick BrU6•A17 normal pair, or BrU^T17 wobble pair, respectively. The e^-_{aq} is represented by a $e^-[H_2O]_6$ anionic cluster. The shown dynamic states are selected by the rule, distance $|e^-_{aq}$ - nucleobase$| < 5$ Å. From the total of 59 states for normal DNA, there are no configurations where e^-_{aq} is close to the central BrU6•A17 base pair. In contrast, in the wobble scDNA from the all 22 states obeying the same selection rule, ~ 65% show close approach to the wobble BrU6^T17 pair. The electron resides most often in the vicinity of the flanking T7 base and less frequently approaches BrU6 and T17. Hydration water and counterions are not shown; BrU•A and BrU^T are in the middle and labeled. Color code: Br-vdW sphere (green); DNA backbone (cyan); nucleotide atoms (standard color); e^-_{aq} (yellow). For details see: Gantchev & Hunting, (2008, 2009).

In addition, the incorporated mismatched pairs (T^T or BU^T) alter the dynamics of the neighboring bases due to incomplete 5'-stacking. Together with the narrowing of the minor groove these phenomena bring the two strands closer which creates conditions for cross-strand (cs) stacking and single and multiple cross-strand (cs) H-bonding not only within the mismatched regions, but also encompassing penultimate nucleotides to create extended "zipper-like" motives (Špačková *et al.*, 2000). The properties of single-mismatch scDNA duplexes, including the effect of the nearest sequence context (*e.g.* presence of T-tract DNA) have been discussed elsewhere (Gantchev *et al.*, 2005). A schematic presentation of the most often formed cross-strand inter-base contacts is given in Fig. 8. The close presence of e_{aq}^{-}, although causes dynamic instability and fluctuations around the mismatched BrdU^dT pair does not abolish, but in contrast, provokes additional frequent cs-H-bonding interactions (Gantchev & Hunting, 2009). All these findings are important in terms of facilitated charge-transfer along UV-, or γ-activated BrdU-scDNA. The intrahelical electron or hole transfer to BrdU and/or •U-yl radical are the next important factor that is largely expected to control the efficiency (and location) of the ensuing DNA damage; the formation of DSB and ICL. Indeed, recently a more effective electron transfer has been reported for mismatched duplexes than for fully complementary DNA (Ito *et al.*, 2009). Using a two electron acceptor DNA model system with incorporated BrdA, BrdG, BrdU and TT-dimer Fazio *et al.* (Fazio *et al.*, 2011) were able to estimate the absolute electron-hoping rates in DNA and have shown that the electron transfer is more efficient in 5′ → 3′ direction. As mentioned, in unsubstituted DNA pyrimidine rather than purine bases have been considered as trapping sites for excess electrons. This is illustrated by resonant free electron attachment experiments (Stokes *et al.*, 2007) which show that both thymine and cytosine form stable valence anions for low energy electrons, *i.e.* both thymine and cytosine possess positive adiabatic electron affinities. However, recently a stabile anionic state of adenine (A^-) has been detected (Haranczyk *et al.*, 2007). Subsequently, this finding has been shown to have a pronounced effect in the ultrafast ET in DNA and on dissociative bond cleavage (Wang *et al.*, 2009), including ET to BrdU from A^- acting as primary trap of radiolysis-generated pre-hydrated electrons (Wang *et al.*., 2010). These new developments in the field add to the existing puzzles of the precise determination of successive chain events leading to multiple BrdU-sensitized damages (DSB and ICL) in wobble scDNA.

Repair of interstrand crosslinks (ICLs) requires multiple strand incisions to separate the two covalently linked DNA strands. It is unclear how these incisions are generated. DNA double-strand breaks (DSBs) have been identified as intermediates in ICL repair, but eukaryotic enzymes responsible for producing these intermediates are not well known (Wang, 2007; Moldovan & D'Andrea, 2009a,b; D'Andrea & Grompe, 2003; Liu *et al.*, 2010; Hanada *et al.*, 2006). Ongoing research shows that in cell free model systems ICLs of different chemical structure exert different effects during repair and some may be difficult to repair. The repair refractive character of a particular ICL resulting from the C4′-AP abasic site and identified to occur as a clustered ICL-SSB lesion (Sczepanski *et al.*, 2008, 2009a) was recently demonstrated to give rise to even more toxic DSBs when subjected to NER (Sczepanski *et al.*., 2009b). Likewise, during UvrABC nucleotide excision repair of the well-defined T[5m-6n]A single-lesion crosslink imbedded in dsDNA (Fig. 6B, Ding *et al.*, 2008), DSB were produced in almost 30% of the excision events (Peng *et al.*, 2010).

DNA packing into chromatin adds to the complexity of DNA damage recognition and removal, because the highly condensed chromatin is, in general, refractory to DNA repair (Hara *et al.*, 2000; Thoma, 2005). In order to grant access to DNA repair machinery, the

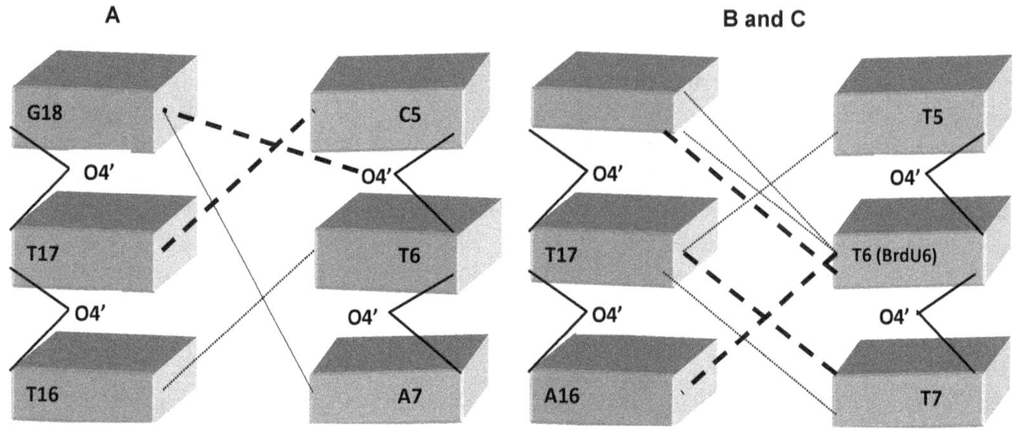

Fig. 8. Nearest-neighbour sequence effects in wobble semi-complementary DNA (scDNA) as observed by MD (adapted from Gantchev *et al.* 2005). Schematic presentation of the frequent cross-strand (cs) inter-base contacts formed in the studied 11-mer DNA duplexes containing a single mismatch: T^T or T^BrU, incorporated in the central triplets: d(CTA)•(TTG) (A), d(TTT)•(ATA) (B) and d(TBrdUT)•(ATA) (C): bold dashed lines (most frequently observed cs H-bons), dotted lines (less frequent cs H-bonds). Note that cs contacts in (C) coincide with those observed also in the presence of e^{-}_{aq} (Gantchev & Hunting, 2009). These data underline the importance of the wobble DNA dynamic structure for both, interstrand ET and high-frequency opposite-strand atom encounter for the generation of (asymmetric) ICL (Fig. 1).

chromatin response to DNA damage involves activation of ATP-dependent chromatin-remodeling complexes and histone post-translational modification pathways (Peterson & Côte, 2004; Nag & Smerdon, 2009; Méndez-Acuña *et al.*, 2010). Again, DSBs recognition and repair in the context of chromatin rearrangement is better studied and understood at the expense of other DNA damages, such as ICLs. One crucial chromatin modification, the phosphorylation of the histone variant H2AX (γH2AX) is perhaps the best example of a histone modification in response to DSB induction in DNA (Van Attikum & Gasser, 2005). Despite the progress achieved in understanding of the repair of certain UV-induced DNA damages (intra-strand crosslinks), *e.g.* cyclobutane pyrimidine dimers (CPD) and 6-4 pyrimidine photoadducts (6-4 PP), or the acetylaminofluorene-guanine (AAF-G) covalent adduct, little is known about the effects of other bulky DNA lesions (*e.g.* ICLs) on the nucleosome structural dynamics and its interplay with the versatile NER pathway (Smerdon & Lieberman, 1978; Pehrson, 1995; Gaillard et al., 2003; Gospodinov & Herceg, 2011). There is a consensus that NER functionality depends primarily on the damage recognition step, which in turn depends on the degree of DNA helix distortion induced by a particular lesion (Cai *et al.*, 2007). It has been hypothesized that structurally different interstrand crosslinks would affect chromatin remodeling and damage recognition in different ways, and some ICLs might retain their refractive character to recognition/repair, or at least will exert an altered repair efficacy. Thus, a recent *in vivo* study (Hlavin *et al.*, 2010) confirmed that the structure of synthetic interstrand crosslinks between mismatched bases affects the repair rate (in this case, transcription coupled NER). It can be further hypothesized that PNA-patches hybridized to DNA (*e.g.*, > 8-10 b.p.; PNA- invaded DNA strands, PNA-DNA triple helices, and/or DNA-PNA covalent adducts) would be difficult to repair without a loss of DNA information, and/or would require major chromatin remodeling. Indeed, Faruqi *et al.* (1998) designed PNAs that bind to the *sup*FG1 mutation reporter gene and found that 8- or 10- b.p. PNA bound to this site induces mutations at frequencies in the range of 0.1%, well above the *in vivo* background. Later, the same group (Kim *et al.*, 2006) demonstrated that a psoralen-*bis*-PNA conjugate directs the formation of a photoadduct at the 5′-TpA step of the PNA binding site to the same *sup*FG1 gene. In mammalian cells, the UV-generated PNA-targeted psoralen phtoadducts induced mutations as high as 0.46%, *i.e.* 6.5-fold above the background.

6. Conclusion

In conclusion, there is a need to better understand the parameters which control the formation and repair of complex DNA lesions, such as interstrand crosslinks. Such complex, repair refractive lesions may offer a means to selectively kill tumor cells by taking advantage of either enhanced formation or reduced repair within the tumor environment.

7. References

Aflatooni K., Gallup G. A., Burrow P.D. (1998) Electron Attachment Energies of the DNA Bases. *Journal of Physical Chemistry A*, 102, 6205–6207.

Cadet J., Douki T., Ravanat J.-L. (2010) Oxidatively generated base damage to cellular DNA. *Free Radical Biology & Medicine* 49, 9–21.

Cai Y., Patel D.J., Geacintov N.E., Broyde S. (2007) Dynamics of benzo[a]pyren-derived guanine DNA lesion in TGT and CGC sequence contexts: Enhanced mobility in TGT explains conformational heterogeneity, flexible bending, and greater susceptibility to nucleotide excision repair. *Journal of Molecular Biology* 374, 292-305.

Cecchini S., Girouard S., Huels M.A., Sanche L., Hunting D.J. (2004) Single strand specific radiosensitization of DNA by Bromodeoxyuridine. *Radiation Research* 162, 604-615.

Cecchini S., Girouard S., Huels M.A., Sanche L., Hunting D.J. (2005a) Interstrand crosslinks: a new type of gamma-ray damage in bromodeoxyuridine-substituted DNA. *Biochemistry* 44, 1932–1940.

Cecchini S., Masson C., La Madeleine C., Huels M.A., Sanche L., Wagner J.R., Hunting D.J. (2005b) Interstrand cross-link induction by UV radiation in bromodeoxyuridine-substituted DNA: Dependence on DNA conformation. *Biochemistry*, 44, 16957-16966.

Chen J., Stubbe JA. (2004) Synthesis and Characterization of Oligonucleotides Containing a 4′-Keto Abasic Site. *Biochemistry* 43, 5278–5286.

Chen T., Cook G.P., Koppisch A.T., Greenberg M.M. (2000) Investigation of the Origin of the Sequence Selectivity for the 5-Halo-2′-deoxyuridine Sensitization of DNA to Damage by UV-Irradiation. *Journal of the American Chemical Society* 122, 3861-3866.

Cutrona G., Carpaneto E.M., Ulivi M., Roncella S., Landt O., Ferrarini M., Boffa L.C. (2000) Effects in live cells of a c-*myc* anti-gene PNA linked to a nuclear localization signal. *Nature Biotechnology* 18, 300-303.

D'Andrea A.D., Grompe M. (2003) The Fanconi anaemia/BRCA pathway. *Nature Reviews Cancer* 3, 23-34.

Dedon P.C. (2008) The Chemical Toxycology of 2-Deoxyribose Oxidation in DNA. *Chemical Research in Toxicology* 21, 206-219.

Demidov V.V., Yavnilovich M.V., Belotserkovskii B.P., Frank-Kamenetskii M.D., Nielsen P.E. (1995) Kinetics and mechanism of polyamide ("peptide") nucleic acid binding to duplex DNA. *Proceedings of the National Academy of Sciences USA* 92, 2637-2641.

Dextraze M.-E., Wagner J.R., Hunting D.J. (2007) 5-Bromodeoxyuridine radiosensitization: conformation-dependent DNA damage. *Biochemistry* 46, 9089–9097.

Dextraze M.-E., Cecchini S., Bergeron F., Girouard S., Turcotte K., Wagner J.R., Hunting D.J. (2009) Reaching for the other side: Generating sequence-dependent interstrand crosslinks with 5-bromodeoxyuridine and γ-rays. *Biochemistry* 48, 2005-2011.

Ding H., Greenberg M.M. (2007) γ-Radiolysis and Hydroxyl Radical Produce Interstrand Cross-Links in DNA Involving Thymidine. *Chemical Research in Toxicology* 20, 1623–1628.

Ding H., Majumdar A., Tolman J.R., Greenberg M.M. (2008) Multinuclear NMR and Kinetic Analysis of DNA Interstrand Cross-Link Formation. *Journal of the American Chemical Society*, 130, 17981–17987.

Ding H., Greenberg M.M. (2010) DNA Damage and Interstrand Cross-Link Formation upon Irradiation of Aryl Iodide C-Nucleotide Analogues. *Journal of Organic Chemistry* 75, 535–544.

Doyle D.F., Braasch D.A., Simmons C.G., Janowski B.A., Corey D.R. (2001) Inhibition of gene expression inside cells by peptide nucleic acids: Effect of mRNA target sequence, mismatched bases, and PNA length. *Biochemistry* 40, 53-64.

Egholm M., Buchardt O., Christensen L., Behrens C., Freir S.M., Driver D.A., Berg R.H., Kim S.K., Norden B., Nielsen P.E. (1993) PNA hybridizes to complementary oligonucleotides obeying the Watson-Crick hydrogen-bonding rules. *Nature* 365, 566-568.

Faruqi F.A., Egholm M., Glazer P.M. (1998) Peptide nucleic acid-targeted mutagenesis of a chromosomal gene in mouse cells. *Proceedings of the National Academy of Sciences U.S.A.* 95, 1398-1403.

Fazio D., Trindler C., Heil K., Chatgilialoglu C., Carell T. (2011) Investigation of Excess-Electron Transfer in DNA Double-Duplex Systems Allows Estimation of Absolute Excess-Electron Transfer and CPD Cleavage Rates. *Chemistry A European Journal* 17, 206-212.

Gaballah S.T., Collier G., Netzel T.L. (2005) Charge Transfer Excited-State Dynamics in DNA Duplexes Substituted with an Ethynylpyrenyldeoxyuridine Electron Source and a Fluorodeoxyuridine Electron Trap. *Journal of Physical Chemistry B*, 109, 12175–12181.

Gaillard H., Fitzgerald D.J., Smith C.L., Peterson C.L., Richmond T.J., Thoma F. (2003) Chromatin remodeling activities act on UV-damaged nucleosomes and modulate DNA damage accessibility to photolyase. *Journal of Biological Chemistry* 278, 17655-17663.

Gantchev T.G., Cecchini S., Hunting D.J. (2005) Dynamic conformational states of DNA containing T•T or BrdU•T mispaired bases: wobble H-bond pairing versus cross-strand inter-atomic contacts. *Journal of Molecular Modeling* 11, 141–159.

Gantchev T.G., Hunting D.J. (2008) Probing the interactions of the solvated electron with DNA by molecular dynamics simulations: bromodeoxyuridine substituted DNA. *Journal of Molecular Modeling* 14, 451–464.

Gantchev T.G., Hunting D.J. (2009) Probing the interactions of the solvated electron with DNA by molecular dynamics simulations: II. Bromodeoxyuridine - thymidine mismatched. *Journal of Molecular Modeling* 15, 9 -23.

Gantchev T.G., Girouard S., Dodd D.W., Wojciechowski F., Hudson R.H.E., Hunting D.J. (2009) γ-Radiation Induced Interstrand Cross-Links in PNA:DNA Heteroduplexes. *Biochemistry* 48, 7032–7044.

Gospodinov A., Herceg Z. (2011) Chromatin: The entry to and exit from DNA repair. *Post-translational Modifications in Health and Disease*, C. Vidal (ed.), Protein Reviews, Springer, v. 13, pp. 387-409.

Guan L., Greenberg M.M. (2009) DNA Interstrand Cross-Link Formation by the 1,4-Dioxobutane Abasic Lesion. *Journal of the American Chemical Society*, 131, 15225–15231.

Hanada K., Budzowska M., Modesti M., Maas A., Wyman C., Essers J., Kanaar R. (2006) The structure-specific endonuclease Mus81–Eme1 promotes conversion of interstrand DNA crosslinks into double-strands breaks. *The EMBO Journal* 25, 4921–4932.

Hara R., Mo, J. Sancar, A. (2000) DNA damage in the nucleosome core is refractory to repair by human excision nuclease. *Molecular Cell Biology* 20, 9173-9181.

Haranczyk M., Gutowski M., Li X., Bowen K.H. (2007) Bound anionic states of adenine. *Proceedings of the National Academy of Sciences* 104, 4804–4807.

Hempel K., Mildenberger E. (1987) Determination of G-values for single and double strand break induction in plasmid DNA using agarose gel electrophoresis and a curve-fitting procedure. *International Journal of Radiation Biology* 52, 125-138.

Higgins G.S., Prevo R., Lee Y.-F., Helleday T., Muschel R.J., Taylor S., Yoshimura M., Hickson I.D., Bernhard E.J., McKenna W.G. (2010) A Small Interfering RNA Screen of Genes Involved in DNA Repair Identifies Tumor-Specific Radiosensitization by POLQ Knockdown. *Cancer Research* 70, 2984–2993.

Hlavin E.M., Smeaton M.B., Noronha A.M., Wilds C.J., Miller P.S. (2010) Cross-Link Structure Affects Replication-Independent DNA Interstrand Cross-Link Repair in Mammalian Cells. *Biochemistry* 49, 3977–3988.

Hong I.S., Ding H., Greenberg M.M. (2006) Radiosensitization by a Modified Nucleotide that Produces DNA Interstrand Cross-Links under Hypoxic Conditions. *Journal of the American Chemical Society* 128, 2230–2231.

Hunting D.J. *et al.*, unpublished.

Ito T., Kondo A., Kamashita, T., Tanabe K., Yamada H., Nishimoto S. (2009) Pathways of excess electron transfer in phenothiazine-tethered DNA containing single-base mismatches, *Organic & Biomolecular Chemistry* 7, 2077–2081.

Jackson S.P. (2002) Sensing and repairing DNA double-strand breaks. Carcinogenesis 23, 687-696.

Kaihatsu K., Jonowski B.A., Corey D.R. (2004) Recognition of chromosomal DNA by PNAs. *Chemistry & Biology* 11, 749-758.

Kim Y., Hong I.S. (2008) PNA/DNA interstrand cross-links from a modified PNA base upon photolysis or oxidative conditions. *Bioorganic and Medicinal Chemistry Letters* 18, 5054-5057.

Kim K.-H. Nielsen P.E., Glazer P.M. (2006) Site-specific gene modification by PNAs conjugated to psoralen. *Biochemistry*, 45, 314-323.

Lin G., Zhang J., Zeng Y., Luo H., Wang Y. (2010) Conformation-Dependent Formation of the G[8-5]U Intrastrand Cross-Link in 5-Bromouracil-Containing G-Quadruplex DNA Induced by UVA Irradiation. *Biochemistry* 49, 2346–2350.

Liu T., Ghosal G., Yuan J., Chen J., Huang J. (2010) FAN1 Acts with FANCI-FANCD2 to Promote DNA Interstrand Cross-Link Repair. *Science* 329, 693- 696.

Mazumder A., Neamati N., Pilon A.A., Sunder S., Pommier Y. (1996) Chemical trapping of ternary complexes of human immunodeficiency virus type I integrase, divalent metal, and DNA substrates containing an abasic site. *Journal of Biological Chemistry* 271, 27330-27338.

Menchise V., De Simone G., Tedeschi T., Corradini R., Sforza S., Marchelli R., Capasso D., Saviano M., Pedone C. (2003) Insights into peptide nucleic acid (PNA) structural features: The crystal structure of a D-lysine-based chiral PNA-DNA duplex. *Proceedings of the National Academy of Sciences USA* 100, 12021-12026.

Méndez-Acuña, L., Di Tomaso M.V., Palitti F., Martínez-López W. (2010) Histone post-translational modifications in DNA damage response. *Cytogenetic and Genome Research* 128, 28-36.

Michaels H.B., Hunt J.W. (1978) A model for radiation damage in cells by direct effect and by indirect effect: A radiation chemistry approach. *Radiation Research* 74, 23-34.

Moldovan G.L., D'Andrea A.D. (2009a) FANCD2 Hurdles the DNA Interstrand Crosslink. *Cell* 139, 1222.

Moldovan G.-L., D'Andrea A.D. (2009b) How the Fanconi Anemia Pathway Guards the Genome. *Annual Review of Genetics* 43, 223.

Nabben F.J., Karman J.Pl., Loman H. (1982) Inactivation of biologically active DNA by hydrated electrons. *International Journal of Radiation Biology* 42, 23-30.

Nag R., Smerdon M.J. (2009) Altering the chromatin landscape for nucleotide excision repair. *Mutation Research: Reviews in Mutation Research* 682, 13-20.

Nese C., Yuan Z., Schuchmann M.N., von Sonntag C. (1992) Electron transfer from nucleobase electron adducts to 5-bromouracil. Is guanine an ultimate sink for the electron in irradiated DNA? *International Journal of Radiation Biology* 62, 527-541.

Nielsen P.E. (1995) DNA analogues with nonphosphodiester backbones. *Annual Review of Biophysics and Biomolecular Structure* 24, 167-183.

Nielsen P.E., Egholm M., Buchardt O. (1994) Sequence-specific transcription arrest by peptide nucleic acid bound to the DNA template strand. *Gene* 149, 139-145.

Op de Beeck M., Madder A. (2011) Unprecedented C-Selective Interstrand Cross-Linking through in Situ Oxidation of Furan-Modified Oligodeoxynucleotides. *Journal of the American Chemical Society* 133, 796–807.

Pehrson, J.R. (1995) Probing the conformation of nucleosome linker DNA in situ with pyrimidine dimer formation. *Journal of Biological Chemistry* 270, 22440-22444.

Pellestor F., Paulasova P., Hamamah S. (2008) Peptide nucleic acids (PNAs) as diagnostic devices for genetic and cytogenetic analysis. *Current Pharmaceutical Design* 14, 2439-2444.

Peng X., Ghosh A.K., Van Houten B., Greenberg M.M. (2010) Nucleotide Excision Repair of a DNA Interstrand Cross-Link Produces Single- and Double-Strand Breaks. *Biochemistry* 49, 11–19.

Peng X., Hong I.S., Li H., Seidman M.M., Greenberg M.M. (2008) Interstrand Cross-Link Formation in Duplex and Triplex DNA by Modified Pyrimidines. *Journal of the American Chemical Society* 130, 10299–10306.

Peterson C.L., Côte J. (2004) Cellular machineries for chromosomal DNA repair. *Genes & Development* 18, 602-616.

Pooga M., Land T., Bartfai T., Langel Ü. (2001) PNA oligomers as tools for specific modulation of gene expression. *Biomolecular Engineering* 17, 183-192.

Porcheddu A. and Giacomelli G. (1996) PNA-nucleic acid complexes. Structure, stability and dynamics. *Quarterly Reviews of Biophysics* 29, 369-394.

Porcheddu A., Giacomelli G. (2005) Peptide nucleic acids (PNAs), A chemical Overview. *Current Medicinal Chemistry* 12, 2561-2599.

Quanz M., Berthault N., Roulin C., Roy M., Herbette A., Agrario C., Alberti C., Josserand V., Coll J.-L., Sastre-Garau X., Cosset J.-M., Larue L., Sun J.-S., Dutreix M. (2009) Small-molecule drugs mimicking DNA damage: A new strategy for sensitizing tumors to radiotherapy. *Clinical Cancer Research* 15, 1308-1316.

Ray A., Norden B. (2000) Peptide nucleic acid (PNA): its medical and biotechnical applications and promise for the future, *FASEB Journal* 14, 1041-1060.

Regulus P., Duroux B., Bayle P.-A., Favier, A., Cadet J., Ravanat J.-L. (2007) Oxidation of the sugar moiety of DNA by ionizing radiation or bleomycin could induce the formation of a cluster DNA lesion. *Proceedings of the National Academy of Sciences* 104, 14032–14037.

Richardson N.A., Gu J., Wang S., Xie Y., Schaefer H.F. III. (2004) DNA Nucleosides and Their Radical Anions: Molecular Structures and Electron Affinities. *Journal of the American Chemical Society*, 126, 4404–4411.

Romanelli A., Pedone C., Saviano M., Bianchi N., Borgatti M., Mischiati C., Gambari R. (2001) Molecular interactions between nuclear factor κB (NF-κB) transcription factors and a PNA-DNA chimera mimicking NF-κB binding sites. *European Journal of Biochemistry* 268, 6066-6075.

Sawada S., Okada S. (1972) Effects of BUdR-labelling on radiation-induced DNA breakage and subsequent rejoining in cultured mammalian cells. *International Journal of Radiation Biology* 21, 599-602.

Sczepanski J.T., Jacobs A.C., Greenberg M.M. (2008) Self-Promoted DNA Interstrand Cross-Link Formation by an Abasic Site. *Journal of the American Chemical Society*, 130, 9646–9647.

Sczepanski J.T., Jacobs A.C., Majumdar A., Greenberg M.M. (2009a) Scope and Mechanism of Interstrand Cross-Link Formation by the C4'-Oxidized Abasic Site. *Journal of the American Chemical Society*, 131, 11132–11139.

Sczepanski J., Jacobs A.C., Van Houten B., Greenberg M.M. (2009b) Double-Strand Break Formation during Nucleotide Excision Repair of a DNA Interstrand Cross-Link. *Biochemistry* 48, 7565–7567.

Sherer C., Cramer C.J. (2004) Structural and dynamic variations in DNA hexamers containing T-T and F-F single and tandem internal mispairs. *Theoretical Chemistry Accounts* 111, 311-327.

Smerdon M.J., Lieberman, M.W. (1978) Nucleosome rearrangement in human chromatin during UV-induced DNA-repair synthesis. *Proceedings of the National Academy of Sciences U.S.A.* 75, 4238-4241.

Špačková N., Berger I., Šponer J. (2000) Nanosecond Molecular Dynamics of Zipper-like DNA Duplex Structures Containing Sheared G·A Mismatch Pairs. *Journal of the American Chemical Society* 122, 7564–7572.

Stokes S.T., Li X., Grubisic A., Ko Y.J., Bowen K.H. (2007) Intrinsic electrophilic properties of nucleosides: Photoelectron spectroscopy of their parent anions. *Journal of Chemical Physics* 127, 084321.

Takata M., Sasaki M.S., Sonoda E., Morrison C., Hashimoto M., Utsumi H., Yamaguchi-Iwai Y., Shinohara A., Takeda S. (1998) Homologous recombination and non-homologous end-joining pathways of DNA double-strand break repair have overlapping roles in the maintenance of chromosomal integrity in vertebrate cells. *EMBO Journal* 17, 5497-5508.

Thoma F. (2005) Repair of UV lesions in nucleosomes - intrinsic properties and remodeling. *DNA Repair* 4, 855-869.

Van Attikum H., Gasser, S.M. (2005) The histone code at DNA breaks: A guide to repair? *Nature Reviews Molecular Cell Biology*. 6, 757-765.

Wang C.-R., Nguyen J., Lu Q.-B. (2009) Bond Breaks of Nucleotides by Dissociative Electron Transfer of Nonequilibrium Prehydrated Electrons: A New Molecular Mechanism for Reductive DNA Damage. *Journal of the American Chemical Society* 131, 11320-11322.

Wang C.-R., Lu Q.-B. (2010) Molecular Mechanism of the DNA Sequence Selectivity of 5-Halo-2'-Deoxyuridines as Potential Radiosensitizers. *Journal of the American Chemical Society* 132, 14710–14713.

Wang W. (2007) Emergence of a DNA-damage response network consisting of Fanconi anaemia and BRCA proteins. *Nature Reviews Genetics* 8, 735-748.

Weng X., Ren L., Weng L., Huang J., Zhu S., Zhou X., Weng L. (2007) Synthesis and Biological Studies of Inducible DNA Cross-Linking Agents. *Angewandte Chemie* 119, 8166–8169.

Yoshioka Y., Kitagawa Y., Takano Y., Yamaguchi K., Nakamura T., Saito I.J. (1999) Experimental and Theoretical Studies on the Selectivity of GGG Triplets toward One-Electron Oxidation in B-Form DNA. *American Chemical Society* 121, 8712-8719.

Zeng Y., Wang Y. (2006) Sequence-dependent formation of intrastrand crosslink products from the UVB irradiation of duplex DNA containing a 5-bromo-20-deoxyuridine or 5-bromo-20-deoxycytidine. *Nucleic Acids Research* 34, 6521–6529.

Zeng Y., Wang Y. (2007) UVB-induced formation of intrastrand cross-link products of DNA in MCF-7 cells treated with 5-bromo-20-deoxyuridine. *Biochemistry* 46, 8189–8195.

Zimbrick J.D., Ward J.F., Myers L.S. Jr. (1969a) Studies on the chemical basis of cellular radiosensitization by 5-bromouracil substitution in DNA. I. Pulse- and steady-state radiolysis of 5-bromouracil and thymine", *International Journal of Radiation Biology* 16, 505-523.

Zimbrick J.D., Ward J.F., Myers L.S. Jr. (1969b) Studies on the chemical basis of cellular radiosensitization by 5-bromouracil substitution in DNA. II. Pulse- and steady-state radiolysis of bromouracil-substituted and unsubstituted DNA, *International Journal of Radiation Biology* 16, 524-534.

8

DNA Damage Protection and Induction of Repair by Dietary Phytochemicals and Cancer Prevention

Alice A. Ramos[1], Cristóvão F. Lima[2] and Cristina Pereira-Wilson[1]
[1]*CBMA – Molecular and Environmental Biology Centre*
[2]*CITAB – Centre for the Research and Technology of Agro-Environmental and Biological Sciences*
Department of Biology, School of Sciences, University of Minho, Campus de Gualtar, Braga, Portugal

1. Introduction

DNA damage accumulates in cells over time as a result of exposure to a variety of exogenous and endogenous agents. These damages, if not repaired properly, can generate mutations in somatic or germline cells, which are involved in the pathogenesis of many diseases, such as cancer. To maintain genomic integrity generation after generation, organisms possess multiple mechanisms such as inhibition of carcinogen uptake into the cells, induction of detoxification enzymes, increased cellular defenses that prevent DNA damage, enhancement of DNA repair, increased anti-inflammatory activity, inhibition of cell proliferation, and modulation of apoptosis through effects on signal transduction pathways (de Kok *et al.*, 2008); (Pan *et al.*, 2008). In the last decades, several dietary constituents have been shown to modulate all these processes. Epidemiological studies as well as laboratory data suggest that consumption of fruits and vegetables is associated with a reduced risk of developing a wide range of cancers. It has been estimated that 30-40% of all tumours can be prevented with a correct lifestyle and diet, in particular colon cancer (Rajamanickam and Agarwal, 2008). Multiple mechanisms have been proposed to explain the chemopreventive effects of phytochemicals. Protection of DNA from damage and modulation of DNA repair assume an important role on prevention of mutations and consequently of the carcinogenic process. The comet assay or single cell gel electrophoresis (SCGE) assay is a rapid, sensitive and relatively simple method for assessing DNA damage and its repair in individual cells. The standard comet assay measures DNA breaks and alkali-labile sites that are converted to strand breaks. With its widespread use, several modifications on the comet assay have been made that allow the quantification of other types of DNA damage as well as DNA repair rates. With the inclusion of an extra step on the comet assay by using specific DNA repair enzymes, different base lesions can be identified by the introduction of breaks at sites of base damage. In this regard, Endonuclease III, FPG and AlkA have been used to detect oxidized pyrimidines, modified purines and alkylpurines bases, respectively. With these modifications the comet assay can be used to estimate oxidative and alkylating DNA damage. Cells' DNA repair capacity can also be measured by using modified protocols of the comet assay, such as following the repair kinetics by the cellular repair assay, or in vitro by using cellular substrates with specific damages to measure base excision repair (BER) and nucleotide excision repair (NER) (Collins *et al.*, 2001b; Collins, 2004). These different modifications of the comet assay have been successfully used to evaluate the chemopreventive potential of several phytochemicals present in our diet. In this review, we will show evidence that dietary agents can protect DNA from oxidative and alkylating agents as well modulate DNA repair in eukaryotic cells, by using the comet assay. Data from different experimental systems, including primary cell cultures, human cell lines, animal models and human biomonitoring studies, will be discussed in order to provide an overview of effects of dietary phytochemicals on DNA damage and repair with particular emphasis on colon cancer chemoprevention. Recently, we have shown that dietary phytochemicals such as quercetin, rutin, rosmarinic acid, luteolin and others not only protect DNA damage but also stimulate DNA repair in liver and colon cell lines (Lima *et al.*, 2006; Ramos *et al.*, 2008; Ramos *et al.*, 2010b; Ramos *et al.*, 2010a). These effects may contribute to their anti-carcinogenic effects. Effects of phytochemicals through DNA repair modulation and their interaction with alkylating agents used as chemotherapeutic drugs will also be referred.

2. DNA damage and genomic stability

Cells of all organisms are under continual attack from reactive oxygen species (ROS) and alkylanting species generated by environmental pollutants, drugs, radiation, cigarette smoke and endogenous metabolism. Theses endogenous and exogenous agents can induce harmful effects if the cell's defense mechanisms are not enough to maintain cellular redox homeostasis. Protection and repair of DNA damage represent two important mechanisms to maintain genomic stability.

2.1 Oxidative DNA damage

Endogenous and exogenous agents can induce disruption of the cellular redox homeostasis in favor of oxidant state. This imbalance is described as oxidative stress. As a consequence, different types of molecules such as proteins, lipids and nucleic acids, can be damaged, resulting in severe metabolic dysfunction (including lipid peroxidation, protein oxidation, membrane disruption and DNA damage) (Aherne *et al.*, 2007). Oxidative stress has been involved in the development of several pathologies such as certain cancers, once it may lead to mutations that activate oncogenes or inactivate tumor suppressor genes (Allen and Tresini, 2000; Maynard *et al.*, 2009). In tumor cells, oxidative stress can act as a selective factor in favour of these cells, through induction of DNA damage that may generate more mutations; activation of growth-promoting transcription factors and modulation of genes involved in apoptosis and proliferation (Allen and Tresini, 2000; Karihtala and Soini, 2007). A significant consequence of oxidative stress is DNA damage, which may result in genomic instability. It has been estimated that around 10^4 lesions are induced in a mammalian cell genome every day (Hegde *et al.*, 2008). There are several types of oxidative DNA damage, such as oxidized bases, abasic sites (also called apurinic/apyrimidinic (AP)) and DNA strand breaks. Hydroxylation of guanine at C-8 position, 8-oxoGua (8-Oxo-7,8-

dihydroguanine) is one of the most abundant forms of DNA oxidation and can cause G to T transversions through mispairing in replication.

Tumor cells are characterized by high levels of ROS. Some studies showed that human tumor cells have an increase of levels of 8-oxoG relative to normal cells. Also, low levels of antioxidant have been found in tumor cells (Maynard et al., 2009).

2.2 Alkylating DNA damage

The removal of oxidative lesions by cellular repair processes is essential for maintaining genome integrity and survival limiting mutagenesis. However, there are a number of studies indicating that oxidative DNA damage could not account entirely by itself for tumor development, since elevated levels of 8-oxoGua have been shown not to reflect reflect increased cancer rates. In fact, oxidative damage is the most studied DNA damage, however, alkylating DNA damage is not less important. Human exposure to alkylating agents can arise from diet (e.g. presence of heterocyclic amines on food), environment (e.g. exposure to cigarette smoke and fuel combustion), or produced endogenously (e.g. nitrosation of amides and amines mediated by enteric bacteria) (Wirtz et al., 2010).

Alkylating agents can cause a wide spectrum of DNA adducts, including N-alkylated adducts, such as N^7-methylguanine (N^7MeG), N^3-methyladenine (N^3MeA) and N^3-methylguanine (N^3MeG), and O-alkylated adducts, such as O^6-methylguanine (O^6MeG) and O^4-methylthymine (O^4MeT). N-alkylated adducts correspond to more than 80% of alkylated bases and exhibit different stabilities. For example, N^7MeG (correspond aprox. 70%) is the most stable N-methylation adduct in vitro with 80hr of half-life. N^3MeA and N^3MeG are less abundant with 9 and 2%, respectively, of total methylation adducts. O^6MeG vary from 0.3% (for methyl methanesulfonate) to 8% (for methylnitrosourea) of the total DNA methyl adducts and it is stable in the absence of the DNA repair protein O^6-methylguanine-DNA methyltransferase (MGMT). O^4MeT is produced in very low amounts (<0.4% of the total DNA methyl adducts) and its mutagenicity and cytotoxicity are unclear. In general, O-alkylations are highly mutagenic and genotoxic, whereas N-alkylations are cytotoxic, but less mutagenic (Drablos *et al.*, 2004; Kondo *et al.*, 2010). O^6MeG is the major pre-mutagenic, pre-carcinogenic and pre-cytotoxic DNA lesion induced by methylating agents (Wirtz et al., 2010).

Prevention of DNA damage and modulation of DNA repair by dietary phytochemicals phytochemicals is the main focus of this review but first a brief overview of DNA repair mechanisms will be presented. Effects on chemoprevention of colon cancer will be addressed.

3. Mechanisms of DNA repair

Maintainance of genomic integrity is complex due to great diversity of damage that can occur in DNA. In contrast to other biomolecules, DNA cannot be replaced, only repaired. To avoid the deleterious consequences of damage accumulation, cells have a variety of DNA repair pathways, each recognize and repair specific types of DNA damage. Base excision repair (BER), nucleotide excision repair (NER), mismatch repair (MMR), homologous recombination (HR), non-homologous end-joining repair (NHEJ) and direct damage reversal repair are some of the most important pathways used by cells to repair oxidative and alkylating DNA damage (Table I). These cellular repair pathways are not completely independent from one another. Some studies have show physical interactions between some repair proteins from different repair pathways, suggesting that regulation of DNA repair involves protein cross-talk (Knudsen *et al.*, 2009). Protein expression, pos-translational modifications and nuclear translocation of DNA repair proteins have been referred as essential in the regulation of DNA repair activity and to maintain genomic stability. However, these subjects need to be clarified in the future (Knudsen *et al.*, 2009; Tudek, 2007). When DNA damage is not repaired, the cell by a complex network that collectively forms the DNA damage response (DDR) machinery delays cell-cycle progression, acting on cell cycle checkpoints. This delay gives the DNA repair machinery more time, allowing correct repair of the damage. DDR machinery can induce other mechanisms such as apoptosis or necrosis to avoid that altered cells continue to proliferate and result in disease (Bartek *et al.*, 2007; Maynard *et al.*, 2009).

3.1 Base Excision Repair

BER is the major pathway involved in the repair of oxidation and alkylation DNA damage and occurs in both the nucleus and mitochondria (D'Errico *et al.*, 2008). BER recognizes and repairs AP sites, DNA SSBs and different types of base modifications, such as oxidized/reduced bases (e.g. 8-oxoG or formamidopyrimidines), alkylated bases, deaminated bases (e.g. uracil) or base mismatches (Maynard et al., 2009). BER pathway involves steps as recognition, excision, filling and ligation that are carried out by four or five enzymes. Briefly, the repair process is initiated by one of several DNA glycosylases, each recognizing a specific DNA lesion (e.g. OGG1, NTH, NEIL and MYH recognize oxidation damage; deamination damages are recognized by UDG, MED1, UNG, and TDG, and MPG initiate alkylation repair) (Knudsen et al., 2009). These DNA glycosylases excise the damaged base (by cleave of N-glycosidic bond between the sugar and the base), generating an AP site. An AP endonuclease, as APE1, cleaves the AP site, to generate 3' OH and 5' deoxyribose phosphate (dRP) terminus. The third step is carried through DNA polymerase that fills the nucleotide gap generated due to lesion base removal. Finally, DNA ligase seals the nick on DNA (Hegde *et al.*, 2008; Evans *et al.*, 2004). Several other protein factors have been identified as interacting with the essential BER proteins and/or the DNA to modulate BER activity. BER pathway is described in detail in the several reviews (Fortini *et al.*, 2003; Hegde *et al.*, 2008; Robertson *et al.*, 2009; Fortini *et al.*, 2003).

Hydroxylation of guanine at C-8 position, 8-oxoGua (8-Oxo-7,8-dihydroguanine) is one of the most abundant forms of DNA oxidation and the most studied because of its mutagenic potential. If not properly repaired, 8-oxoG can pair with cytosine or adenine. Replication of 8-oxoG paired with C by DNA polymerases is a non-mutagenic process. However, replication of 8-oxoG paired with A results in GC to TA or TA to GC transversions that are strong mutagenic DNA lesions (Pastoriza Gallego and Sarasin, 2003). In mammalian cells 8-oxoGua is predominantly recognized and excised by a specific DNA glycosylases. hOGG1 removes 8-oxoG when paired with a cytosine and the glycosylase hMYH removes adenine when mispaired with 8-oxoG, both through the BER pathway. Activity of OGG1 is enhanced by cofactors such as human apurinic/apyrimidinic endonuclease (APE1), Xeroderma Pigmentosum complementation group C (XPC) and human endonuclease VIII-like (NEIL1) (D'Errico et al., 2008).

N^7alkylG adducts can be repaired by spontaneous depurination resulting in abasic sites that are often correctly repaired by BER. If not repaired, abasic sites may result in single-stranded gaps that can stall replication forks resulting in double stranded breaks. N^7alkylG adducts are also recognized and removed from DNA by N-methylpurine-DNAglycoslase

(MPG). MPG is responsible for enzymatic hydrolysis of the N-glycosylic bond resulting an abasic site in the DNA that is repaired by other enzymes of BER pathway. Over expression of MPG may produce an imbalance between abasic sites formation and repair in favor of abasic sites formation leading an increase of alkylating agents cytotoxicity (Doak et al., 2008).

It has been estimated that a large number of AP sites are generated per cell per day. AP sites are unstable and are highly mutagenic because they result in non-template DNA and RNA synthesis. However, the number of mutations is extremely low, which demonstrate the efficient repair of this damage by the repair mechanisms (Jaiswal and Narayan, 2008). The ability of one glycosylase to recognize more than one type of damage, and the fact that each damage may be recognized by more than one type of glycosylases, give a degree of redundancy in the DNA repair processes which contribute to efficient damage repair (Maynard et al., 2009). Several studies have been showed that post-translational modifications, such as phosphorylation, acetylation and sumoylation may modulate repair activity of BER enzymes, influencing repair efficiencies (Tudek, 2007).

Decrease on BER activity can predispose humans to development of certain cancers, such as colon cancer (Jaiswal and Narayan, 2008; Wilson and Bohr, 2007). Otherwise, an increase of BER activity has been associated with resistance to certain cancer treatments (Liu and Gerson, 2006; Marchesi *et al.*, 2007). Nevertheless, the functional significance of BER in prevention, development and treatment of disease remains unclear.

DNA Repair pathway	DNA damage	Reviews
Base Excision Repair (BER)	Base modifications (e.g. oxidized and alkylated bases; AP sites; SSBs	Hegde, M. L., et al., 2008 Robertson, A.B., et al., 2009
Nucleotide Excision Repair (NER)	DNA adducts (e.g. thymidine dimers and 6-4 photoproducts) induced by UV radiation or electrophilic chemicals	Hanawalt, P.C., 2002 Nouspikel, T., 2009
Mismatch Repair (MMR)	Mispaired nucleotides and insertion/deletion loops (IDLs)	Jiricny J., 2006
Direct damage reversal repair	O^6MeG lesions	Kondo N., et al., 2010 Kaina, B., et al., 2007 and 2010
Homologous recombination (HR) and non-homologous end-joining repair (NHEJ)	Double strand breaks	Dudas and Chovanec, 2004 Helleday et al., 2007

Table 1. The main DNA repair pathways and types of DNA damage repaired.

3.2 Nucleotide Excision Repair

NER is another important repair pathway involved in DNA adduct repair (e.g. thymidine dimers and 6-4 photoproducts) that are induced by ultraviolet radiation, chemicals or ROS (Benhamou and Sarasin, 2000). These adducts change the normal structure of the DNA helix, breaking transcription and replication processes. Two distinct NER sub-pathways, transcription coupled repair (TCR) and global genomic repair (GGR), have been described. Briefly, TCR repair transcription-blocking lesions present in transcribed DNA strands; and GGR pathway repairs lesions over the bulk genome including non-transcribed strands of active genes (Knudsen et al., 2009). Lesions like thymidine dimmers are usually repaired by

TCR, while other lesions as 6-4 photoproducts are efficiently repaired by GGR (for review see Hanawalt, 2002; Nouspikel, 2009).

3.3 Mismatch Repair

MMR is a post-replicative DNA repair mechanism that mainly corrects base-base mismatches which are caused by errors of DNA polymerases and insertion/deletion loops (IDLs). Two complexes are responsible for the repair initiation, MutSα (MSH2/MSH6) and MutSβ (MSH2/MSH3) complexes. MutSα recognize base-base mismatches and small IDLs (with one or two extrahelical nucleotides) while MutSβ recognize the larger IDLs. Repair of the new synthesized strand give the DNA polymerase the chance to generate an error-free copy of the template sequence, protecting cells from point mutations and possibly cancer development (Jiricny, 2006; Knudsen *et al.*, 2009). Loss of MMR function prevents the correction of replicative errors, leading to instability of the genome (Davis and Milner, 2007). As more details about NER and MMR pathways are known, relation between deficiencies on these pathways and cancer become stronger (Hegde et al., 2008).

DNA repair pathways have an important role during all carcinogenic process and in its treatment. Defects in DNA-repair pathways, like MMR, BER and NER, lead to an accumulation of mutations and consequently to carcinogenesis (Jiricny and Marra, 2003). Some of these pathways are inactivated due to mutation or epigenetic modifications in some human cancer, for instance, loss of MMR is observed in 15% of sporadic colorectal cancers (Casorelli *et al.*, 2008).

3.4 Direct damage reversal repair

Human cells have several DNA repair mechanisms that are capable of correcting specific types of alkylating damage. O^6MeG lesions are repaired by direct damage reversal repair carried out by MGMT also referred to as alkylguanine transferase (AGT). Cells with deficient repair of O^6MeG by MGMT are hypersensitive to chromosome aberration induced by alkylating agents (Armstrong and Galloway, 1997). MGMT is a key suicide enzyme that efficiently repairs O^6MeG before replication, through direct transfer of the adducted methyl group from the oxygen in the guanine to a cysteine residue in the catalytic site of MGMT. O^6MeG is highly mutagenic and carcinogenic because it possess a high potential to mispair with thymine during replication. This lesion is read as adenine by DNA polymerases causing GC-AT transitions (Eker *et al.*, 2009). The toxicity of the O^6MeG lesion is attributed to the recognition of O^6MeG:T mispairs by the MMR pathway that remove the new thymine. In the next round of replication another thymine mispairs with O^6MeG that will be removed by MMR. Recognition by MMR creates a gap in DNA by incision on the new replicated strand. If O^6MeG remains in one of the template strands the repair process will be repeated, creating a "futile repair loop". This loop will eventually result in toxic double-strand breaks leading to chromosomal aberrations, cell-cycle arrest or apoptosis (Bugni *et al.*, 2009; Kaina *et al.*, 2007; Kaina *et al.*, 2010; Kondo *et al.*, 2010). When both of these systems fail to repair, O^6MeG results in point mutations that can possibly initiate the carcinogenic process. Beyond the ability to remove methyl adducts, MGMT can also remove larger adducts such as, ethyl, propyl and butyl adducts, however at a lower efficiency (Doak et al., 2008).

Some authors mention the important role of MGMT in protection against sporadic human colorectal cancer, once that epigenetic silencing of MGMT gene was observed in 50% of these cancers (Lind et al., 2004). MGMT expression in tumor cells have been related with the resistance of tumors to alkylating agents toxicity (Eker *et al.*, 2009; Nystrom and Mutanen, 2009). Removal of the methyl group from O^6MeG by MGMT is dependent on the rate of MGMT syntheses which is induced in response to DNA damage (Doak et al., 2008). Depletion of MGMT by reducing MGMT activity or decreasing gene expression can occur using a specific inhibitor O^6-benzylguanine (BG) or through epigenetic silencing, (Eker et al., 2009). Inhibition of MGMT with BG in rats increases azoxymethane (AOM)-induced colon tumors, and transgenic expression of MGMT in mice protects against AOM-induced aberrant crypt foci (ACF) (Bugni *et al.*, 2009; Wali *et al.*, 1999).

3.5 Homologous recombination and Non-homologous end-joining repair

In mammalian cells double strand breaks (DSBs), one of the most deleterious damage, can be repaired by two different types of mechanism: 1) non-homologous end-joining (NHEJ) that rejoins the two broken ends in a template independent way with concomitant loss of sequence information. After overlapping of the two DNA ends, the ligase IV complex start the ligation process of the two broken ends; and 2) homologous recombination repair (HR) that uses a homologue undamaged DNA sequence (sister-chromatid or homologous chromosome) to repair the missing sequence between the two DNA ends. HR is an error-free process (Dudas and Chovanec, 2004; Helleday *et al.*, 2007).

If not properly repaired DSB can cause loss of chromosomes and consequently generate mutations with or without induction of cell death (Dudas and Chovanec, 2004). Single-strand breaks repair (SSBR) is a DNA repair pathway extremely important to avoid the deleterious effects of single-strand breaks (for more detail see the review Caldecott, 2007). Since DNA damage is recognized as the initial step in chemical carcinogenesis, inhibition of DNA damage and/or induction of repair would be the first line of defense against cancer caused by carcinogens. Chemoprevention by diet and dietary constituints against oxidative and alkylating agents will be covered by this review.

4. Chemopreventive activities of dietary phytochemicals

Diet and lifestyle play crucial roles in cancer aetiology. Nowadays, the idea that prevention of any disease is preferable over treatment is accepted by all. In this context, in the last decades, several studies suggest that regular consumption of fruits, vegetables and spices have health benefits including risk reduction of developing a cancer, namely, colon cancer (Terry et al., 2001). Much of the protective effects have been attributed to phytochemicals such as polyphenols, terpenes and alkaloids, present in low levels in plants (Barth et al., 2005). For instance, flavonoids (polyphenolic compounds) have been reported to possess potential on prevention of several cancers specially cancers of gastrointestinal tract, like oral cavity and colon cancer (Kuo, 1996). The World Cancer Research Fund (WCRF) in its report about diet and prevention of cancer in 2007, mentioned that fruits and vegetables in general probably protect against cancers of the mouth, pharynx, larynx, oesophagus, lung, and stomach and there are limited evidences that suggest protective effects of fruits against cancers of the nasopharynx, pancreas, liver, and colorectum (WCRF, 2007).

The use of plants for the prevention of diseases is an ancient practice. However, it was in the last decades that scientific community started to show interest in the medicinal properties of plants. The first scientific evidences showing that vegetables and fruits might be protective against some cancers emerged in the 1990s. Nevertheless, twenty year on no consensus exists about the real role of diet on cancer prevention, and many questions remain to be answered. Which component(s) of the diet is (are) responsible for the protective effects? Are the protective effects the result of the interactions between different components? What type of interactions exists between them (e.g. synergistic, antagonistic interaction)? What is the mechanism by which they prevent cancer?

Dietary agents have different structural features that are responsible for a great variety of biological activities such as anti-inflammatory, antioxidant, free radical scavenging, anti-mutagenic and enzyme modulating activities. These activities may be responsible for the possible chemopreventive effects of natural compound. Modulation of diet can be used as a possible cancer chemoprevention strategy (Heo *et al.*, 2001; WCRF, 2007).

Chemoprevention is the process of using natural or synthetic compounds to block, reverse, or prevent the development of cancers through the action on multiple cellular mechanisms. Generally, these cellular mechanisms can be grouped in two: 1) Anti-mutagenesis, that includes the inhibition of the uptake, formation/activation of carcinogens, their detoxification, the blockage of carcinogen–DNA binding, and the enhancement of fidelity of DNA repair; 2) Anti-proliferation/anti-progression, that includes modification of signal transduction pathways, inhibition of oncogene activity, promotion of the cellular differentiation, enhancement of apoptosis, inhibition of inflammation and angiogenesis, and modulation of hormone/growth factor activity (Davis, 2007; Moon Y. Yeo et al., 2001). Phytochemicals may alter multiple molecular targets within a specific biological process related with cancer and when in combination with other natural compounds can have an additive or synergistic effect as well as antagonistic interactions. Nowadays, it is accepted that the combination of foods and/or multiple natural compounds may offer increased chemoprevention against cancer as compared to isolated compounds. However, the interactions between the different compounds within the food or with other foods need to be clarified. Furthermore, active compounds of many plants remain uncharacterized, which restrict the knowledge about the role of diet on cancer prevention (Davis and Milner, 2007; Mehta *et al.*, 2010).

In chemoprevention studies several experimental models can be used. However, experience shows that the results may be different depending on the experimental model used and whether the whole plants evaluated or only isolated compounds. Data from cultured cells and animal models may not reflect the response in humans. Also, plants and their isolated compounds may not have similar biological effects (Davis and Milner, 2007; Mehta *et al.*, 2010). Chemopreventive effect of food and/or its compounds depend on absorption, metabolism, distribution and excretion of phytochemicals. Phytochemicals' absorption is dependent on source and the method of food processing. In the same plant species the phytochemicals contents may change depending on the plant genotype, the season of the year and the place where the plant was grown. Intensity and duration of the exposure to dietary components also influence the cellular response. Thus, dose and duration of exposure become fundamental considerations in interpreting findings from nutritional studies (Davis and Milner, 2007).

During the last decades, some long-term intervention studies have been performed to understand the contribution of diet on prevention of diseases. However, this type of studies has the inconvenience of the high time consumption and cost. Several biomarkers have been validated to predict cancer risk and to evaluate the potential chemopreventive effect of food and/or its compounds (Davis and Milner, 2007). In general, biomarkers can be divided in three major types: biomarkers of exposure, which allow the evaluation of whether the intake of dietary components is sufficient to lead to a certain biological response; biomarkers of effect, which give information about the mechanisms of action of dietary components; and biomarkers of susceptibility, which indicate which individuals are susceptible to specific dietary exposures (Davis and Milner, 2007). In this review, we will be focus in one biomarker of exposure assessed by comet assay.

5. The comet assay

The comet assay, also called the single cell gel electrophoresis (SCGE) assay was first introduced by Ostling and Johanson in 1984 as a microelectrophoretic technique for the direct visualization of DNA damage in individual cells. In this assay, cells embedded in agarose are placed on a microscope slide, lysed by detergents in high salt solution and submitted to electrophoresis under neutral conditions. It usually accepted that, in neutral condition, DNA migration is due to presence of double-strand breaks (DSB). However, it was demonstrated that DSB as well as single strand breaks (SSB) were detected in this conditions (Collins *et al.*, 1997a; Gedik *et al.*, 1992; Ostling and Johanson, 1984). Singh *et al.*, (1988) introduced the electrophoresis under alkaline (pH >13) conditions for detecting DNA damage in single cells. At alkaline conditions, DNA migration is associated with the presence of strand breaks (single and/or double strand), SSB associated with incomplete excision repair sites, and alkali-labile sites (ALS). The alkaline version of comet assay had more success because it allows the detection of a wide spectrum of damages, and in fact almost all genotoxic agents induce more SSB and/or ALS than DSB (Fairbairn *et al.*, 1995; Tice et al., 2000).

Among the several methods to measure DNA damage including classical cytogenetic tests such as chromosome aberrations, micronuclei and sister chromatid exchanges, the comet assay has become the most commonly used. This assay shows some advantages relatively to other genotoxicity assays such as: 1) evaluates DNA damage at individual cell; 2) requires a small number of cells per sample; 3) any animal tissue can be used, since single cell/nucleus suspension can be obtained; 4) proliferating or non-proliferating cells can be used; 5) detects low levels of DNA damage (high sensitivity); 6) needs small amounts of a test substance; 7) detects several classes of DNA damage such as DSB, SSB, ALS, incomplete repair of a-basic sites and cross-links; 8) low costs; 9) simple and fast tool (Hartmann et al., 2003; Speit *et al.*, 2003). Despite great advantages, some limitations have been attributed to the comet assay: it does not detect high level of DNA damage and DNA fragments smaller than 50 kb, and therefore apoptotic cells detection is very difficult (Nossoni, 2008). The comet assay done with lymphocytes is an important biomarker for early biological effects of exposure to environmental mutagenic agents (Dusinska and Collins, 2008). Angerer *et al.*, (2007) in a review about human biomonitoring refer, however, some problems that should be kept in mind when lymphocytes are used. The major difficulty is the interpretation of data, because the damage levels and capacity to repair of these cells may be different from cells of others tissues. Usually lymphocytes repair their damage very slowly and not all the damage to cells and organs are detectable using lymphocytes. Furthermore, a great intra-individual and inter-individual variability of the basal level of DNA damage it was found that is influenced by a variety of factors such as lifestyle, diet, medication, air pollution, season, climate or exercise. Lymphocytes also show limited survival in vitro, requiring incubation with a mitogen such as phytohaemagglutinin (Collins et al., 2008).

In the last decade, scientific community demonstrated an increasing interest in the alkaline version of comet assay that has brought a rapid increase in the number of papers and reports published using this assay. Comet assay is now used in different research areas such as human and environmental biomonitoring, mechanistic studies of DNA repair, genetic toxicology, nutrition and clinical studies. Below is a detailed description of the standard comet assay and new modifications to detect different DNA damages and DNA repair capacities (fig.1).

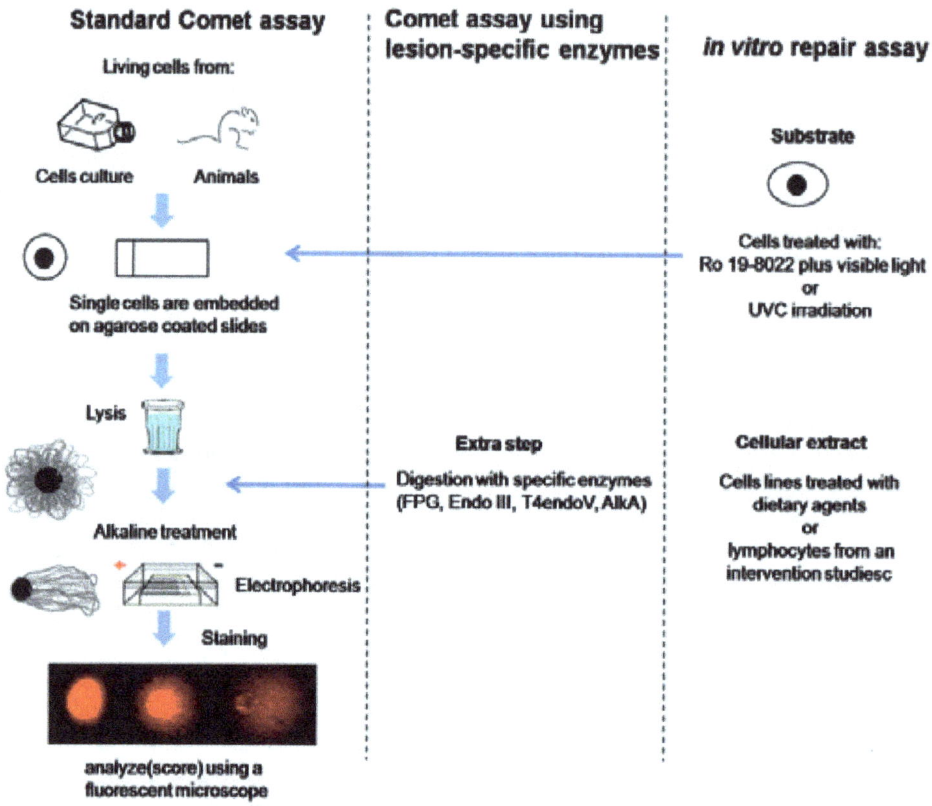

Fig. 1. General steps of the standard comet assay and its modifications.

5.1 Standard comet assay

Among the various versions of the comet assay, the alkaline (pH of the unwinding and electrophoresis buffer >13) is the most used.The first step is to cover microscope slides with 1% of normal melting point (NMP) agarose and dry it at room temperature. A second layer composed by cells embedded in 0.5% LMP agarose (at 37ºC) is spread above the first layer, covering it with a cover glass and keeping at 4ºC during few minutes. After removing cover glass, slides are lysed at least for one hour up to 24h in lysing solution containing detergent and high molarity NaCl (2.5M NaCl, 100mM Na2EDTA, 10mM Tris Base, pH 10 plus 1% Triton X-100). This solution removes membranes and soluble cellular (300mM NaOH, 1mM Na2EDTA, pH >13) constituents, as well as histones, producing nucleoids of supercoiled DNA attached to the nuclear matrix. DNA unwinding occur in alkaline conditions (pH>13) immersing slides in alkaline buffer at 4ºC. The time required for unwinding changes based on the cells being examined. In this step, breaks in the DNA relax the supercoiling and allow DNA loops to expand. Electrophoresis occurs under alkaline condition at 0.8V/cm and 300 mA for 20 min.

During electrophoresis, DNA loops containing breaks migrate towards the anode forming in the end DNA structures like a comet, with a head (the nuclear region) and a tail that contain DNA loops that extended during electrophoresis due to breaks. DNA migration is dependent of several parameters, such as, concentration of agarose in the gel, pH, temperature and duration of alkaline unwinding, temperature, voltage, and duration of electrophoresis.
After electrophoresis, slides are neutralized using neutralization buffer, stained with fluorescent agent (e.g. ethidium bromide, SYBRGold), and analyzed (scored) using a fluorescent microscope. The scoring may be done by visual scoring or by computer programs. In visual scoring the researcher scores at least one hundred comets using the following classification: 0 to comet without DNA in tail; 1, 2 and 3 with increasing amount of DNA in tail and 4 to comet were DNA is almost all in the tail. In the end the score of each sample changes between 0 and 400 (arbitrary units). An alternative methodology are the computer programs that allow to measure different parameters of the comets such as tail intensity, tail length, intensity of head, and tail moment. Tail intensity corresponds to the percentage of DNA in the tail of the comet and is the most used parameter. Intensity of tail fluorescence indicates the extent of damage. It is important to use positive and negative controls as well as to blind scoring (Collins et al., 2008; Nossoni, 2008).
Comet assay under standard conditions reflects endogenous DNA damage such as single and double strand breaks and apurinic/apyrimidinic (AP) sites in almost any eukaryotic cell population. There are other modifications that make it even more sensitive and allow to measure oxidised pyrimidines and purines and alkylation DNA damage. These modifications will be explained below.

5.2 The use of lesion-specific enzymes

Alkaline version (described above) measures strand DNA breaks and AP sites (that are converted to strand breaks). However, genotoxic agents not only induce breaks and AP sites, but also DNA damage such as base oxidation and others base modifications, that are generated in large scale in cells. Several DNA repair enzymes recognize damaged bases, introducing breaks at sites of the base damage. Thus, inclusion of an extra step of nucleoid DNA digestion with lesion-specific enzymes following lysis, allow detection of modified bases increasing the sensitivity and specificity of the comet assay (Collins, 2009; Hoelzl et al., 2009).
Endonuclease III (EndoIII) was the first enzyme used to recognize oxidized pyrimidines in DNA and to remove them, leaving an AP site that is subsequently converted in breaks at pH13. These breaks that occur at sites of base oxidation increase comet tail intensity (Collins *et al.*, 1993). Formamidopyrimidine DNA glycosylase (FPG) recognizes and breaks modified purines as well as 8-oxoguanine and also ring-opened purines, or formamidopyrimidines (Fapy) (Dusinska and Collins, 1996). T4 endonuclease V recognise UV-induced cyclobutane pyrimidine dimers (Collins *et al.*, 1997b). AlkA is a bacterial repair enzyme whose main substrate is the N^3-MeA, an alkylated base and converts it to AP sites (Collins *et al.*, 2001a).
The use of repair enzymes has been particularly useful in estimating oxidative damage of certain pollutants and drugs in several experimental models and in biomonitoring studies, for example to evaluate the role of dietary agents in protection against oxidative DNA damage. However, the specificity of the enzymes is limited, for instance FPG recognizes 8-oxoGua but also detects alkylation damage (N^7 MeG) (Speit *et al.*, 2004).
After lysis, in parallel with a slide incubated with a lesion-specific enzyme, a slide incubated without enzyme (only with buffer) is used as a control. Subtraction of control (which contain

SBs and AP sites) to the condition treated with enzyme gives a value that correspond to the damage recognized by the enzyme and is usually referred as 'netenzyme-sensitive sites'.

5.3 DNA repair assays

Beside effects on protection against DNA damage, comet assay was also developed to assess DNA repair ability of the cells and effects of diet on DNA damage repair rates. For that, two different methodologies are frequently used:

1. The "cellular repair assay" that measures the ability of cells to rejoin strand breaks induced by a DNA damaging agent. In this assay two different treatment regimens can be used: (A) Pretreatment of cells with dietary agent followed by exposure to DNA damaging agent, and cells allowed to recover in fresh culture medium at 37ºC. At different time points, samples are taken for analysis with the standard comet assay. Thus, we evaluate the effect of preincubation with test extract/compound on the ability of cells to rejoin SBs; and (B) treatment with DNA damaging agent treatment is done before cells are incubated with the test extract/compounds. In this case the aim is to test effects on nonenzymatic repair. Inclusion of lesion-specific enzymes allow to assess repair ability of others damages beyond strand breaks and AP sites.
2. The "in vitro repair assay" was developed by (Collins *et al.*, 2001b) to measure excision repair activity of cell extracts, such as lymphocytes collected in dietary intervention studies or from cells treated with dietary agents. These cell extracts are used as an extra step (similar to the use of lesion-specific enzymes) in DNA substrates containing a specific damage. The first application of this assay was the measurement of repair rates of oxidized bases, called "in vitro BER assay". In this case substrate cells are treated with the photosensitiser Ro 19-8022 (Roche) plus visible light to induce 8-oxoGua, and then cells are embedded in agarose on a slide. After lysis, substrate nucleoids are incubated with a cell extract (e.g. cells incubated with dietary agent) that have enzymes that recognize 8-oxoGua and cut at the place of the lesion. This assay allows to measure the activity of the repair enzyme 8-oxoguanine DNA glycosylase OGG1present in cell extract. A modification of the "in vitro repair assay" was introduced by Langie et al., (2006) to assess nucleotide excision repair (NER), the "in vitro NER assay". In this version cells were treated with benzo(a)pyrene diolepoxide and bulky adducts were formed. In 2009, Gaivao *et al.*, (2009) exposed cells to UVC irradiation inducing cyclobutane pyrimidine dimers and 6-4 photoproducts. Irradiated cells are embedded in agarose on a slide, and lysed to expose the DNA, which is then incubated with the cell extract. Incision at damage sites is detected using the alkaline comet assay and indicates repair ability. In these assays, higher DNA intensity in the tail indicates higher DNA repair activity of the cell extracts. Cell extracts of cells incubated with vehicle are used as control (basal) repair abilities.

5.4 Other modifications

The format of comet assay most used is 2 gels per slide. To large numbers of samples new formats have been developed, such as 12 gels per slide, that have several advantages: 1) reduces the number of cells required for each gel (approx. 200 cells/gel); 2) allows different conditions in the same slide (different genotoxic chemicals; enzymes or cell extracts); 3) requires low volume of solutions; 4) increases the number of samples processed at one time. This new format has been used in human biomonitoring studies with a great number of samples, and also when is necessary to use several repair enzymes to detect different kinds of damage (Shaposhnikov et al., 2010).

6. Application of the comet assay in chemoprevention studies

Application of the comet assay to the study of the protective effects of diet against oxidative/alkylating DNA damage and repair will be summarized bellow. For more details see the following revisions, (Hoelzl et al., 2009; Moller and Loft, 2002; Wasson *et al.*, 2008 and Wong *et al.*, 2005).

6.1 Effect of diet on prevention of oxidative DNA damage

Prevention of DNA damage is one of the cellular mechanisms that may prevent cancer. Diet plays an important role in regulating DNA damage for instance by modulating the antioxidant/oxidant balance. The protective effect observed in many studies could be due, in part, to the presence of phenolic and/or non-phenolic constituents that have ability to act as antioxidant by free radical scavenging and chelating metal ions (Anderson *et al.*, 2000); (Ross and Kasum, 2002). They can also act as indirect antioxidant by increasing levels of antioxidants such as glutathione (GSH) and/or by increasing the activity of antioxidant enzymes such as catalase (CAT), glutathione peroxidase (GPX) and superoxide dismutase (SOD) (Alia *et al.*, 2005; Lima *et al.*, 2005; Lima *et al.*, 2006; Frei and Higdon, 2003). Phytochemicals can also modulate phase I (activating) enzymes and phase II (detoxifying) enzymes involved in xenobiotic metabolism (Chen and Kong, 2004; Ferguson *et al.*, 2004; Moon *et al.*, 2006; Ross and Kasum, 2002).

Phytochemicals are bioactive compounds present in plants where they are produced as secondary metabolites to protect themselves from several pathogenic agents. Their consumption by humans confers protection against some diseases. Most bioactive phytochemicals belong to one of 5 groups: polyphenols, carotenoids, alkaloids, nitrogen-containing compounds, and organosulfur compounds. Polyphenols and carotenoids include several hundreds of compounds and are the most studied groups. Polyphenols may be further classified into 4 groups, according with the number of phenol rings that they contain: Flavonois, phenolic acids, stilbenes, and lignans. The flavonoids may themselves be classified into the follow subgroups: flavonols, flavones, isoflavones, flavanones, flavanols and anthocyanidins (Fig.2).

6.1.1 Polyphenols

Numerous studies have shown the antioxidant and DNA protective properties of polyphenols. Quercetin is a flavonoid found in a variety of foods including apples, onions, wine and tea. Several studies, including our own showed the protective effects of quercetin against oxidative DNA damage in HepG2 cells (Lima et al., 2006; Ramos et al., 2008), Caco-2 cells (Aherne and O'Brien, 1999), HMB-2 cells (Horvathova *et al.*, 2005), human macrophage (U-937 cells) (Kanupriya et al., 2006; Moon et al., 2006); human lymphocytes (healthy volunteers) (Wilms *et al.*, 2007), and murine leukemia L1210 cells (Horvathova *et al.*, 2003). Wilms *et al.*, (2005) reported the protective effects of quercetin against the formation of oxidative DNA damage and bulky DNA adducts in human lymphocytes, induced by H_2O_2 and benzo(a)pyrene (B(a)P, respectively. In the same study, results obtained in an in vivo experiments showed that four weeks of quercetin-rich blueberry/apple juice mixture

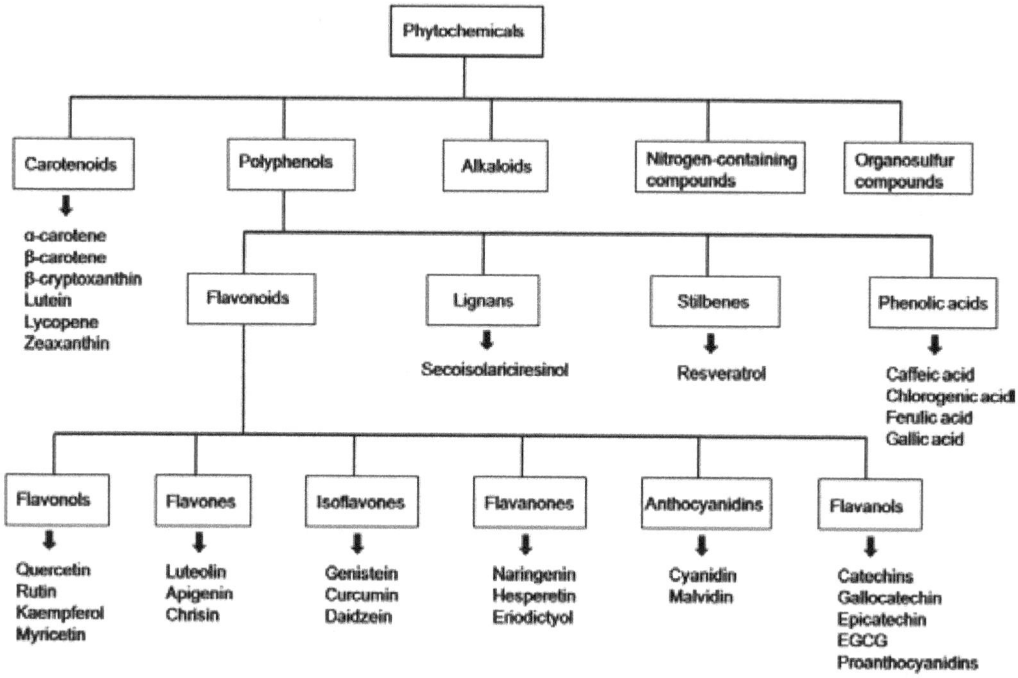

Fig. 2. Classification of phytochemicals and the main natural compounds in each group.

consumption led to a decrease of oxidative DNA damage and BPDE-DNA adduct levels by 41% and 11%, respectively, although the results were not statistically significant. Increases in the total antioxidant capacity of plasma and in plasma quercetin content were observed. Others flavonoids, such as luteolin (Cai *et al.*, 1997; Horvathova et al., 2005; Lima et al., 2006; Min and Ebeler, 2008; Ramos *et al.*, 2010b), rutin (Moon et al., 2006; Ramos et al., 2008), genistein (Cai et al., 1997), catechin and epicatechin (Kanupriya et al., 2006), showed antigenotoxic effects against oxidative DNA damage in several cell models.

In an ex vivo study, lymphocytes from three healthy subjects were pre-incubated with several dietary antioxidants. Quercetin and caffeic acid (a phenolic acid) protected against H_2O_2-induced DNA damage, however in this study no effect was observed when cells were treated with catechin, epicatechin, catechin gallate and epicatechin gallate (Szeto and Benzie, 2002).

Besides quercetin and rutin, we reported that ursolic acid (a triterpenoid) protect against DNA damage induced by tert-butyl hydroperoxide (t-BHP) in HepG2 cells (Ramos et al., 2008). Other reports showed that ursolic acid and/or luteolin protect DNA from damage induced by H_2O_2, t-BHP or AZT (3_-azido-3_-dideoxythymidine) in several cell lines, such as leukemic cells, HEI-OC1 auditory cells and PC12 cells (Horvathova et al., 2003; Horvathova *et al.*, 2004; Ovesna *et al.*, 2006; Yu et al., 2009; Noroozi *et al.*, 1998; Silva *et al.*, 2008). Rosmarinic acid (RA), reduced the frequency of micronuclei and the extent of DNA damage induced by doxorubicin in V79 cells (Furtado *et al.*, 2009). Caffeic acid (3,4-dihydroxy cinnamic acid), also a dietary phenolic compound, showed a photoprotective effect (Devipriya *et al.*, 2008; Benkovic et al., 2009). Human blood lymphocytes irradiated with UVB (280-320) after pretreatment with caffeic acid exhibited lower levels of lipid peroxidation markers such as thiobarbituric acid reactive substance (TBARS) and lipid hydroperoxide (LPH) and also a decrease of UVB-induced DNA damage (Prasad *et al.*, 2009).

Naringin, a citrus grapefruit flavonone, showed antigenotoxic properties in V79 cells (Jagetia *et al.*, 2007). 4-Coumaric acid, a phenolic acid present in many foods and drinks, such as wine, tea, berries, apples, spinach and cereals reduced basal oxidative DNA damage in rat colonic mucosa when evaluated by comet assay (Guglielmi *et al.*, 2003). Resveratrol, found in substantial amounts in several types of beverages including red wine and fruits, showed genoprotective effects under conditions of oxidative stress induced by H_2O_2 in C6 glioma cells (Quincozes-Santos et al., 2007). Apigenin, a flavonoid widely distributed in many herbs, fruits, and vegetables, has shown chemopreventive activities in several biological systems. Jeyabal *et al.*, (2005) reported the protective role of apigenin against the oxidative stress caused by N-nitrosodiethylamine and phenobarbital in Wistar albino rats. Rusak et al., (2010), showed genoprotective effects of apigenin and other flavonoids (luteolin and kaempferol) in human peripheral lymphocytes against oxidative damage induced by hydrogen peroxide.

6.1.2 Carotenoids

Tomato is one of the main sources of lycopene, a carotenoid with antioxidant properties. Pretreatment of rat hepatocytes with lycopene (1.86, 9.31 and 18.62 μM) in culture, showed a significant decrease in the levels of TBARS and DNA damage induced by gamma-radiation. Antioxidant enzymes such as superoxide dismutase (SOD), catalase (CAT) and glutathione peroxidase (GPx), as well as, the levels of GSH, vitamins A, E, C, increased significantly when hepatocytes were pretreated with the carotenoid (Srinivasan et al., 2007). At physiological concentrations (0.3-10 μM) lycopene and beta-carotene also protect Chinese hamster lung fibroblasts against DNA damage induced by 3-morpholinosydnonimine (SIN-1) (Muzandu et al., 2006). In a human intervention study, healthy volunteers were submitted to a supplementation with lycopene during 8 weeks. Consumption of lycopene decreased oxidative DNA damage in lymphocytes and urinary 8-hydroxy deoxoguanosine levels when compared with the basal levels (Devaraj et al., 2008). Also, Zhao *et al.*, (2006) evaluated the protective effect of lycopene and others carotenoids against DNA damage in humans. Here, thirty-seven healthy, nonsmoking postmenopausal women consumed for 56 days a daily dose of mixed carotenoids (lycopene, lutein and beta-carotene; 4 mg each), 12 mg of a single carotenoid (lycopene, lutein or beta-carotene), or placebo. At the end the lymphocytes were isolated and DNA damage measured by comet assay. The results showed that all groups that consumed carotenoids had significantly lower endogenous DNA damage than that found on baseline measurements. No differences were found in placebo group. Lutein also decreased DNA damage induced by cisplatin in mice when evaluated by comet assay and increased GSH levels when compared with a negative control group (Serpeloni *et al.*, 2010). Lorenzo *et al.*, (2009) reported that β-cryptoxanthin at low concentrations, close to those found in plasma, protects Caco-2 and HeLa cells from oxidative DNA damage induced by H_2O_2 or by visible light in the presence of a photosensitizer. Consumption of β-carotene decreased the number of strand breaks induced by H_2O_2 in lymphocytes (Panayiotidis and Collins, 1997).

Pre-treatment with astaxanthin, a red carotenoid used as a dietary additive, at 12.5, 25 and 50 mg/kg/day for 5 days before cyclophosphamide treatment resulted in the amelioration of antioxidant defenses (glutathione and superoxide dismutase) in the liver and decreased DNA damage evaluated by standard comet assay and using specific-enzymes (FPG and EndoIII) in bone marrow cells and peripheral blood lymphocytes isolated from mice. This carotenoid also reduced the frequency of chromosomal breakage and micronucleus formation in the mouse bone marrow cells and peripheral blood. Astaxanthin, also showed antigenotoxic effects against cyclophosphamide in germ cell from male mice (Tripathi and Jena, 2008).

6.1.3 Whole foods

Several studies, including our own with colon cancer cells, have found that polyphenol rich plant extracts inhibit formation of SBs and 8-oxoGua induced by oxidantive agents (Ramos *et al.*, 2010a). Some plants, such as *Salvia officinalis L.* (sage), *Rosmarinus officinalis L.* (rosemary) and *Origanum vulgare L.* (oregano) have antioxidant properties that confer protection against oxidative DNA damage in colon cells as demonstrated by Aherne et al., (2007).

Green tea is rich in polyphenolic antioxidants and their effects on health are the subject of several studies. Green tea decreased DNA oxidation in lymphocytes, colonocytes and hepatocytes when rats ingested 6.5 mg/kg bw per day, 5 days of tea extract (Kager et al., 2010). Evidences of genoprotective effects of green tea appear not only from in vitro and in vivo studies, but also from human supplementation trials. Human lymphocytes isolated from healthy volunteers that took 2 x 150 ml/d of 1% (w/v) green tea showed a decrease of basal oxidation-induced DNA damage with and without FPG enzyme (Han *et al.*, 2011). One of the main constituents of green tea is (-)-epigallocatechin-3-gallate (EGCG) that could be responsible for their beneficial effects. In human peripheral leucocytes treatement with low EGCG concentrations (2-100μM) decreased both bleomycin-induced breaks and endonuclease III sensitive sites (Glei and Pool-Zobel, 2006).

Apple is one of the most consumed fruit, therefore is an important source of polyphenols in humans. Their chemoprotective effects have been shown in vitro and in vivo studies (Koch et al., 2009; Veeriah et al., 2008). Apple juice has been found to possess antioxidant and antiproliferative activities as well as the ability to increase the expression of phase II gene glutathione S-transferase T2 (GSTT2) in human colon cells (Petermann et al., 2009). Apple extract can also protect against oxidative-induced DNA damage in human colon cells, such as LT97 (Miene (Miene *et al.*, 2009), HT29, HCT115 and CaCo-2 cells (McCann et al., 2007; Schaefer et al., 2006). Also, grape juices exhibit antigenotoxic activity (Dani et al., 2009).

The anticarcinogenic properties of olive oil have been attributed to the presence of phenolic compounds. Fabiani et al., (2008) reported that some of its isolated compounds (e.g. hydroxytyrosol, [3,4-dyhydroxyphenyl-ethanol (3,4-DHPEA)] and a complex mixture of phenols extracted from virgin olive oil) protected against H2O2 in human peripheral blood mononuclear cells and promyelocytic leukemia cells (HL60). These results have a great impact not only because of the high level of protection observed (between 80 and 90%) but also because, according to the authors, the concentrations tested could easily be reached with normal intake of olive oil.

Annatto is a native shrub from Tropical America, whose seeds are a rich source of carotenoids, such as bixin, norbixin and phytoene and have antigenotoxic effects against oxidative DNA damage (Kovary et al., 2001).

Results from human intervention trials have demonstrated the protective effect of isolated compounds as well as fruits and vegetables in peripheral lymphocytes. Pool-Zobel *et al.*, (1997) showed a decrease in pyrimidine oxidation during supplementation with carrot juice. Porrini and Riso, (2000) reported that supplementation with tomato that is rich in lycopene, increase protection against H_2O_2-induced DNA damage in lymphocytes. Also a diet rich in fruit and vegetables for 14 days showed a DNA protection from oxidative damage in lymphocytes (Thompson et al., 1999). Broccoli intake also decreases oxidative DNA damage in smokers and nonsmokers (Riso *et al.*, 2009). In a recent study, Sprague-Dawley rats fed with a wild-blueberry diet or a control diet for four or eight weeks were used to assess the effect of the consumption of this fruit on the resistance to H_2O_2-induced DNA damage. After treatment period, lymphocytes were exposed, ex vivo, to H_2O_2 and it was observed that wild-blueberry diet did not change antioxidant capacity in lymphocytes after eight weeks of treatment, but increased DNA protection against oxidative damage (Del Bo et al., 2010). Dulebohn et al., (2008) using the same animal model, reported that blueberries consumption for 3 weeks increase GST activity and decrease oxidative DNA damage in the liver. However, contrarily to in vitro studies, blueberries consumption did not significantly increase phase II enzyme activities in short-term supplementation times.

As described above, many isolated compounds and some plants showed genoprotective effects in several experimental models, however it is important to keep in mind that these dietary agents can also induce DNA damage in certain conditions. The balance between the genoprotective and genotoxic effects of dietary agents is dependent on their concentration, incubation period and types of cells (Rusak et al., 2010).

6.2 Effect of diet on prevention of alkylating DNA damage

Alkylation of DNA can be an important initial step in cancer formation. High levels of alkylating damage have been found in human colorectal DNA where high incidence of tumours have been observed (Hall *et al.*, 1991; Povey *et al.*, 2000). To assess antigenotoxic effects of diet against alkylating damage, several experimental models have been developed. Among them, colon tumours induction in rodent models, with carcinogenic chemicals such as 1,2-dimethylhydrazine (DMH) or azoxymethane (AOM) are the most used, and they are believed to be representative of colon carcinogenesis in humans (Barth et al., 2005).

6.2.1 Phytochemicals

Dolara et al., (2005) reported that red wine polyphenols (50 mg/kg) administered to F344 rats for 16 weeks inhibited colon carcinogenesis induced by AOM or DMH. Wine polyphenols also decreased basal level of DNA oxidative damage of the colon mucosa. Supplementation of Wistar male rats with resveratrol showed to significantly decrease DMH-induced leukocyte DNA damage. In this study, an increase of levels of enzymic and non-enzymic antioxidant defense and a decrease in the extent of lipid peroxidation markers were also observed (Sengottuvelan *et al.*, 2009). Other chemopreventive agents, such as quercetin, rutin, curcumin, silymarin, lycopene and farnesol, with antioxidant properties, have been found to inhibit DMH- and AOM-induced colon carcinogenesis and DNA damage in animal models (Kim et al., 1998; Volate *et al.*, 2005). Lupeol, a pentacyclic triterpene present in mango, also protected against DMBA induced DNA alkylation damage in Swiss albino mice (Nigam *et al.*, 2007).

6.2.2 Whole foods

Many whole foods and plant crude extracts have also been found to protect against alkylating damage. The water extract of *Salvia officinalis* prevent formation of aberrant crypt foci (ACFs, a pre-carcinogenic lesion) induced by AOM in rat colon and also protected DNA of colonocytes (unpublished observations). Using the same experimental model, Sengupta *et al.*, (2004 and 2003) reported that tomato and garlic prevent ACFs, induced by AOM in rat colon. Tomato also decreased incidence and progression of 9,10-dimethyl benzanthracene (DMBA)-induced mouse skin tumours (De and Das, 2001). Intake of beer reduced ACF formation and protected against DNA damage induced by AOM in the rat colon mucosa (Nozawa et al., 2004). de Lima *et al.*, (2005) evaluated the effect of aqueous extract of propolis on the formation of DMH-induced ACF and DNA damage in rat colon. Propolis had no effect on ACF formation, however, modulation of DMH-induced DNA damage in colon cells was observed. At lower concentrations (12, 34 and 108 mg/Kg bw/day) aqueous extract of propolis decrease the level of DNA damage. However, the highest concentration (336mg/Kg bw/day) induced DNA damage in rat colon. Dietary agents such as, ginseng, lemon grass and propolis, have been found to inhibit DMH- and AOM-induced colon carcinogenesis and DNA damage in animal model (Bazo et al., 2002; Suaeyun *et al.*, 1997; Volate et al., 2005). Consumption of onion, blueberries (Boateng et al., 2007), and garbanzo beans (Murillo *et al.*, 2004) also decreased the number of AOM-induced ACFs in rats and mice, respectively.

Some studies reported antigenotoxic effects of diet against alkylating DNA damage using cytogenetic assays (micronucleus assay) (Azevedo Bentes Monteiro Neto et al., 2011; Gurbuz *et al.*, 2009). Edenharder *et al.*, (1998) reported that sweet cherries, strawberries, cucumber, tomatoes, bananas, oranges, asparagus, yellow red peppers and specially spinach had a protective effect against clastogenicity of cyclosphosphamide (an alkylating drug) in mice.

Using comet assay some in vivo studies have shown the antigenotoxic effects of dietary agents, namely, artepillin C (a polyphenolic acid found in Brazilian green propolis and Baccharis dracunculifolia) (Azevedo Bentes Monteiro Neto et al., 2011), safranal, (a constituent of Crocus sativus L. stigmas) (Hosseinzadeh and Sadeghnia, 2007), orange juice (Franke *et al.*, 2005b) and vitamin C (Franke *et al.*, 2005a) against DNA damage induced by methyl methanesulfonate (MMS). Also lemongrass protected leukocytes from DNA damage induced by N-methyl-N-nitrosurea (MNU) (Bidinotto *et al.*, 2010). Data from application of comet assay in the assessment of genoprotective effects of diet against alkylating DNA damage is limited. First, AlkA is, as far as we know, the only repair enzyme used for detection of alkylating DNA damage by the comet assay (Collins *et al.*, 2001a). Alk A recognises 3-MeA in DNA, but its specificity is low, detecting other modified bases, some of which are also other alkylated bases. Furthermore, 3-MeA is not the most abundant alkylating damage and it does not represent the alkylating damage with more mutagenic/carcinogenic potential. Other alkylating lesions, like N^7MeG, the most abundant lesion, and O^6MeG, the most mutagenic, are until now undectectable by comet assay.

6.3 Effect of diet on induction of DNA repair

DNA damage can arrest cell cycle progression to allow DNA repair, preventing, therefore, replication of errors, or to induce apoptosis to eliminate cells severely damaged. Defective DNA repair is usually linked to human cancer development. Therefore, enhancement of DNA repair can be understood as a prevention strategy against cancer and an important molecular target for dietary phytochemicals (Davis and Milner, 2007). However, few studies have investigated whether DNA repair activity can be modified by diet in humans.

New modifications of the comet assay have been developed to assess effects of dietary agents on DNA repair ability (as described above). Briefly, the "cellular repair assay" measures the ability of cells to rejoin strand breaks induced by a DNA damaging agent; while the "in vitro repair assay" measures the excision repair activity of a protein extract prepared from cells treated with dietary agents, incubating with a DNA substrate containing a specific type of damage.

6.3.1 Polyphenols

Recently, we reported that luteolin and luteolin-7-glucoside increased rejoining of strand breaks after treatment with H_2O_2 in Caco-2 cells. Luteolin-7-glucoside also had a BER inductive effect increasing incision activity in Caco-2 cells (Ramos *et al.*, 2010a; Ramos *et al.*, 2010b). Quercetin also increased rejoining of strand breaks induced by *t*-BHP in HepG2 (Ramos et al., 2008). Moreover, dietary agents such as flavonoids, vitamins E and C had been reported as inducers of oxidative DNA damage repair activity (Davis and Milner, 2007).

6.3.2 Carotenoids

An in vitro study using HeLa and Caco-2 cells reported that β-cryptoxanthin increased rejoining of strand breaks induced by H_2O_2 and increase the repair of oxidised bases. However, increase of repair activity was not related with increase of hOGG1 or APE1expression (Lorenzo et al., 2009). The lack of correlation between activity and mRNA expression of OGG1 and APE1 has also been demonstrated in other studies (Collins *et al.*, 2003; Silva *et al.*, 2009). β-carotene, lutein and lycopene also enhanced strand breaks rejoining in lymphocytes (Fillion *et al.*, 1998; Torbergsen and Collins, 2000). Paz-Elizur *et al.*, (2007) measured OGG1 activity and mRNA expression in 120 healthy individuals and a poor correlation between activity and mRNA was found.

6.3.3 Whole foods

Water extracts of Salvia species increased rejoining of strand breaks after treatment with H_2O_2 in Caco-2 cells. These water extracts also increased incision activity of a Caco-2 cell extract on a DNA substrate containing specific oxidative damage (8-oxoGua) (Ramos *et al.*, 2010a). Nakamura et al., (2000) reported that aqueous fractions of Fushimi sweet pepper increase repair against ultraviolet-induced cyclobutane pyrimidine dimers in human fibroblasts.

Collins et al., (2003), in a human intervention study, showed that 3 weeks of a dietary supplementation with kiwifruit increased DNA repair capacity measured by "in vitro repair assay". Also Freese, (2006) showed that kiwifruit consumption increased DNA repair capacity in human lymphocytes. Brevik *et al.*, (2011) in a human biomonitoring study, reported that consumption of kiwifruits and antioxidant-rich plant products reduced DNA strand breaks in lymphocytes. Increase of BER activity was observed in the group that consumed antioxidant-rich plant products. However, a reduction of NER activity was observed in both groups. No explanations have been found for this decrease in NER pathway. Diet supplementation with cooked carrots, during 3 weeks, increased in vitro repair activity and strand break rejoining in lymphocytes (Astley *et al.*, 2004).

High dietary folate intake has been associated with a decreased risk of cancer development, such as colorectal cancer. In vitro, rodent and human studies demonstrated that low folate intake increases uracil misincorporation leading to increase of DNA damage, chromosomal breakage and malignant transformation; modulates DNA repair by inhibiting thymidine and purine biosynthesis and induces epigenetic changes leading to global DNA hypomethylation and/or changes in gene-specific methylation and protooncogene activation (Duthie and McMillan, 1997; Duthie, 2010; Duthie *et al.*, 2000; Melnyk et al., 1999). In vivo, folate deficiency induced DNA repair, such as increase of OGG1 and MGMT (Duthie *et al.*, 2010). However, remains unclear if increasing folate intake improve DNA repair. Generaly, the protective role of folate against carcinogenesis is not completely understood.

7. Effects of phytochemicals through DNA repair modulation and their interaction with alkylating agents used as chemotherapeutic

Some DNA-damaging agents (specially alkylating agents) are used in cancer therapy due to their ability to induce DNA damage and subsequently apoptosis of tumor cells (Maynard et al., 2009). The efficacy of DNA damage-based cancer therapy is modulated by DNA repair pathways. Therefore these pathways may, attenuate the therapeutic effects of alkylating agents. These drugs are usually classified in two classes: monofunctional (e.g., N-methyl-N_-nitro-N-nitrosoguanidine [MNNG], temozolomide [TMZ] and dacarbazine) and bifunctional alkylating agents (e.g., carmustine [BCNU], cyclophosphamide, lomustine [CCNU] and fotemustine).

BCNU, induces several kinds of DNA damage such as cross-linking, strand breaks and modified bases (Kondo et al., 2010). Between alkylation damage, N^7 alkyl-guanine is the most abundant (around 90% of the total alkylation events) and O^6 alkyl-guanine is the less frequent. O^6 alkyl-guanine, if not repaired before cell division, can form base pairs with T, generating GC→AT transitions mutations by action of MMR pathway. O^6 alkyl-guanine is the lesion mainly responsible for the cytotoxic and mutagenic effects of these alkylating drugs. However O^6 alkyl-guanine can be repaired by MGMT. In human colorectal adenoma, reduced MGMT activity has been found. Therefore, more mutations occur when cells are treated with alkylating agent (Lees *et al.*, 2004; Lees *et al.*, 2002). However, high levels of MGMT where found in some other tumors (Baer et al., 1993). In the context of therapy with alkylating agents, inhibition of MGMT activity in tumor cells is desirable. The coadjuvant drug O^6-benzylguanine (O^6-BG) inactivates MGMT, acting as a pseudosubstrate. Effect of O^6-BG has been investigated when in combination with an alkylating drug to increase its efficacy (Liu *et al.*, 2002).

N^7-alkylG is the most frequent alkylation damage however is not considered to be as mutagenic as O^6-alkylG because it is efficiently repaired by BER pathway. N-methylpurine-DNAglycoslase (MPG), the only glycosylase that recognizes alkylation lesions in animal cells, removes N^7-alkylG by hydrolysis of the N-glycosylic bond creating an AP site that is repaired by the other enzymes of BER pathway (Drablos et al., 2004). An overexpression of MPG increases the production of AP sites. If the levels of the other enzymes of BER pathway remain unaltered, repair of AP sites is low and accumulation of these lesions becomes cytotoxic and mutagenic. Therefore, an overexpression of MPG or a decrease in other enzymes involved in the subsequent steps in BER pathway, increases cytotoxicity of alkylating drugs. This cytoxicity becomes more relevant when cells are resistant to cytotoxicity from O^6-alkylation.

MGMT and MMR have contrasting effects on DNA O6-alkylG. While MGMT is an efficient mechanism of repair, MMR in contrast, does not remove the alkylated base but introduce more lesions like strand break in an attempt to repair the mismatch. Accumulation of strand breaks may activate apoptotic pathways, leading to cell death. In some cells, resistance to alkylating agents can be mediated by MGMT and MMR. Active MGMT and loss of MMR pathway protect cells against the cell death induced by methylating chemotherapeutic drugs (Allan and Travis, 2005). Depletion of MGMT activity (for example, by O^6-BG or by epigenetic silencing of the MGMT gene) and intact MMR system results in reversion of resistance with high sensitivity to the cytotoxic effects of alkylating drugs (Casorelli et al., 2008; Esteller et al., 2000; Hegi et al., 2005). Tumors with low MGMT level are more sensitive to alkylating chemotherapy (Bandres et al., 2005). Therefore,DNA repair mechanisms may be understood as a promising target to develop new cancer treatments (Helleday *et al.*, 2008; Jiricny, 2006). Different strategies have been developed to enhance the efficacy of chemotherapy using alkylating agents. In tumor cells, inhibition of MGMT activity and/or BER pathway decreases resistance to alkylating drugs (Drablos et al., 2004; Jaiswal et al., 2011; Middleton and Margison, 2003). Downregulation of DNA repair pathways (except MMR) may increase efficacy of alkylating agents, decreasing the amount of drug needed for chemotherapy and consequently reduction of the side effects (Kondo et al., 2010).

Dietary agents that modulate MGMT expression and/or BER pathway may play an important role in chemotherapy when in combination with alkylating agents. However this subject, in contrast to chemoprevention, has received little attention. Some studies have been that dietary agents may increase MGMT activity. Niture *et al.*, (2006), investigated the potential ability of some Indian medicinal plants extracts to modulate MGMT activity and expression in human peripheral blood lymphocytes and cancer cell lines. The results showed that both the ethanolic and aqueous extracts from neem (*Azadirachta indica*), holy basil (*Ocimum sanctum*), winter cherry (*Withania somnifera*), and oregano (*Origanum majorana*) increased MGMT expression and its activity. Extracts from gooseberry (*Emblica officinalis*), common basil (*Ocimum basilicum*), and spearmint (*Mentha viridis*) also increased MGMT levels, however to a smaller extent. Later, the same author reported that some phytochemicals such as curcumin, silymarin and resveratrol increase protein expression as well as activity of MGMT in lymphocytes and cancer cell lines (Niture *et al.*, 2007). In tumor cells a number of genes are abnormally methylated. Some dietary agents, such as genistein and epigallocatechin-3-gallate showed the ability to reactivate some methylation-silenced genes in cancer cells like MGMT due to a direct inhibition of DNA methyltransferase (Fang et al., 2005; Fang et al., 2003). Recently, Billson et al., (2009), demonstrated that a high vegetable intake in humans decreases MGMT activity in normal colorectal mucosa. To understand the real role of dietary agents on chemotherapy when in combination with alkylating drugs more studies are need.

8. Conclusion

Prevention of DNA damage and/or enhanced DNA repair activity by dietary agents constitute an important strategy to prevent mutations and consequently inhibit the carcinogenic process. Diet supplementation with phytochemicals, with beneficial effects, increases their concentrations in the organism. However, effects of supra-physiological concentrations need to be evaluated in each case since a safe phytochemical at physiological concentrations can be toxic at higher concentrations.

The comet assay is a powerful tool to assess the effects of diet on DNA. The immense literature (more than 5500 papers in Pubmed since 1995) that use comet assay (standard and modified versions) demonstrates the real potential of this assay. Some dietary agents have shown ability to prevent DNA damage (oxidative and/or alkylanting) in several experimental models from in vitro to human intervention studies. Less is known about the effect of diet on DNA repair modulation. However, the modifications of comet assay (e.g. use specific-enzymes) gives an opportunity to enhance the knowledge in this field. In spite of the large number of publications much remains to be done. An emergent field is the effect of combinations between diet and drugs used in chemotherapy. In our view, comet assay can be a useful approach also to understand the role of dietary constituents on chemotherapy.

9. Acknowledgment

Ramos A.A. is supported by the Foundation for Science and Technology, Portugal, grant SFRH/BD/35672/2007.

10. References

Aherne, S. A., Kerry, J. P. & O'Brien, N. M. (2007). Effects of plant extracts on antioxidant status and oxidant-induced stress in Caco-2 cells. Br J Nutr, 97, 321-328.

Aherne, S. A. & O'Brien, N. M. (1999). Protection by the flavonoids myricetin, quercetin, and rutin against hydrogen peroxide-induced DNA damage in Caco-2 and Hep G2 cells. Nutr Cancer, 34, 160-166.

Alia, M., Ramos, S., Mateos, R., Bravo, L. & Goya, L. (2005). Response of the antioxidant defense system to tert-butyl hydroperoxide and hydrogen peroxide in a human hepatoma cell line (HepG2). J Biochem Mol Toxicol, 19, 119-128.

Allan, J. M. & Travis, L. B. (2005). Mechanisms of therapy-related carcinogenesis. Nat Rev Cancer, 5, 943-955.

Allen, R. G. & Tresini, M. (2000). Oxidative stress and gene regulation. Free Radic Biol Med, 28, 463-499.

Anderson, R. F., Amarasinghe, C., Fisher, L. J., Mak, W. B. & Packer, J. E. (2000). Reduction in free-radical-induced DNA strand breaks and base damage through fast chemical repair by flavonoids. Free Radic Res, 33, 91-103.

Angerer, J., Ewers, U. & Wilhelm, M. (2007). Human biomonitoring: state of the art. Int J Hyg Environ Health, 210, 201-228.

Armstrong, M. J. & Galloway, S. M. (1997). Mismatch repair provokes chromosome aberrations in hamster cells treated with methylating agents or 6-thioguanine, but not with ethylating agents. Mutat Res, 373, 167-178.

Astley, S. B., Elliott, R. M., Archer, D. B. & Southon, S. (2004). Evidence that dietary supplementation with carotenoids and carotenoid-rich foods modulates the DNA damage: repair balance in human lymphocytes. Br J Nutr, 91, 63-72.

Azevedo Bentes Monteiro Neto, M., Souza Lima, I. M., Furtado, R. A., Bastos, J. K., Silva Filho, A. A. & Tavares, D. C. (2011). Antigenotoxicity of artepillin C in vivo evaluated by the micronucleus and comet assays. J Appl Toxicol.

Baer, J. C., Freeman, A. A., Newlands, E. S., Watson, A. J., Rafferty, J. A. & Margison, G. P. (1993). Depletion of O6-alkylguanine-DNA alkyltransferase correlates with potentiation of temozolomide and CCNU toxicity in human tumour cells. Br J Cancer, 67, 1299-1302.

Bandres, E., Andion, E., Escalada, A., Honorato, B., Catalan, V., Cubedo, E., Cordeu, L., Garcia, F., Zarate, R., Zabalegui, N. & Garcia-Foncillas, J. (2005). Gene expression profile induced by BCNU in human glioma cell lines with differential MGMT expression. J Neurooncol, 73, 189-198.

Bartek, J., Bartkova, J. & Lukas, J. (2007). DNA damage signalling guards against activated oncogenes and tumour progression. Oncogene, 26, 7773-7779.

Barth, S. W., Fahndrich, C., Bub, A., Dietrich, H., Watzl, B., Will, F., Briviba, K. & Rechkemmer, G. (2005). Cloudy apple juice decreases DNA damage, hyperproliferation and aberrant crypt foci development in the distal colon of DMH-initiated rats. Carcinogenesis, 26, 1414-1421.

Bazo, A. P., Rodrigues, M. A., Sforcin, J. M., de Camargo, J. L., Ribeiro, L. R. & Salvadori, D. M. (2002). Protective action of propolis on the rat colon carcinogenesis. Teratog Carcinog Mutagen, 22, 183-194.

Benhamou, S. & Sarasin, A. (2000). Variability in nucleotide excision repair and cancer risk: a review. Mutat Res, 462, 149-158.

Benkovic, V., Knezevic, A. H., Orsolic, N., Basic, I., Ramic, S., Viculin, T., Knezevic, F. & Kopjar, N. (2009). Evaluation of radioprotective effects of propolis and its flavonoid constituents: in vitro study on human white blood cells. Phytother Res, 23, 1159-1168.

Bidinotto, L. T., Costa, C. A., Salvadori, D. M., Costa, M., Rodrigues, M. A. & Barbisan, L. F. (2010). Protective effects of lemongrass (Cymbopogon citratus STAPF) essential oil on DNA damage and carcinogenesis in female Balb/C mice. J Appl Toxicol.

Billson, H. A., Harrison, K. L., Lees, N. P., Hall, C. N., Margison, G. P. & Povey, A. C. (2009). Dietary variables associated with DNA N7-methylguanine levels and O6-alkylguanine DNA-alkyltransferase activity in human colorectal mucosa. Carcinogenesis, 30, 615-620.

Boateng, J., Verghese, M., Shackelford, L., Walker, L. T., Khatiwada, J., Ogutu, S., Williams, D. S., Jones, J., Guyton, M., Asiamah, D., Henderson, F., Grant, L., DeBruce, M., Johnson, A., Washington, S. & Chawan, C. B. (2007). Selected fruits reduce azoxymethane (AOM)-induced aberrant crypt foci (ACF) in Fisher 344 male rats. Food Chem Toxicol, 45, 725-732.

Brevik, A., Karlsen, A., Azqueta, A., Tirado, A. E., Blomhoff, R. & Collins, A. (2011). Both base excision repair and nucleotide excision repair in humans are influenced by nutritional factors. Cell Biochem Funct, 29, 36-42.

Bugni, J. M., Meira, L. B. and Samson, L. D. (2009) Alkylation-induced colon tumorigenesis in mice deficient in the Mgmt and Msh6 proteins. Oncogene, 28, 734-741.

Cai, Q., Rahn, R. O. & Zhang, R. (1997). Dietary flavonoids, quercetin, luteolin and genistein, reduce oxidative DNA damage and lipid peroxidation and quench free radicals. Cancer Lett, 119, 99-107.

Caldecott, K. W. (2007). Mammalian single-strand break repair: mechanisms and links with chromatin. DNA Repair (Amst), 6, 443-453.

Casorelli, I., Russo, M. T. & Bignami, M. (2008). Role of mismatch repair and MGMT in response to anticancer therapies. Anticancer Agents Med Chem, 8, 368-380.

Chen, C. and Kong, A. N. (2004). Dietary chemopreventive compounds and ARE/EpRE signaling. Free Radic Biol Med, 36, 1505-1516.

Collins, A. R. (2004). The comet assay for DNA damage and repair: principles, applications, and limitations. Mol Biotechnol, 26, 249-261.

Collins, A. R. (2009). Investigating oxidative DNA damage and its repair using the comet assay. Mutat Res, 681, 24-32.

Collins, A. R., Dobson, V. L., Dusinska, M., Kennedy, G. & Stetina, R. (1997a). The comet assay: what can it really tell us? Mutat Res, 375, 183-193.

Collins, A. R., Dusinska, M. & Horska, A. (2001a). Detection of alkylation damage in human lymphocyte DNA with the comet assay. Acta Biochim Pol, 48, 611-614.

Collins, A. R., Dusinska, M., Horvathova, E., Munro, E., Savio, M. & Stetina, R. (2001b). Inter-individual differences in repair of DNA base oxidation, measured in vitro with the comet assay. Mutagenesis, 16, 297-301.

Collins, A. R., Duthie, S. J. & Dobson, V. L. (1993). Direct enzymic detection of endogenous oxidative base damage in human lymphocyte DNA. Carcinogenesis, 14, 1733-1735.

Collins, A. R., Harrington, V., Drew, J. & Melvin, R. (2003). Nutritional modulation of DNA repair in a human intervention study. Carcinogenesis, 24, 511-515.

Collins, A. R., Mitchell, D. L., Zunino, A., de Wit, J. & Busch, D. (1997b). UV-sensitive rodent mutant cell lines of complementation groups 6 and 8 differ phenotypically from their human counterparts. Environ Mol Mutagen, 29, 152-160.

Collins, A. R., Oscoz, A. A., Brunborg, G., Gaivao, I., Giovannelli, L., Kruszewski, M., Smith, C. C. & Stetina, R. (2008). The comet assay: topical issues. Mutagenesis, 23, 143-151.

D'Errico, M., Parlanti, E. & Dogliotti, E. (2008). Mechanism of oxidative DNA damage repair and relevance to human pathology. Mutat Res, 659, 4-14.

Dani, C., Oliboni, L. S., Umezu, F. M., Pasquali, M. A., Salvador, M., Moreira, J. C. & Henriques, J. A. (2009). Antioxidant and antigenotoxic activities of purple grape juice--organic and conventional--in adult rats. J Med Food, 12, 1111-1118.

Davis, C. D. (2007). Nutritional interactions: credentialing of molecular targets for cancer prevention. Exp Biol Med (Maywood), 232, 176-183.

Davis, C. D. & Milner, J. A. (2007). Biomarkers for diet and cancer prevention research: potentials and challenges. Acta Pharmacol Sin, 28, 1262-1273.

de Kok, T. M., van Breda, S. G. & Manson, M. M. (2008). Mechanisms of combined action of different chemopreventive dietary compounds: a review. Eur J Nutr, 47 Suppl 2, 51-59.

de Lima, R. O., Bazo, A. P., Said, R. A., Sforcin, J. M., Bankova, V., Darros, B. R. & Salvadori, D. M. (2005). Modifying effect of propolis on dimethylhydrazine-induced DNA damage but not colonic aberrant crypt foci in rats. Environ Mol Mutagen, 45, 8-16.

De, S. & Das, S. (2001). Protective Effects of Tomato Juice on Mouse Skin Carcinogenesis. Asian Pac J Cancer Prev, 2, 43-47.

Del Bo, C., Martini, D., Vendrame, S., Riso, P., Ciappellano, S., Klimis-Zacas, D. & Porrini, M. (2010). Improvement of lymphocyte resistance against H(2)O(2)-induced DNA damage in Sprague-Dawley rats after eight weeks of a wild blueberry (Vaccinium angustifolium)-enriched diet. Mutat Res, 703, 158-162.

Devaraj, S., Mathur, S., Basu, A., Aung, H. H., Vasu, V. T., Meyers, S. & Jialal, I. (2008). A dose-response study on the effects of purified lycopene supplementation on biomarkers of oxidative stress. J Am Coll Nutr, 27, 267-273.

Devipriya, N., Sudheer, A. R. & Menon, V. P. (2008). Caffeic acid protects human peripheral blood lymphocytes against gamma radiation-induced cellular damage. J Biochem Mol Toxicol, 22, 175-186.

Doak, S. H., Brusehafer, K., Dudley, E., Quick, E., Johnson, G., Newton, R. P. & Jenkins, G. J. (2008). No-observed effect levels are associated with up-regulation of MGMT following MMS exposure. Mutat Res, 648, 9-14.

Dolara, P., Luceri, C., De Filippo, C., Femia, A. P., Giovannelli, L., Caderni, G., Cecchini, C., Silvi, S., Orpianesi, C. & Cresci, A. (2005). Red wine polyphenols influence carcinogenesis, intestinal microflora, oxidative damage and gene expression profiles of colonic mucosa in F344 rats. Mutat Res, 591, 237-246.

Drablos, F., Feyzi, E., Aas, P. A., Vaagbo, C. B., Kavli, B., Bratlie, M. S., Pena-Diaz, J., Otterlei, M., Slupphaug, G. & Krokan, H. E. (2004). Alkylation damage in DNA and RNA--repair mechanisms and medical significance. DNA Repair (Amst), 3, 1389-1407.

Dudas, A. & Chovanec, M. (2004). DNA double-strand break repair by homologous recombination. Mutat Res, 566, 131-167.

Dulebohn, R. V., Yi, W., Srivastava, A., Akoh, C. C., Krewer, G. & Fischer, J. G. (2008). Effects of blueberry (Vaccinium ashei) on DNA damage, lipid peroxidation, and phase II enzyme activities in rats. J Agric Food Chem, 56, 11700-11706.

Dusinska, M. & Collins, A. R. (1996). Detection of oxi-dised purines and UV-induced photoproducts in DNA of single cells, by inclusion of lesion-specific enzymes in the comet assay. Alternative Laboratory Animal, 24, 405-411.

Dusinska, M. & Collins, A. R. (2008). The comet assay in human biomonitoring: gene-environment interactions. Mutagenesis, 23, 191-205.

Duthie, S. J. (2010) Folate and cancer: how DNA damage, repair and methylation impact on colon carcinogenesis. J Inherit Metab Dis, 34, 101-109.

Duthie, S. J., Grant, G., Pirie, L. P., Watson, A. J. and Margison, G. P. (2010) Folate deficiency alters hepatic and colon MGMT and OGG-1 DNA repair protein expression in rats but has no effect on genome-wide DNA methylation. Cancer Prev Res (Phila), 3, 92-100.

Duthie, S. J. and McMillan, P. (1997) Uracil misincorporation in human DNA detected using single cell gel electrophoresis. Carcinogenesis, 18, 1709-1714.

Duthie, S. J., Narayanan, S., Blum, S., Pirie, L. and Brand, G. M. (2000) Folate deficiency in vitro induces uracil misincorporation and DNA hypomethylation and inhibits DNA excision repair in immortalized normal human colon epithelial cells. Nutr Cancer, 37, 245-251.

Edenharder, R., Frangart, J., Hager, M., Hofmann, P. and Rauscher, R. (1998) Protective effects of fruits and vegetables against in vivo clastogenicity of cyclosphosphamide or benzo[a]pyrene in mice. Food Chem Toxicol, 36, 637-645.

Eker, A. P., Quayle, C., Chaves, I. and van der Horst, G. T. (2009) DNA repair in mammalian cells: Direct DNA damage reversal: elegant solutions for nasty problems. Cell Mol Life Sci, 66, 968-980.

Esteller, M., Garcia-Foncillas, J., Andion, E., Goodman, S. N., Hidalgo, O. F., Vanaclocha, V., Baylin, S. B. and Herman, J. G. (2000) Inactivation of the DNA-repair gene MGMT and the clinical response of gliomas to alkylating agents. N Engl J Med, 343, 1350-1354.

Evans, M. D., Dizdaroglu, M. and Cooke, M. S. (2004) Oxidative DNA damage and disease: induction, repair and significance. Mutat Res, 567, 1-61.

Fabiani, R., Rosignoli, P., De Bartolomeo, A., Fuccelli, R., Servili, M., Montedoro, G. F. and Morozzi, G. (2008) Oxidative DNA damage is prevented by extracts of olive oil, hydroxytyrosol, and other olive phenolic compounds in human blood mononuclear cells and HL60 cells. J Nutr, 138, 1411-1416.

Fairbairn, D. W., Olive, P. L. and O'Neill, K. L. (1995) The comet assay: a comprehensive review. Mutat Res, 339, 37-59.

Fang, M. Z., Chen, D., Sun, Y., Jin, Z., Christman, J. K. and Yang, C. S. (2005) Reversal of hypermethylation and reactivation of p16INK4a, RARbeta, and MGMT genes by genistein and other isoflavones from soy. Clin Cancer Res, 11, 7033-7041.

Fang, M. Z., Wang, Y., Ai, N., Hou, Z., Sun, Y., Lu, H., Welsh, W. and Yang, C. S. (2003) Tea polyphenol (-)-epigallocatechin-3-gallate inhibits DNA methyltransferase and reactivates methylation-silenced genes in cancer cell lines. Cancer Res, 63, 7563-7570.

Ferguson, L. R., Philpott, M. and Karunasinghe, N. (2004) Dietary cancer and prevention using antimutagens. Toxicology, 198, 147-159.

Fillion, L., Collins, A. and Southon, S. (1998) Beta-carotene enhances the recovery of lymphocytes from oxidative DNA damage. Acta Biochim Pol, 45, 183-190.

Fortini, P., Pascucci, B., Parlanti, E., D'Errico, M., Simonelli, V. and Dogliotti, E. (2003) The base excision repair: mechanisms and its relevance for cancer susceptibility. Biochimie, 85, 1053-1071.

Franke, S. I., Pra, D., da Silva, J., Erdtmann, B. and Henriques, J. A. (2005a) Possible repair action of Vitamin C on DNA damage induced by methyl methanesulfonate, cyclophosphamide, FeSO4 and CuSO4 in mouse blood cells in vivo. Mutat Res, 583, 75-84.

Franke, S. I., Pra, D., Erdtmann, B., Henriques, J. A. and da Silva, J. (2005b) Influence of orange juice over the genotoxicity induced by alkylating agents: an in vivo analysis. Mutagenesis, 20, 279-283.

Freese, R. (2006) Markers of oxidative DNA damage in human interventions with fruit and berries. Nutr Cancer, 54, 143-147.

Frei, B. and Higdon, J. V. (2003) Antioxidant activity of tea polyphenols in vivo: evidence from animal studies. J Nutr, 133, 3275S-3284S.

Furtado, R. A., de Araujo, F. R., Resende, F. A., Cunha, W. R. and Tavares, D. C. (2009) Protective effect of rosmarinic acid on V79 cells evaluated by the micronucleus and comet assays. J Appl Toxicol, 30, 254-259.

Gaivao, I., Piasek, A., Brevik, A., Shaposhnikov, S. and Collins, A. R. (2009) Comet assay-based methods for measuring DNA repair in vitro; estimates of inter- and intra-individual variation. Cell Biol Toxicol, 25, 45-52.

Gedik, C. M., Ewen, S. W. and Collins, A. R. (1992) Single-cell gel electrophoresis applied to the analysis of UV-C damage and its repair in human cells. Int J Radiat Biol, 62, 313-320.

Glei, M. and Pool-Zobel, B. L. (2006) The main catechin of green tea, (-)-epigallocatechin-3-gallate (EGCG), reduces bleomycin-induced DNA damage in human leucocytes. Toxicol In Vitro, 20, 295-300.

Guglielmi, F., Luceri, C., Giovannelli, L., Dolara, P. and Lodovici, M. (2003) Effect of 4-coumaric and 3,4-dihydroxybenzoic acid on oxidative DNA damage in rat colonic mucosa. Br J Nutr, 89, 581-587.

Gurbuz, N., Ozkul, A. and Burgaz, S. (2009) Effects of vitamin C and N-acetylcysteine against cyclophosphamide-induced genotoxicity in exfoliated bladder cells of mice in vivo. J BUON, 14, 647-652.

Hall, C. N., Badawi, A. F., O'Connor, P. J. and Saffhill, R. (1991) The detection of alkylation damage in the DNA of human gastrointestinal tissues. Br J Cancer, 64, 59-63.

Han, K. C., Wong, W. C. and Benzie, I. F. (2011) Genoprotective effects of green tea (Camellia sinensis) in human subjects: results of a controlled supplementation trial. Br J Nutr, 105, 171-179.

Hanawalt, P. C. (2002) Subpathways of nucleotide excision repair and their regulation. Oncogene, 21, 8949-8956.

Hartmann, A., Agurell, E., Beevers, C., Brendler-Schwaab, S., Burlinson, B., Clay, P., Collins, A., Smith, A., Speit, G., Thybaud, V. and Tice, R. R. (2003) Recommendations for conducting the in vivo alkaline Comet assay. 4th International Comet Assay Workshop. Mutagenesis, 18, 45-51.

Hegde, M. L., Hazra, T. K. and Mitra, S. (2008) Early steps in the DNA base excision/single-strand interruption repair pathway in mammalian cells. Cell Res, 18, 27-47.

Hegi, M. E., Diserens, A. C., Gorlia, T., Hamou, M. F., de Tribolet, N., Weller, M., Kros, J. M., Hainfellner, J. A., Mason, W., Mariani, L., Bromberg, J. E., Hau, P., Mirimanoff, R. O., Cairncross, J. G., Janzer, R. C. and Stupp, R. (2005) MGMT gene silencing and benefit from temozolomide in glioblastoma. N Engl J Med, 352, 997-1003.

Helleday, T., Lo, J., van Gent, D. C. and Engelward, B. P. (2007) DNA double-strand break repair: from mechanistic understanding to cancer treatment. DNA Repair (Amst), 6, 923-935.

Helleday, T., Petermann, E., Lundin, C., Hodgson, B. and Sharma, R. A. (2008) DNA repair pathways as targets for cancer therapy. Nat Rev Cancer, 8, 193-204.

Heo, M. Y., Sohn, S. J. and Au, W. W. (2001) Anti-genotoxicity of galangin as a cancer chemopreventive agent candidate. Mutat Res, 488, 135-150.

Hoelzl, C., Knasmuller, S., Misik, M., Collins, A., Dusinska, M. and Nersesyan, A. (2009) Use of single cell gel electrophoresis assays for the detection of DNA-protective effects of dietary factors in humans: recent results and trends. Mutat Res, 681, 68-79.

Horvathova, K., Chalupa, I., Sebova, L., Tothova, D. and Vachalkova, A. (2005) Protective effect of quercetin and luteolin in human melanoma HMB-2 cells. Mutat Res, 565, 105-112.

Horvathova, K., Novotny, L., Tothova, D. and Vachalkova, A. (2004) Determination of free radical scavenging activity of quercetin, rutin, luteolin and apigenin in H2O2-treated human ML cells K562. Neoplasma, 51, 395-399.

Horvathova, K., Novotny, L. and Vachalkova, A. (2003) The free radical scavenging activity of four flavonoids determined by the comet assay. Neoplasma, 50, 291-295.

Hosseinzadeh, H. and Sadeghnia, H. R. (2007) Effect of safranal, a constituent of Crocus sativus (saffron), on methyl methanesulfonate (MMS)-induced DNA damage in mouse organs: an alkaline single-cell gel electrophoresis (comet) assay. DNA Cell Biol, 26, 841-846.

Jagetia, A., Jagetia, G. C. and Jha, S. (2007) Naringin, a grapefruit flavanone, protects V79 cells against the bleomycin-induced genotoxicity and decline in survival. J Appl Toxicol, 27, 122-132.

Jaiswal, A. S., Banerjee, S., Aneja, R., Sarkar, F. H., Ostrov, D. A. and Narayan, S. (2011) DNA polymerase beta as a novel target for chemotherapeutic intervention of colorectal cancer. PLoS One, 6, e16691.

Jaiswal, A. S. and Narayan, S. (2008) A novel function of adenomatous polyposis coli (APC) in regulating DNA repair. Cancer Lett, 271, 272-280.

Jeyabal, P. V., Syed, M. B., Venkataraman, M., Sambandham, J. K. and Sakthisekaran, D. (2005) Apigenin inhibits oxidative stress-induced macromolecular damage in N-nitrosodiethylamine (NDEA)-induced hepatocellular carcinogenesis in Wistar albino rats. Mol Carcinog, 44, 11-20.

Jiricny, J. (2006) The multifaceted mismatch-repair system. Nat Rev Mol Cell Biol, 7, 335-346.

Jiricny, J. and Marra, G. (2003) DNA repair defects in colon cancer. Curr Opin Genet Dev, 13, 61-69.

Kager, N., Ferk, F., Kundi, M., Wagner, K. H., Misik, M. and Knasmuller, S. (2010) Prevention of oxidative DNA damage in inner organs and lymphocytes of rats by green tea extract. Eur J Nutr, 49, 227-234.

Kaina, B., Christmann, M., Naumann, S. and Roos, W. P. (2007) MGMT: key node in the battle against genotoxicity, carcinogenicity and apoptosis induced by alkylating agents. DNA Repair (Amst), 6, 1079-1099.

Kaina, B., Margison, G. P. and Christmann, M. (2010) Targeting O-methylguanine-DNA methyltransferase with specific inhibitors as a strategy in cancer therapy. Cell Mol Life Sci, 67, 3663-3681.

Kanupriya, Dipti, P., Sharma, S. K., Sairam, M., Ilavazhagan, G., Sawhney, R. C. and Banerjee, P. K. (2006) Flavonoids protect U-937 macrophages against tert-butylhydroperoxide induced oxidative injury. Food Chem Toxicol, 44, 1024-1030.

Karihtala, P. and Soini, Y. (2007) Reactive oxygen species and antioxidant mechanisms in human tissues and their relation to malignancies. APMIS, 115, 81-103.

Kim, J. M., Araki, S., Kim, D. J., Park, C. B., Takasuka, N., Baba-Toriyama, H., Ota, T., Nir, Z., Khachik, F., Shimidzu, N., Tanaka, Y., Osawa, T., Uraji, T., Murakoshi, M., Nishino, H. and Tsuda, H. (1998) Chemopreventive effects of carotenoids and curcumins on mouse colon carcinogenesis after 1,2-dimethylhydrazine initiation. Carcinogenesis, 19, 81-85.

Knudsen, N. O., Andersen, S. D., Lutzen, A., Nielsen, F. C. and Rasmussen, L. J. (2009) Nuclear translocation contributes to regulation of DNA excision repair activities. DNA Repair (Amst), 8, 682-689.

Koch, T. C., Briviba, K., Watzl, B., Fahndrich, C., Bub, A., Rechkemmer, G. and Barth, S. W. (2009) Prevention of colon carcinogenesis by apple juice in vivo: impact of juice constituents and obesity. Mol Nutr Food Res, 53, 1289-1302.

Kondo, N., Takahashi, A., Ono, K. and Ohnishi, T. (2010) DNA damage induced by alkylating agents and repair pathways. J Nucleic Acids, 2010, 543531.

Kovary, K., Louvain, T. S., Costa e Silva, M. C., Albano, F., Pires, B. B., Laranja, G. A., Lage, C. L. and Felzenszwalb, I. (2001) Biochemical behaviour of norbixin during in vitro DNA damage induced by reactive oxygen species. Br J Nutr, 85, 431-440.

Kuo, S. M. (1996) Antiproliferative potency of structurally distinct dietary flavonoids on human colon cancer cells. Cancer Lett, 110, 41-48.

Langie, S. A., Knaapen, A. M., Brauers, K. J., van Berlo, D., van Schooten, F. J. and Godschalk, R. W. (2006) Development and validation of a modified comet assay to phenotypically assess nucleotide excision repair. Mutagenesis, 21, 153-158.

Lees, N. P., Harrison, K. L., Hall, C. N., Margison, G. P. and Povey, A. C. (2004) Reduced MGMT activity in human colorectal adenomas is associated with K-ras GC->AT transition mutations in a population exposed to methylating agents. Carcinogenesis, 25, 1243-1247.

Lees, N. P., Harrison, K. L., Hill, E., Hall, C. N., Margison, G. P. and Povey, A. C. (2002) Longitudinal variation in O(6)-alkylguanine DNA-alkyltransferase activity in the human colon and rectum. Br J Cancer, 87, 168-170.

Lima, C. F., Andrade, P. B., Seabra, R. M., Fernandes-Ferreira, M. and Pereira-Wilson, C. (2005) The drinking of a Salvia officinalis infusion improves liver antioxidant status in mice and rats. J Ethnopharmacol, 97, 383-389.

Lima, C. F., Fernandes-Ferreira, M. and Pereira-Wilson, C. (2006) Phenolic compounds protect HepG2 cells from oxidative damage: relevance of glutathione levels. Life Sci, 79, 2056-2068.

Lind, G. E., Thorstensen, L., Lovig, T., Meling, G. I., Hamelin, R., Rognum, T. O., Esteller, M. and Lothe, R. A. (2004) A CpG island hypermethylation profile of primary colorectal carcinomas and colon cancer cell lines. Mol Cancer, 3, 28.

Liu, L. and Gerson, S. L. (2006) Targeted modulation of MGMT: clinical implications. Clin Cancer Res, 12, 328-331.

Liu, L., Schwartz, S., Davis, B. M. and Gerson, S. L. (2002) Chemotherapy-induced O(6)-benzylguanine-resistant alkyltransferase mutations in mismatch-deficient colon cancer. Cancer Res, 62, 3070-3076.

Lorenzo, Y., Azqueta, A., Luna, L., Bonilla, F., Dominguez, G. and Collins, A. R. (2009) The carotenoid beta-cryptoxanthin stimulates the repair of DNA oxidation damage in addition to acting as an antioxidant in human cells. Carcinogenesis, 30, 308-314.

Marchesi, F., Turriziani, M., Tortorelli, G., Avvisati, G., Torino, F. and De Vecchis, L. (2007) Triazene compounds: mechanism of action and related DNA repair systems. Pharmacol Res, 56, 275-287.

Maynard, S., Schurman, S. H., Harboe, C., de Souza-Pinto, N. C. and Bohr, V. A. (2009) Base excision repair of oxidative DNA damage and association with cancer and aging. Carcinogenesis, 30, 2-10.

McCann, M. J., Gill, C. I., G, O. B., Rao, J. R., McRoberts, W. C., Hughes, P., McEntee, R. and Rowland, I. R. (2007) Anti-cancer properties of phenolics from apple waste on colon carcinogenesis in vitro. Food Chem Toxicol, 45, 1224-1230.

Mehta, R. G., Murillo, G., Naithani, R. and Peng, X. (2010) Cancer chemoprevention by natural products: how far have we come? Pharm Res, 27, 950-961.

Melnyk, S., Pogribna, M., Miller, B. J., Basnakian, A. G., Pogribny, I. P. and James, S. J. (1999) Uracil misincorporation, DNA strand breaks, and gene amplification are associated with tumorigenic cell transformation in folate deficient/repleted Chinese hamster ovary cells. Cancer Lett, 146, 35-44.

Middleton, M. R. and Margison, G. P. (2003) Improvement of chemotherapy efficacy by inactivation of a DNA-repair pathway. Lancet Oncol, 4, 37-44.

Miene, C., Klenow, S., Veeriah, S., Richling, E. and Glei, M. (2009) Impact of apple polyphenols on GSTT2 gene expression, subsequent protection of DNA and modulation of proliferation using LT97 human colon adenoma cells. Mol Nutr Food Res, 53, 1254-1262.

Min, K. and Ebeler, S. E. (2008) Flavonoid effects on DNA oxidation at low concentrations relevant to physiological levels. Food Chem Toxicol, 46, 96-104.

Moller, P. and Loft, S. (2002) Oxidative DNA damage in human white blood cells in dietary antioxidant intervention studies. Am J Clin Nutr, 76, 303-310.

Moon, H. K., Yang, E. S. and Park, J. W. (2006) Protection of peroxynitrite-induced DNA damage by dietary antioxidants. Arch Pharm Res, 29, 213-217.

Murillo, G., Choi, J. K., Pan, O., Constantinou, A. I. and Mehta, R. G. (2004) Efficacy of garbanzo and soybean flour in suppression of aberrant crypt foci in the colons of CF-1 mice. Anticancer Res, 24, 3049-3055.

Muzandu, K., Ishizuka, M., Sakamoto, K. Q., Shaban, Z., El Bohi, K., Kazusaka, A. and Fujita, S. (2006) Effect of lycopene and beta-carotene on peroxynitrite-mediated cellular modifications. Toxicol Appl Pharmacol, 215, 330-340.

Nakamura, Y., Tomokane, I., Mori, T., Tanaka, A., Koutani, J., Matsuo, T., Okamoto, S., Sato, K. and Ohtsuki, K. (2000) DNA repair effect of traditional sweet pepper Fushimi-togarashi: seen in suppression of UV-induced cyclobutane pyrimidine dimer in human fibroblast. Biosci Biotechnol Biochem, 64, 2575-2580.

Nigam, N., Prasad, S. and Shukla, Y. (2007) Preventive effects of lupeol on DMBA induced DNA alkylation damage in mouse skin. Food Chem Toxicol, 45, 2331-2335.

Niture, S. K., Rao, U. S. and Srivenugopal, K. S. (2006) Chemopreventative strategies targeting the MGMT repair protein: augmented expression in human lymphocytes and tumor cells by ethanolic and aqueous extracts of several Indian medicinal plants. Int J Oncol, 29, 1269-1278.

Niture, S. K., Velu, C. S., Smith, Q. R., Bhat, G. J. and Srivenugopal, K. S. (2007) Increased expression of the MGMT repair protein mediated by cysteine prodrugs and chemopreventative natural products in human lymphocytes and tumor cell lines. Carcinogenesis, 28, 378-389.

Noroozi, M., Angerson, W. J. and Lean, M. E. (1998) Effects of flavonoids and vitamin C on oxidative DNA damage to human lymphocytes. Am J Clin Nutr, 67, 1210-1218.

Nossoni, F. (2008) Single-Cell Gel Electrophoresis (Comet Assay): Methodology, Potential Applications, and Limitations in Cancer Research. MMG 445 Basic Biotechnology eJournal, 4, 30-35.

Nouspikel, T. (2009) DNA repair in mammalian cells : Nucleotide excision repair: variations on versatility. Cell Mol Life Sci, 66, 994-1009.

Nozawa, H., Yoshida, A., Tajima, O., Katayama, M., Sonobe, H., Wakabayashi, K. and Kondo, K. (2004) Intake of beer inhibits azoxymethane-induced colonic carcinogenesis in male Fischer 344 rats. Int J Cancer, 108, 404-411.

Nystrom, M. and Mutanen, M. (2009) Diet and epigenetics in colon cancer. World J Gastroenterol, 15, 257-263.

Ostling, O. and Johanson, K. J. (1984) Microelectrophoretic study of radiation-induced DNA damages in individual mammalian cells. Biochem Biophys Res Commun, 123, 291-298.

Ovesna, Z., Kozics, K. and Slamenova, D. (2006) Protective effects of ursolic acid and oleanolic acid in leukemic cells. Mutat Res, 600, 131-137.

Pan, M. H., Ghai, G. and Ho, C. T. (2008) Food bioactives, apoptosis, and cancer. Mol Nutr Food Res, 52, 43-52.

Panayiotidis, M. and Collins, A. R. (1997) Ex vivo assessment of lymphocyte antioxidant status using the comet assay. Free Radic Res, 27, 533-537.

Pastoriza Gallego, M. and Sarasin, A. (2003) Transcription-coupled repair of 8-oxoguanine in human cells and its deficiency in some DNA repair diseases. Biochimie, 85, 1073-1082.

Paz-Elizur, T., Elinger, D., Leitner-Dagan, Y., Blumenstein, S., Krupsky, M., Berrebi, A., Schechtman, E. and Livneh, Z. (2007) Development of an enzymatic DNA repair assay for molecular epidemiology studies: distribution of OGG activity in healthy individuals. DNA Repair (Amst), 6, 45-60.

Petermann, A., Miene, C., Schulz-Raffelt, G., Palige, K., Holzer, J., Glei, M. and Bohmer, F. D. (2009) GSTT2, a phase II gene induced by apple polyphenols, protects colon epithelial cells against genotoxic damage. Mol Nutr Food Res, 53, 1245-1253.

Pool-Zobel, B. L., Bub, A., Muller, H., Wollowski, I. and Rechkemmer, G. (1997) Consumption of vegetables reduces genetic damage in humans: first results of a human intervention trial with carotenoid-rich foods. Carcinogenesis, 18, 1847-1850.

Porrini, M. and Riso, P. (2000) Lymphocyte lycopene concentration and DNA protection from oxidative damage is increased in women after a short period of tomato consumption. J Nutr, 130, 189-192.

Povey, A. C., Hall, C. N., Badawi, A. F., Cooper, D. P. and O'Connor, P. J. (2000) Elevated levels of the pro-carcinogenic adduct, O(6)-methylguanine, in normal DNA from the cancer prone regions of the large bowel. Gut, 47, 362-365.

Prasad, N. R., Jeyanthimala, K. and Ramachandran, S. (2009) Caffeic acid modulates ultraviolet radiation-B induced oxidative damage in human blood lymphocytes. J Photochem Photobiol B, 95, 196-203.

Quincozes-Santos, A., Andreazza, A. C., Nardin, P., Funchal, C., Goncalves, C. A. and Gottfried, C. (2007) Resveratrol attenuates oxidative-induced DNA damage in C6 Glioma cells. Neurotoxicology, 28, 886-891.

Rajamanickam, S. and Agarwal, R. (2008) Natural products and colon cancer: current status and future prospects. Drug Dev Res, 69, 460-471.

Ramos, A. A., Azqueta, A., Pereira-Wilson, C. and Collins, A. R. (2010a) Polyphenolic compounds from Salvia species protect cellular DNA from oxidation and stimulate DNA repair in cultured human cells. J Agric Food Chem, 58, 7465-7471.

Ramos, A. A., Lima, C. F., Pereira, M. L., Fernandes-Ferreira, M. and Pereira-Wilson, C. (2008) Antigenotoxic effects of quercetin, rutin and ursolic acid on HepG2 cells: evaluation by the comet assay. Toxicol Lett, 177, 66-73.

Ramos, A. A., Pereira-Wilson, C. and Collins, A. R. (2010b) Protective effects of ursolic acid and luteolin against oxidative DNA damage include enhancement of DNA repair in Caco-2 cells. Mutat Res, 692, 6-11.

Riso, P., Martini, D., Visioli, F., Martinetti, A. and Porrini, M. (2009) Effect of broccoli intake on markers related to oxidative stress and cancer risk in healthy smokers and nonsmokers. Nutr Cancer, 61, 232-237.

Robertson, A. B., Klungland, A., Rognes, T. and Leiros, I. (2009) DNA repair in mammalian cells: Base excision repair: the long and short of it. Cell Mol Life Sci, 66, 981-993.

Ross, J. A. and Kasum, C. M. (2002) Dietary flavonoids: bioavailability, metabolic effects, and safety. Annu Rev Nutr, 22, 19-34.

Rusak, G., Piantanida, I., Masic, L., Kapuralin, K., Durgo, K. and Kopjar, N. (2010) Spectrophotometric analysis of flavonoid-DNA interactions and DNA damaging/protecting and cytotoxic potential of flavonoids in human peripheral blood lymphocytes. Chem Biol Interact, 188, 181-189.

Schaefer, S., Baum, M., Eisenbrand, G., Dietrich, H., Will, F. and Janzowski, C. (2006) Polyphenolic apple juice extracts and their major constituents reduce oxidative damage in human colon cell lines. Mol Nutr Food Res, 50, 24-33.

Sengottuvelan, M., Deeptha, K. and Nalini, N. (2009) Resveratrol ameliorates DNA damage, prooxidant and antioxidant imbalance in 1,2-dimethylhydrazine induced rat colon carcinogenesis. Chem Biol Interact, 181, 193-201.

Sengupta, A., Ghosh, S. and Das, S. (2003) Tomato and garlic can modulate azoxymethane-induced colon carcinogenesis in rats. Eur J Cancer Prev, 12, 195-200.

Sengupta, A., Ghosh, S. and Das, S. (2004) Modulatory influence of garlic and tomato on cyclooxygenase-2 activity, cell proliferation and apoptosis during azoxymethane induced colon carcinogenesis in rat. Cancer Lett, 208, 127-136.

Serpeloni, J. M., Grotto, D., Mercadante, A. Z., de Lourdes Pires Bianchi, M. and Antunes, L. M. (2010) Lutein improves antioxidant defense in vivo and protects against DNA damage and chromosome instability induced by cisplatin. Arch Toxicol, 84, 811-822.

Shaposhnikov, S., Azqueta, A., Henriksson, S., Meier, S., Gaivao, I., Huskisson, N. H., Smart, A., Brunborg, G., Nilsson, M. and Collins, A. R. (2010) Twelve-gel slide format optimised for comet assay and fluorescent in situ hybridisation. Toxicol Lett, 195, 31-34.

Silva, J. P., Gomes, A. C. and Coutinho, O. P. (2008) Oxidative DNA damage protection and repair by polyphenolic compounds in PC12 cells. Eur J Pharmacol, 601, 50-60.

Silva, J. P., Gomes, A. C., Proenca, F. and Coutinho, O. P. (2009) Novel nitrogen compounds enhance protection and repair of oxidative DNA damage in a neuronal cell model: comparison with quercetin. Chem Biol Interact, 181, 328-337.

Singh, N. P., McCoy, M. T., Tice, R. R. and Schneider, E. L. (1988) A simple technique for quantitation of low levels of DNA damage in individual cells. Exp Cell Res, 175, 184-191.

Speit, G., Schutz, P., Bonzheim, I., Trenz, K. and Hoffmann, H. (2004) Sensitivity of the FPG protein towards alkylation damage in the comet assay. Toxicol Lett, 146, 151-158.

Speit, G., Witton-Davies, T., Heepchantree, W., Trenz, K. and Hoffmann, H. (2003) Investigations on the effect of cigarette smoking in the comet assay. Mutat Res, 542, 33-42.

Srinivasan, M., Sudheer, A. R., Pillai, K. R., Kumar, P. R., Sudhakaran, P. R. and Menon, V. P. (2007) Lycopene as a natural protector against gamma-radiation induced DNA damage, lipid peroxidation and antioxidant status in primary culture of isolated rat hepatocytes in vitro. Biochim Biophys Acta, 1770, 659-665.

Suaeyun, R., Kinouchi, T., Arimochi, H., Vinitketkumnuen, U. and Ohnishi, Y. (1997) Inhibitory effects of lemon grass (Cymbopogon citratus Stapf) on formation of azoxymethane-induced DNA adducts and aberrant crypt foci in the rat colon. Carcinogenesis, 18, 949-955.

Szeto, Y. T. and Benzie, I. F. (2002) Effects of dietary antioxidants on human DNA ex vivo. Free Radic Res, 36, 113-118.

Terry, P., Giovannucci, E., Michels, K. B., Bergkvist, L., Hansen, H., Holmberg, L. and Wolk, A. (2001) Fruit, vegetables, dietary fiber, and risk of colorectal cancer. J Natl Cancer Inst, 93, 525-533.

Thompson, H. J., Heimendinger, J., Haegele, A., Sedlacek, S. M., Gillette, C., O'Neill, C., Wolfe, P. and Conry, C. (1999) Effect of increased vegetable and fruit consumption on markers of oxidative cellular damage. Carcinogenesis, 20, 2261-2266.

Tice, R. R., Agurell, E., Anderson, D., Burlinson, B., Hartmann, A., Kobayashi, H., Miyamae, Y., Rojas, E., Ryu, J. C. and Sasaki, Y. F. (2000) Single cell gel/comet assay: guidelines for in vitro and in vivo genetic toxicology testing. Environ Mol Mutagen, 35, 206-221.

Torbergsen, A. C. and Collins, A. R. (2000) Recovery of human lymphocytes from oxidative DNA damage; the apparent enhancement of DNA repair by carotenoids is probably simply an antioxidant effect. Eur J Nutr, 39, 80-85.

Tripathi, D. N. and Jena, G. B. (2008) Astaxanthin inhibits cytotoxic and genotoxic effects of cyclophosphamide in mice germ cells. Toxicology, 248, 96-103.

Tudek, B. (2007) Base excision repair modulation as a risk factor for human cancers. Mol Aspects Med, 28, 258-275.

Veeriah, S., Balavenkatraman, K. K., Bohmer, F., Kahle, K., Glei, M., Richling, E., Scheppach, W. and Pool-Zobel, B. L. (2008) Intervention with cloudy apple juice results in altered biological activities of ileostomy samples collected from individual volunteers. Eur J Nutr, 47, 226-234.

Volate, S. R., Davenport, D. M., Muga, S. J. and Wargovich, M. J. (2005) Modulation of aberrant crypt foci and apoptosis by dietary herbal supplements (quercetin, curcumin, silymarin, ginseng and rutin). Carcinogenesis, 26, 1450-1456.

Wali, R. K., Skarosi, S., Hart, J., Zhang, Y., Dolan, M. E., Moschel, R. C., Nguyen, L., Mustafi, R., Brasitus, T. A. and Bissonnette, M. (1999) Inhibition of O(6)-methylguanine-DNA methyltransferase increases azoxymethane-induced colonic tumors in rats. Carcinogenesis, 20, 2355-2360.

Wasson, G. R., McKelvey-Martin, V. J. and Downes, C. S. (2008) The use of the comet assay in the study of human nutrition and cancer. Mutagenesis, 23, 153-162.

WCRF (2007) Food, Nutrition, Physical Activity and the Prevention of Cancer: A Global Perspective. American Institute for Cancer Research, London.

Wilms, L. C., Claughton, T. A., de Kok, T. M. and Kleinjans, J. C. (2007) GSTM1 and GSTT1 polymorphism influences protection against induced oxidative DNA damage by quercetin and ascorbic acid in human lymphocytes in vitro. Food Chem Toxicol, 45, 2592-2596.

Wilms, L. C., Hollman, P. C., Boots, A. W. and Kleinjans, J. C. (2005) Protection by quercetin and quercetin-rich fruit juice against induction of oxidative DNA damage and formation of BPDE-DNA adducts in human lymphocytes. Mutat Res, 582, 155-162.

Wilson, D. M., 3rd and Bohr, V. A. (2007) The mechanics of base excision repair, and its relationship to aging and disease. DNA Repair (Amst), 6, 544-559.

Wirtz, S., Nagel, G., Eshkind, L., Neurath, M. F., Samson, L. D. and Kaina, B. (2010) Both base excision repair and O6-methylguanine-DNA methyltransferase protect against methylation-induced colon carcinogenesis. Carcinogenesis, 31, 2111-2117.

Wong, V. W. C., Szeto, Y. T., Collins, A. R. and Benzie, I. F. F. (2005) THE COMET ASSAY: a biomonitoring tool for nutraceutical research. Current Topics in Nutraceutical Research, 3, 1-14.

Yu, H. H., Hur, J. M., Seo, S. J., Moon, H. D., Kim, H. J., Park, R. K. and You, Y. O. (2009) Protective effect of ursolic acid from Cornus officinalis on the hydrogen peroxide-induced damage of HEI-OC1 auditory cells. Am J Chin Med, 37, 735-746.

Zhao, X., Aldini, G., Johnson, E. J., Rasmussen, H., Kraemer, K., Woolf, H., Musaeus, N., Krinsky, N. I., Russell, R. M. and Yeum, K. J. (2006) Modification of lymphocyte DNA damage by carotenoid supplementation in postmenopausal women. Am J Clin Nutr, 83, 163-169.

9

SiDNA and Other Tools for the Indirect Induction of DNA Damage Responses

Maria Quanz[1,2], Amélie Croset[1,2] and Marie Dutreix[1]
[1]*Institut Curie, Centre National de Recherche Scientifique (CNRS) UMR3347, Institut National de la Santé et de Recherche Médicale (INSERM) U1021, Université Paris-Sud 11, Centre Universitaire, 91405 Orsay*
[2]*DNA Therapeutics SA, 91058 Evry*
France

1. Introduction

Cells respond to DNA damage by activating an intricate signaling network leading to DNA repair, cell cycle arrest or apoptosis. In recent years, progress has been made in the discovery and characterization of a number of DNA repair pathways, and it has become apparent that the inhibition of specific components of these pathways could offer new targets for combating the resistance of tumors to chemotherapy or radiotherapy. A thorough understanding of the various DNA repair pathways and their regulation is therefore essential. The DNA damage response (DDR) is of great importance in determining cell fate decisions. It includes many signal amplification steps and several steps that are partly redundant due to the ability of different kinases to phosphorylate the same target. Furthermore, the timing and origin of the damage play an important role in determining the DNA repair pathway activated. All this makes it difficult to study the role of one particular protein in DNA damage signaling. In addition, the available tools for activating DNA repair pathways are mostly agents that systematically produce more than one type of DNA damage. Even if the damage caused is initially of one predominant type (as for topoisomerase inhibitors, alkylators or the I-SceI endonuclease system), the damage may rapidly be transformed by normal cellular processes, such as DNA replication, or specific nuclease activities. Studies of the DDR become even more complicated if the agent used to create DNA lesions also damages other cellular components, as is the case for ionizing radiation (IR), alkylators and hydrogen peroxide. Furthermore, the damage is transient, as DNA damage signaling is rapid and lesions are quickly repaired. The signal induced by the damage therefore disappears rapidly, soon after the induction of damage. In some cells, the DNA may not be successfully repaired, leading to apoptosis or senescence. These aspects make it difficult to study the signaling network induced by a given type of damage.

In this chapter, we will provide an overview of the response of the cell to DNA damage and possible ways of inducing a DDR in cells without actually damaging chromatin. We will focus on stabilized short interfering DNA molecules (siDNA), which mimic different types of damage and induce a pure damage-specific response.

2. DNA-damaging treatments induce multiple and dynamic responses

DNA is a stable material, as required for the storage of genetic information, but it is also susceptible to spontaneous changes under normal cellular conditions. It has been estimated that each cell spontaneously loses about 5000 purine bases (depurination) every day (Friedberg, 1995). The deamination of cytosine to uracil also occurs spontaneously. In addition to this inherent instability, our genomes are exposed to numerous endogenous or environmental agents, including reactive metabolites, environmental chemicals and ultraviolet radiation, capable of inducing a wide diversity of DNA lesions (Figure 1). The large number of different lesions possible – more than 100 different oxidative modifications

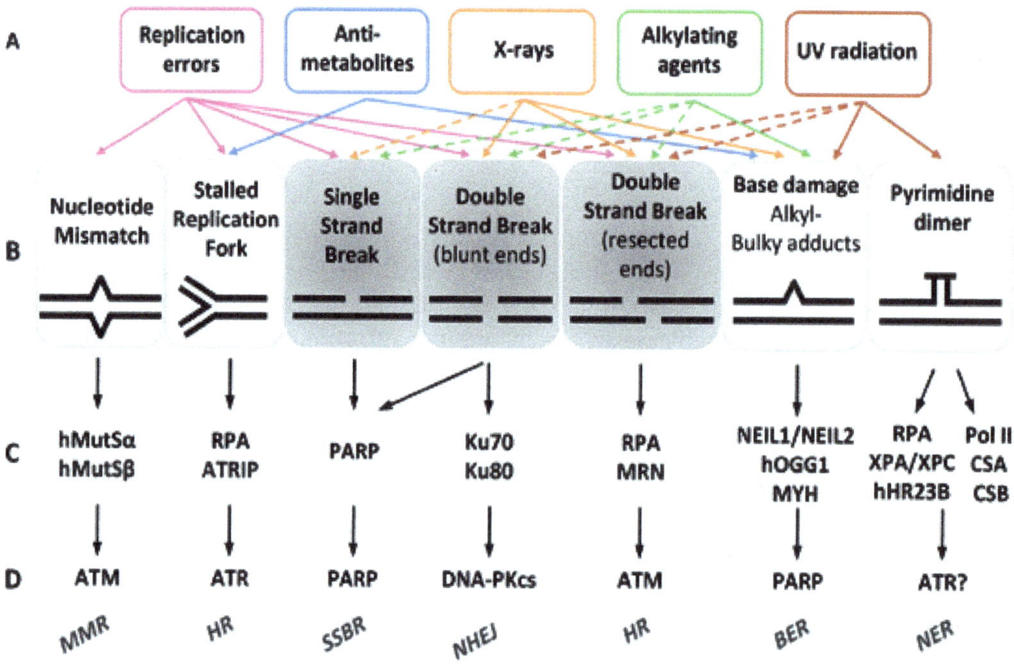

Fig. 1. DNA-damaging treatments induce multiple and dynamic responses mediated by DNA damage sensors and transducers. Common DNA-damaging agents (A) induce several types of DNA damage (B) directly (solid line) or indirectly (dotted line). Single- and double-strand breaks (highlighted in gray) are the most frequent end products of unrepaired damage. DNA damage is recognized by sensor proteins (C) that recruit and/or activate transducers (D), initiating a signal transduction cascade (not shown). Abbreviations: ATM, ataxia telangiectasia mutated; ATR, ataxia and rad3-related; ATRIP, ATR-interacting protein; BER, base excision repair; CSA or CSB, Cockayne Syndrome A or B; DNA-PKcs, DNA-dependent protein kinase catalytic subunit; hOGG1, human 8-hydroxyguanine DNA-glycosylase; HR, homologous recombination repair; hHR23B, human Rad23 homolog B; MMR, mismatch repair; MRN, Mre11-RAD50-Nbs1; MYH, MutY glycosylase homologue; NEIL1, nei endonuclease VIII-like 1; NER, nucleotide excision repair; NHEJ, non-homologous end joining; PARP, poly(ADP-ribose) polymerase; RPA, replication protein A; SSBR, single-strand break repair; UV, ultraviolet; XPC, xeroderma pigmentosum group C.

alone have been identified in DNA (Cadet et al., 1997) – has led to the evolution of many different repair pathways for sensing and repairing the various types of damage.
The complete signaling network for each damage type and its individual contribution to the cellular damage response are not fully understood, but the essential repair mechanisms have been elucidated (reviewed for example by Fortini & Dogliotti (2007); Friedberg (1995; 2001); Helleday et al. (2008); Li (2008); Wyman & Kanaar (2006)). Figure 1 summarizes the main pathways and highlights the sensors (DNA binding proteins that recognize specific DNA lesions) and transducers (enzymes that amplify the damage signal by posttranslational modification of downstream targets) involved in repair and signaling for particular types of damage. The main DNA damage transducers are the phosphoinositide 3-kinase-like kinase (PIKK) family members ATM (ataxia telangiectasia mutated), ATR (ataxia telangiectasia and Rad3-related) and DNA-PK (DNA-dependent protein kinase). A DNA break signal can also be transduced by poly(ADP-ribose) polymerases 1 or 2 (here both designated PARP), which use NAD^+ to catalyze the modification of their targets with negatively charged, long and branched ADP-ribose polymers. We provide below a brief description of the DNA repair pathways, the subsets of damage they repair and the transducers that are activated.

2.1 Repair processes that do not directly activate transducers

The direct repair of certain alkylation adducts and other uncomplicated base modifications by specialized single enzymes is probably the simplest repair mechanism. O6-alkylguanine DNA alkyltransferase (AGT) is a major enzyme involved in direct repair. It is encoded by the O6-methylguanine-DNA-methyltransferase (MGMT) gene and transfers the alkyl adducts produced by alkylating agents, such as temozolomide, dacarbazine or nitrosourea compounds, from O6-methylguanine, O4-methylthymine, O6-ethylguanine or O6-chloroethylguanine to a cysteine residue within the active site of the enzyme, thereby inactivating the enzyme (Gerson, 2004). Other direct repair enzymes include the DNA dioxygenases ABH2 and ABH3, which can convert 1-methyladenine and 3-methylcytosine back into adenine and cytosine, respectively (Duncan et al., 2002). The repair of alkylated lesions is a rapid process, with most alkylated sites successfully repaired within an hour (Zhu et al., 2009). The types of damage targeted by direct repair processes do not seem to be associated with the activation of damage signaling kinases, probably due to the rapid repair kinetics and the absence of intermediate strand break generation during the repair process.

2.2 Repair mechanisms that activate mainly PARP as a transducer

The base excision repair (BER) pathway recognizes and removes bases carrying non-bulky modifications that have been damaged by nonenzymatic alkylation, oxidation, ring saturation, or IR (Chan et al., 2006). BER also eliminates deaminated bases and DNA single-strand breaks (SSBs). As a first step in BER, a damage-specific DNA glycosylase (e.g. hOOG1, NEIL1 or NEIL2) recognizes and excises the damaged base, leading to the formation of a potentially cytotoxic intermediate apurinic or apyrimidinic site (AP site) (Bandaru et al., 2002; Boiteux & Radicella, 2000). The abasic sugar is cleaved by an AP endonuclease (APE1), which generates a strand break that is further processed by PARP, DNA polymerase β and ligase III in either short-patch or long-patch pathways (Fortini & Dogliotti, 2007). PARP not only recognizes the intermediate SSB but also acts as a damage transducer amplifying the damage signal by linking poly(ADP-ribose) (PAR) chains to its substrates, including itself. These polymers bind specific proteins, including XRCC1, DNA ligase III, p53 and DNA-PK, affecting the repair process as well as downstream responses to DNA damage (Malanga & Althaus, 2005).

2.3 Repair pathways that lead to PIKK activation

Most repair pathways involve the activation of PIKKs as transducers, especially if DNA breaks persist. Since PARPs can also sense DNA breaks, an implication of these enzymes in the pathways described in the following cannot be excluded.

2.3.1 Nucleotide excision repair

The nucleotide excision repair (NER) pathway senses and repairs various bulky, helix-distorting lesions that block DNA replication and transcription (Hanawalt, 2002). These lesions may arise, for example, following exposure to genotoxic compounds, such as polycyclic aromatic hydrocarbons or cisplatin. Two major repair mechanisms are known to be involved in this pathway: transcription-coupled repair, which specifically targets lesions blocking RNA polymerase II, and global genome repair, which deals with lesions in the rest of the genome (Cleaver, 2005). The damage sensors involved in transcription-coupled repair include, in addition to RNA polymerase II, Cockayne Syndrome A and B proteins. By contrast, XPA, Rpa and the XPC-hHR23B complex recognize lesions during global genome NER (Brown et al., 2010; Reardon & Sancar, 2005). NER is a complex multistep process involving the recognition of disrupted base pairing followed by unwinding of the DNA helix around the lesion and dual incision. The oligonucleotide patch carrying the lesion is excised, and the remaining gap is filled by regular DNA replication, using the intact complementary strand as a template. The main transducer kinase activated by the NER pathway is probably ATR, in response to UV-induced DNA damage in particular (Shell et al., 2009).

2.3.2 Mismatch repair

Mismatch repair (MMR) targets mispaired bases and nucleotides and insertion-deletion loops that arise through errors in DNA replication. The mechanisms by which eukaryotic cells distinguish mismatched from correctly matched bases in non replicating DNA remain unclear, but it is thought that recognition involves the contact of MMR proteins with the replication machinery. The eukaryotic mismatch sensors are the heterodimeric hMutSα (MSH2-MSH6) and hMutSβ (MSH2-MSH3) complexes. Whereas hMutSα preferentially recognizes base-base mismatches and insertion/deletion mispairs of one or two nucleotides, hMutSβ recognizes larger insertion/deletion mispairs (Li, 2008). The removal of mismatched bases and the restoration of strand integrity resemble the processes occurring in BER and NER. MMR proteins can interact with proteins in other repair pathways, such as BER, NER and homologous recombination, suggesting coordinated crosstalk between these processes (Kunkel & Erie, 2005). hMutSα and hMutSβ may directly activate DNA damage signaling by physical interaction with ATM, ATR-ATRIP, c-Abl, and the p53-related transcription factor p73 (Kim et al., 2007; Shimodaira et al., 2003; Yoshioka et al., 2006). Consistently, hMutSα and hMutSβ-deficient cells are defective in cell cycle arrest in response to multiple types of DNA damaging agents (Li, 2008). Another model proposes that a DDR could be activated by DNA breaks that are produced during "futile" DNA repair cycles. This model suggests that strand-specific MMR, which targets only newly replicated DNA, engages in repetitive repair cycles when it encounters a DNA lesion in the template strand, and this futile cycling activates ATR and/or ATM signaling leading to cell cycle arrest and apoptosis (Li, 1999; 2008).

2.3.3 Double-strand break repair pathways

It is generally accepted that the DNA double-strand break (DSB) is one of the most toxic and mutagenic DNA lesions occurring in human cells. A single DSB can, if left unrepaired, lead to the loss of a chromosome fragment and, thus, the death of the cell. However, despite the potential danger posed by DSBs, eukaryotic cells have evolved ways of improving biological processes based on the controlled induction of a DSB. Examples of this include the generation of variation during meiosis (Inagaki et al., 2010) and in the immune system (Fugmann et al., 2000), and the relaxation of supercoiled DNA by topoisomerases. Another endogenous source of DSBs are reactive oxygen species (ROS) produced by normal cellular processes, such as oxidative respiration, cytochrome P450 metabolism, peroxisomes and inflammatory responses. Examples of exogenous sources of DSBs will be described below.

DSB repair occurs via two main pathways: non homologous end-joining (NHEJ) and homologous recombination (HR) repair (Wyman & Kanaar, 2006). In mammalian cells, NHEJ is the major pathway for repairing breaks not associated with replication. This process may occur in all phases of the cell cycle, but predominantly in G1 phase. NHEJ involves the direct rejoining of two damaged DNA ends in a sequence-independent manner (Helleday et al., 2007; Weterings & van Gent, 2004). This end-joining mechanism is very precise for blunt ends and other simple end structures (van Heemst et al., 2004). However, the processing of incompatible ends may result in sequence alterations, such as deletions, occurring at "complicated" breaks. DNA double-strand breaks are first sensed by the ring-shaped Ku70/80 heterodimer. This DNA-Ku70/80 complex then attracts and activates the serine/threonine kinase activity of the DNA-PK catalytic subunit (DNA-PKcs). Following correct end alignment, DNA-PKcs is autophosphorylated (Weterings & Chen, 2007) and makes the ends available for ligation by ligase IV/XRCC4. Another essential NHEJ factor involved in the ligation of DSBs is XLF/Cernunnos (Ahnesorg et al., 2006; Buck et al., 2006). The MRN (Mre11 (Meiotic recombination 11)-Rad50-Nbs1 (Nijmegen breakage syndrome 1)) complex may facilitate the alignment of the two DNA ends, particularly when end processing is required (de Jager et al., 2001; Moreno-Herrero et al., 2005). The processing of "complex" lesions, such as hairpins, damaged backbone sugar residues, damaged bases, aberrant 5′ hydroxyl groups or 3′ phosphate groups, may involve polynucleotide kinase (Chappell et al., 2002; Koch et al., 2004), the RecQ helicase WRN (Perry et al., 2006), DNA polymerases μ and λ (Nick McElhinny et al., 2005) and the structure-specific nuclease Artemis (Ma et al., 2002; Moshous et al., 2001).

It has recently been suggested that there is an alternative or "backup"-NHEJ (B-NHEJ) pathway that functions in conditions in which the NHEJ pathway is compromised (Iliakis, 2009). The B-NHEJ pathway seems to be dependent principally on histone H1 (Rosidi et al., 2008), PARP, which binds to DSBs with an even greater affinity than that with which it binds SSBs (D'Silva et al., 1999), and DNA ligase III/XRCC1 (Audebert et al., 2004).

Whereas NHEJ repairs DNA in a template-independent fashion by rejoining two broken ends, HR can accurately resynthesize damaged or missing sequence information at the break site, using homologous sequences as a template, preferably the adjacent sister chromatid in S or G2 phase. Several mechanisms of HR have been identified (reviewed for example by Helleday et al. (2007) and Hartlerode & Scully (2009)). All are initiated by 5′→3′ resection at the DSB end, facilitated by the MRN complex (Paull & Gellert, 1998), which plays a critical role in the sensing of DSBs for HR. The MRN complex also recruits and helps to activate ATM (Lee & Paull, 2004; 2005). In addition to MRN, other factors, including CtIP (CTBP-interacting protein), Exo1 and BLM (Bloom's syndrome protein), are required for 5'-end resection in mammalian cells (Hartlerode & Scully, 2009; Sartori et al., 2007; Yun & Hiom, 2009). After resection, single-stranded DNA (ssDNA) rapidly binds the ssDNA-binding protein RPA, which is then replaced by multimers of the Rad51 recombinase, forming a nucleoprotein filament at the end of the ssDNA. Rad51 loading involves direct interaction with BRCA2 (Pellegrini et al., 2002) and other factors (Hartlerode & Scully, 2009; Sy et al., 2009). The Rad51 nucleoprotein filament then captures double-stranded DNA (dsDNA) and scans it for homology (Bianco et al., 1998). When a homologous region is encountered, the 3'-end of the invading strand is extended by a polymerase, using the duplex DNA as a template. From this stage on, the repair pathway may diverge. The DSBR (DNA double-strand break repair pathway, also known as the double Holliday junction model) pathway mostly results in chromosomal crossover, whereas the SDSA (synthesis-dependent strand annealing) pathway ends with non crossover products (Johnson & Jasin, 2000; Liu & West, 2004; Van Dyck et al., 2001).

2.4 Dynamics and heterogeneity of DNA damage

One challenge in the study of the cellular response to DNA damage is the multitude of lesions introduced by most genotoxic agents. For instance, the exposure of cells to IR results in damage to all components of the cell, including lipids, proteins and nucleic acids. IR acts directly on the DNA, causing breaks in its phosphodiester backbone. This process accounts for about 30% of the DNA damage induced by IR (Chapman et al., 1973). The radicals produced by the indirect effects of radiation may account for as much as 70% of the DNA damage induced by IR (Chapman et al., 1973). These radicals damage DNA, resulting in a wide diversity of DNA lesions, such as damage to bases and the backbone sugar (oxidation, rearrangement, adducts), intrastrand crosslinks, the formation of abasic sites, single- and double-strand breaks and DNA-protein crosslinks (Jeggo & Lavin, 2009). Complex lesions, such as clustered DSBs and LMDS (locally multiply damaged sites) may also occur. After these complex lesions, DSBs are the most harmful lesions to the cell (Ward, 1975). It has been shown, in rodent cells, that the extent of cell death is directly correlated with the yield of DSB under various X-ray irradiation conditions (Radford, 1985). IR is therefore often used in investigations of the cellular response to DSBs. However, DSBs are not the most frequent type of lesion induced by IR. A dose of 1 Gy, for example, induces about 1000 SSBs and 150 protein-DNA crosslinks, but only 40 DSBs (Friedberg, 1995).

The reaction of various alkylating agents with DNA leads to the formation of highly heterogeneous products. Some agents may preferentially produce certain alkylation products, but the DNA damage generated is never limited to a single type (De Bont & van Larebeke, 2004). Furthermore, as for IR, other cell components, including proteins and ribonucleic acids, may be modified. Cellular responses to these modifications, such as activation of the proteasomal degradation pathway, may interfere with DDR pathways, or be involved in crosstalk with these pathways.

One type of damage can be transformed into another by inefficient repair and DNA replication or transcription (Figure 2). As described above, DNA repair pathways, such as BER, MMR and NER, generate intermediate SSBs. These SSBs may result in DSBs, if the repair is incomplete and the lesion persists (Bonner et al., 2008). The transformation of SSBs into DSBs occurs, for example, when replication forks encounter a SSB on the template and collapse (Strumberg et al., 2000) (Figure 2). Common types of DNA damage interfering with replication fork

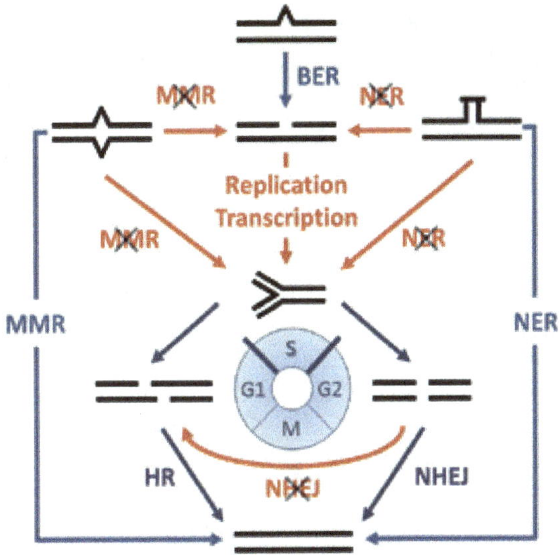

Fig. 2. Transformation of DNA damage. DNA lesions are normally repaired by the corresponding repair pathways. However, deficient repair may result in SSBs or DSBs. If a lesion persists during S-Phase (blue circle), stalled replication forks may arise. The collapse of a stalled replication fork results frequently in DSBs. DNA damage symbols and abbreviations are as for Figure 1.

progression are adducts of DNA bases (Helleday et al., 2008). By the same mechanism, inhibitors of DNA synthesis may also indirectly cause DSBs, as they impair replication fork progression (Lundin et al., 2002). Such inhibitors include aphidicolin, which inhibits DNA polymerases (Ikegami et al., 1978) and hydroxyurea, an inhibitor of ribonucleotide reductase (Bianchi et al., 1986). Topoisomerase inhibitors induce DSBs by exploiting the natural activity of topoisomerases during DNA replication. Topoisomerases resolve the DNA torsions induced during replication, by introducing a transient break in the DNA. Inhibitors of topoisomerases prevent the resealing of the break, by trapping the enzyme in a complex with the DNA (Hsiang et al., 1989; Kohn et al., 1987).

Thus, DSBs are the final outcome of unrepaired damage at the end of all these transformation processes (Figure 2). It is therefore not surprising that redundant and well regulated mechanisms have evolved for detecting, in particular, the presence of this toxic lesion and for activating DDR. DSBs can activate DNA-PK directly and they also activate ATM and ATR after end resection (Lopez-Contreras & Fernandez-Capetillo, 2010; Smith et al., 2010). Under certain conditions, PARP may also signal the presence of a DSB (Iliakis, 2009). The direct precursors of DSBs – SSBs and stalled replication forks – may themselves induce DDR, but there is less redundancy in the detection of these structures. SSBs are probably recognized and signaled to damage checkpoints mostly by PARP (Bouchard et al., 2003) and aberrant replication forks induce ATR activity through the recognition of RPA-coated stretches of ssDNA (Lopez-Contreras & Fernandez-Capetillo, 2010). The lack of redundancy in the signaling of these structures may account for their frequent transformation into DSBs.

2.5 Cellular DNA damage response

DNA breaks, including DSBs in particular, induce a highly coordinated DDR process leading to signal amplification, enhanced repair functions, cell cycle arrest or apoptosis. Many proteins are implicated in the DDR, which involves complex spatial and temporal coordination and many dynamic interactions between repair proteins and DNA.

2.5.1 Spatiotemporal organization of the DNA damage response

The components of the DDR pathway may be classified roughly as DNA-damage sensors, mediators, transducers and effectors (Figure 3A). After the sensing of a DNA break, mediator and repair proteins rapidly accumulate on the chromatin surrounding the lesion, to form subnuclear repair foci (Fernandez-Capetillo et al., 2003) (Figure 3B). Protein recruitment to DSBs normally occurs in a hierarchical manner and involves multiple posttranslational modifications, such as phosphorylation, ubiquitination, PARylation or acetylation (Essers et al., 2002; Lukas et al., 2004; Polo & Jackson, 2011). The massive accumulation of DNA repair and signaling factors may lead to structural stabilization of the break. The amplification and maintenance of the DNA-damage signal through the recruitment of multiple copies of transducer kinases to sites of damage is probably an even more important function (Misteli & Soutoglou, 2009).

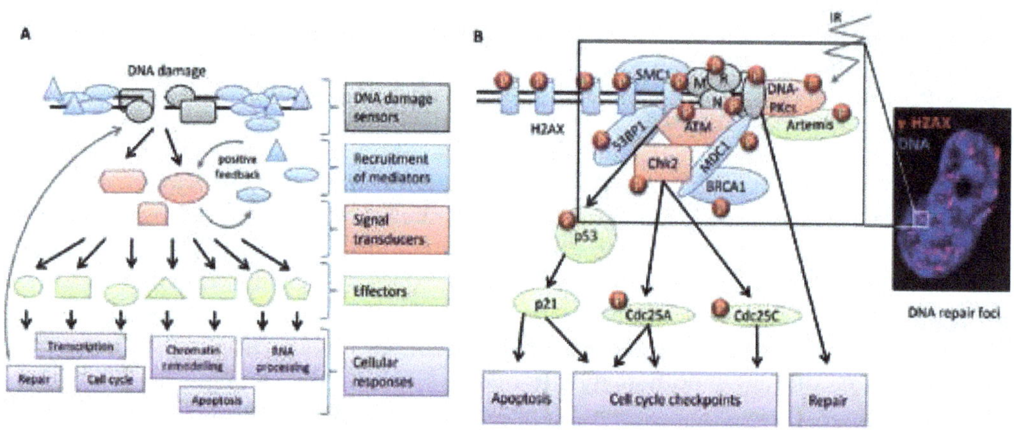

Fig. 3. The DDR signal transduction cascade. (A) DNA damage is first physically recognized by sensor proteins (gray). Mediator proteins (blue) facilitate the recruitment and activation of transducer kinases (red). A positive feedback loop between mediators and transducers leads to the maintenance and amplification of the signal. The transducer kinases then phosphorylate various effector proteins (green), including kinases, transcription factors and repair proteins. Depending on the severity of the damage, this can lead to various cellular responses (purple). (B) Formation of multiprotein complexes at the sites of DSBs (Ward & Chen, 2004) and microscopic visualization of the formation of γ-H2AX foci in response to IR. The exposure of cells to IR results in the rapid recruitment of numerous proteins to the sites of DNA lesions. The signal transducing kinases ATM and the related DNA-PK initiate a cascade of phosphorylation events (P), amplifying the signal to activate, if necessary, cell cycle checkpoint pathways or apoptosis, in situations in which the damage is too great to be repaired.

DNA break sensors include the MRN complex (Rupnik et al., 2008), Ku70/80, PARP and RPA. Break recognition by these sensors leads to the activation of transducer kinases, such as the PIKKs ATM, ATR and DNA-PK as well as PARP (Iliakis, 2009; Stiff et al., 2004; Ward & Chen, 2001). ATM, DNA-PK and ATR can phosphorylate the serine 139 residue of the histone variant H2AX (yielding γ-H2AX), at nucleosomes around the lesion. H2AX phosphorylation is probably the earliest posttranslational modification in DDR and may be considered the initial signal amplification step. γ-H2AX formation is followed by binding of the mediator protein MDC1 (mediator of DNA damage checkpoint 1) to the DSB-flanking chromatin (Jungmichel & Stucki, 2010). Mediator or adaptor proteins help to transmit, enhance and sustain the signaling between sensors and transducers, leading to the spread of the repair machinery along the chromosome. Other mediators include 53BP1 (p53-binding protein 1) and BRCA1 (Li & Zou, 2005; Misteli & Soutoglou, 2009). The recruitment of 53BP1 and BRCA1 to the DSB is indirect, requiring the activity of the E3 ubiquitin ligases RNF8 (Huen et al., 2007; Kolas et al., 2007) and RNF168 (Doil et al., 2009; Stewart et al., 2009). ssDNA compartments may be bound by RPA, which subsequently recruits ATR (Lobrich & Jeggo, 2007) and Rad51. Foci of Rad51 binding colocalize with Rad52 (Liu & Maizels, 2000), Rad54 (Essers et al., 2002), RPA (Raderschall et al., 1999), BRCA1 (Scully et al., 1997) and BRCA2 (Chen et al., 1998). Sustained activation of the transducers results in the transmission of the damage signal to effectors, which relay the signal to downstream pathways with endpoints in different cellular processes, such as checkpoint arrest or apoptosis (Kastan & Bartek, 2004) (Figure 3).

Not all the actors in DNA damage signaling and repair form characteristic foci. Unlike ATM, MDC1, 53BP1, BRCA1/BARD1 and MRN, the central NHEJ proteins Ku70/80 and DNA-PK do not spread to the adjacent chromatin upon recruitment to the break, presumably because they are required at low copy number at sites of damage (Bekker-Jensen et al., 2006; Lukas et al., 2003). The same is true for the effector kinases Chk1 and Chk2, and for p53, which interact only transiently with damage sites, subsequently diffusing rapidly to relay the signal to their soluble downstream targets.

One endpoint of the described signaling cascade in response to DNA damage is the activation of checkpoints to provide the cell with more time for DNA repair. DDR checkpoints have been identified at the G1/S and G2/M boundaries, and during S phase and, potentially, in mitosis (reviewed by Lukas et al. (2004)). After activation, the transducer kinases ATM, ATR or DNA-PK phosphorylate p53 either directly or via ATM-induced activation of the effector kinase Chk (checkpoint kinase) 2. Phosphorylated p53 then induces transcription of the gene encoding the Cdk inhibitor p21, which ultimately prevents transition from G1 to S-phase. Both Chk 1 and 2 activate the G2/M and intra-S checkpoints (Smith et al., 2010). It was long thought that ATM principally phosphorylated Chk1 and that ATR preferentially phosphorylated Chk2. However, this view has been modified by the discovery of various crosstalk between these kinases (Bartek & Lukas, 2003). The precise role of DNA-PK in this regulation remains unclear. PARP may contribute to checkpoint signaling by activation of p53. p53 exhibits high affinity for automodified PARP (Malanga et al., 1998) and p53 functions are impaired in PARP-deficient cells (Wang et al., 1998; Wieler et al., 2003). Furthermore, PARP activation in response to excessive DNA damage leads to extensive NAD^+ consumption. The cellular NAD^+ depletion can induce cell death through several mechanisms, depending on the cellular context (reviewed by Rouleau et al. (2010)).

2.5.2 Complexity of DNA damage response regulation

The outcomes of DNA damage signaling are, literally, a matter of life or death. Depending on the severity of DNA damage, the cell will either repair the damage to enable it to continue dividing or enter apoptosis. Complex, redundant signaling pathways converging on several central node proteins have emerged to ensure that this signaling remains under tight control. These node proteins must obtain input signals from several sources, in the form of protein modifications, before they can relay the signal to downstream effectors. This has a protective effect, greatly reducing the risk of important cell fate decisions, such as entry into apoptosis, occurring in response to a single erroneous input signal (Yarosh, 2001). The nodes in DDR include checkpoint proteins, such as Chk1 and Chk2, which control cell cycling and require input signals from several sources for full activation (McAdams & Arkin, 1999). Another prominent example for a node protein in DNA damage signaling is p53 (Kohn, 1999). The p53 protein has 11 sites for phosphorylation and acetylation, and can theoretically assume about 2000 modification states, if all the possible independent combinations are taken into account. Twelve different kinases can phosphorylate p53, and activated p53 can interact with at least 15 downstream proteins (Yarosh, 2001). The kinases that phosphorylate p53 in response to DNA damage include DNA-PK, ATM and ATR. Full p53 activity requires phosphorylation by both DNA-PK and ATM, at least (Wang et al., 2000). It is therefore now thought that p53 plays a key role in determining the degree of damage, through the assessment of input signals, on which the decision as to whether apoptosis is necessary is based (Kohn, 1999). There is a need to determine the specific conditions under which individual PIKKs become activated. Which (genotoxic) stresses lead to the activation of all transducer kinases? Is it possible to activate a single PIKK specifically, without affecting the others, and what are the cellular consequences of this?

There is also direct interplay between the transducer kinases (Chen et al., 2007). PIKKs can phosphorylate each other in response to DNA damage, resulting in mutual control of their activities. In addition to mediating posttranslational modifications, the kinases seem to regulate each other, either directly or indirectly (Peng et al., 2005). Studies on mutants and siRNA experiments have shown that a decrease in the amount of one of these kinases often leads to a decrease in the amounts of the PIKK sister kinases. The location of the kinases also seems to play an important role. For ATM, for example, the concentration of multiple copies in repair foci plays an important role in kinase activation, whereas DNA-PK does not need such an accumulation of multiple copies for full activation.

Another layer of complexity is added by the partially overlapping substrate specificities of the transducers ATM, DNA-PK and ATR (reviewed by Durocher & Jackson (2001) and Yang et al. (2003)). These transducers signal different types of DNA damage, but it was recently shown that the PIKK-mediated signaling network is highly extensive, with hundreds of phosphorylation events at ATR, ATM and DNA-PK consensus target sites induced by IR (Matsuoka et al., 2007). As discussed above, the plethora of types of damage induced by IR results in the activation of all three PIKKs. It remains to be determined which substrates are specific or overlapping for which transducer kinases in this long list of potential PIKK targets. Further insight into the contributions of individual repair signaling pathways has been provided by studies of the responses induced by damage signals in the absence of chromatin damage. This aspect will be discussed below.

3. Methods and mechanisms for inducing a damage response in the absence of chromatin damage

The induction of DNA damage repair pathways by exogenous DNA was first reported in bacteria, into which UV-irradiated lambda bacteriophages (D'Ari & Huisman, 1982; George et al., 1974) or plasmids (Bailone et al., 1984) were introduced. This indirect response is controlled by activation at the sites of exogenous DNA damage of the RecA protein, the key enzyme of the bacterial damage signaling response known as the "SOS response" (see Schlacher & Goodman (2007)). No such mechanism was initially found in mammals, despite a few publications reporting that UV-irradiated H-1 parvovirus or SV40 simian virus induced an "SOS-like" repair pathway in infected mammalian cells (Cornelis et al., 1982). Elucidation of the mechanisms underlying the response to damaged DNA or RNA in the cell took much longer in mammals. We review here the mammalian cell response to oligonucleotides, viral and immunostimulatory DNA and the insight into DDR gained from the analysis of artificial repair foci.

3.1 Cellular response to DNA oligonucleotides

In bacteria, ssDNA has been identified as the signal triggering the bacterial SOS repair response. The RecA protein (Rad51 in humans) is directly stimulated by ssDNA, inactivating the LexA repressor and triggering the repair response (Craig & Roberts, 1981). It has been suggested that ssDNA (at SSBs, stalled replication forks or resected DSBs) acts also as the major stimulatory signal for DNA damage responses in eukaryotic cells (Li & Deshaies, 1993; Nur et al., 2003). Several studies based on transfection or the microinjection of synthetic DNA oligonucleotides have analyzed the response of the cell to ssDNA. Studies by Nur et al. (2003) have shown that ssDNA acts upstream from ATM/p53 in DNA damage signaling. The transfection of cells with short (as few as 5 bases) ssDNA molecules with random sequences induced ATM activation and apoptosis, whereas very short (8 bp) dsDNA molecules did not (Nur et al., 2003). The induction of apoptosis by ssDNA is consistent with earlier studies, in which transfection with randomly fragmented DNA (Schiavone et al., 2000) or the nuclear injection of linearized plasmid DNA, circular DNA containing a gap, or single-stranded circular phagemids induced cell cycle arrest or apoptosis (Huang et al., 1996). The activation of ATM by fragmented DNA requires the MRN-assisted assembly of short, linear ssDNA fragments into high-molecular weight complexes, as shown by experiments in *Xenopus laevis* extracts (Costanzo et al., 2004).

So, if ssDNA can activate ATM directly, how is ATM activated in response to DNA double-strand breaks? When DNA double-strand breaks are sensed by the MRN complex, MRN partially unwinds the ends to expose ssDNA (Lee & Paull, 2005). It has been shown in *Xenopus laevis* egg extracts that 70 bp synthetic double-stranded molecules are rapidly resected in an MRN-dependent manner to generate ssDNA oligonucleotides, which activate ATM (Jazayeri et al., 2008). Consistent with these findings, the injection of small synthetic ssDNA oligomers into undamaged cells also induces ATM activation, and the elimination of ssDNA oligomers results in the rapid extinction of ATM activity. In summary, the results obtained from experiments with single-stranded or long double-stranded DNA fragments suggest that short ssDNA molecules are the essential signal for the induction of ATM-dependent cell cycle arrest and apoptosis.

The cellular response to single-stranded oligonucleotides may also have consequences for targeted gene repair with synthetic oligonucleotides. In gene targeting processes, ssDNA molecules are transported to the nucleus, where they align with their complementary sequence in the target gene, facilitating nucleotide exchange (Brachman & Kmiec, 2002). However, the introduction of large amounts of oligonucleotides into cells may induce cell cycle arrest and stalled DNA replication in the corrected cells, due to the ATM activation by the mechanism described above. Ferrara & Kmiec (2006) showed that the transfection of human colorectal cancer cells with 47-mer single-stranded oligonucleotides mostly activated Chk1 and Chk2 in corrected cells. As a consequence, uncorrected cells may outgrow corrected cells. The uncorrected cells probably contain fewer oligonucleotides, too few indeed to generate a local ssDNA concentration high enough to activate ATM. This may account for previous reports of the decline of corrected populations over time (Igoucheva et al., 2004).

3.2 Synthetic interstrand crosslinks

The cytotoxic activity of many chemotherapeutic agents, including cisplatin, nitrogen mustards and mitomycin C, is due to the induction of interstrand crosslinks (ICLs) in DNA. These lesions block the strand separation necessary for essential DNA functions, such as transcription and replication. ICLs affect both strands of the chromosome, and their repair is particularly complex. It involves factors from multiple repair pathways and the mechanisms may differ at different stages of the cell cycle. Nucleotide-excision repair, homologous recombination repair, the Fanconi anemia repair pathway, MMR and translesion synthesis have all been shown to participate in ICL repair.

Oligonucleotides containing synthetic ICLs are a valuable tool for the study of ICL repair (Guainazzi & Scharer, 2010). The advantage of such molecules over cell treatment with a cross-linking agent is that it is possible to study the components involved in the repair of specific interstrand crosslink products one at a time. This has mostly involved the ligation of the synthetic ICL-containing DNA fragments into plasmids, followed by analysis of their repair in cell-free extracts or cells (Orelli et al., 2010; Raschle et al., 2008; Wang et al., 2001). The repair of the specific ICL can be analyzed with reporter genes or by enzymatic digestion followed by Southern blotting. Studies with synthetic DNA ICLs have contributed to our understanding of the mechanism of replication-coupled DNA ICL repair (Wang et al., 2001) and the role of the Fanconi anemia pathway in this repair process (Knipscheer et al., 2009).

3.3 Viral infection

The highly organized cellular response to DNA damage may be disorganized or hijacked during viral infection (Lilley et al., 2007; Weitzman et al., 2004). Viruses often produce large amounts of exogenous DNA during infection, and generate proteins that interfere with DNA repair pathways and cell cycle checkpoints. Recent studies have suggested that the cellular DNA repair machinery can recognize viral nucleic acids as damage (Lilley et al., 2007). In some cases, the host DNA repair response is inactivated by viruses, whereas in others, the maintenance of a functional host DNA repair machinery seems to increase viral replication. Studies of the interaction of viruses with the host cell DNA repair machinery have improved our understanding of normal cellular DNA repair functions, and viruses may be useful model systems for studying certain aspects of DNA repair (Weitzman & Ornelles, 2005). In this section, we provide an overview of the ways in which viral infection can activate the DDR in cells, thereby focusing on the response to viral genomic material. For a detailed description of the ways in which viral proteins can manipulate the host DNA repair machinery and cell cycle checkpoints, we refer the reader to Chaurushiya & Weitzman (2009), Davy & Doorbar (2007) and Weitzman et al. (2004).

3.3.1 DDR induction by DNA viruses

Adenoviruses (Ad), which belong to the parvovirus family, are probably the most thoroughly investigated DNA viruses. Their genome consists of a linear, 36 kb dsDNA molecule, with inverted terminal repeats (ITRs) at each end and origins for DNA replication (Weitzman & Ornelles, 2005). Viral proteins synthesized before viral DNA replication prevent the recognition of the Ad genome by host DNA repair factors. This may involve the targeting, by these proteins, of cellular damage sensors and repair effectors, such as the MRN complex or DNA ligase IV, for degradation and relocalization (Carson et al., 2003; Stracker et al., 2002). Infection with Ad lacking the proteins required for blockade of the host DNA repair machinery results in partial DDR activation. DNA damage mediator proteins accumulate at sites of viral replication (Stracker et al., 2002) and γ-H2AX is formed at the periphery of viral centers, in a process dependent on host cell PIKK activity (Carson et al., 2003). Despite the interference of viral proteins with the cellular DNA repair system during infection with wild-type Ad, the cellular DDR does not seem to be completely abolished. The foreign DNA induces H2AX phosphorylation during later stages of infection, after the onset of viral DNA replication (Nichols et al., 2009). H2AX phosphorylation follows a pan-nuclear pattern, suggesting that all the H2AX on the host chromatin is phosphorylated by ectopic kinase activation, contrasting with the localized γ-H2AX formation observed in response to DSBs in the chromatin. Viral replication seems to be required for this phosphorylation, because infection with a nonreplicating virus does not induce γ-H2AX (Nichols et al., 2009) production. ATR may be the principal kinase phosphorylating H2AX in these conditions, although ATM and DNA-PK also seem to be involved (Nichols et al., 2009).

Pan-nuclear H2AX phosphorylation has also been observed in cells infected with the adeno-associated virus (AAV) (Collaco et al., 2009; Fragkos et al., 2008; Schwartz et al., 2009). The AAV genome, like that of Ad, consists of an ssDNA molecule with ITRs at both ends, resulting in the formation of double-hairpin structures (Brown, 2010). AAV infection requires helper functions, which may be supplied by Ad or other viruses (Geoffroy & Salvetti, 2005), and components of the host cell DNA replication machinery (Nash et al., 2009). Viral replication takes place in the nucleus, where cellular proteins, including RPA, colocalize with viral proteins in replication centers (Stracker et al., 2004). AAV replication in the presence of minimal Ad helper proteins induces a robust DDR-like response. This response is independent of the MRN complex and seems to be mediated principally by DNA-PKcs and, to a lesser extent, by ATM (Collaco et al., 2009; Schwartz et al., 2009). The response involves the accumulation of DNA-PK in compartments in which viral replication is occurring, and the pan-nuclear phosphorylation, not only of H2AX, but also of Smc1 and ATM (Schwartz et al., 2009). In another study, the phosphorylation of RPA, Nbs1 and Chk1/2 was observed, but the phosphorylation pattern was not investigated (Collaco et al., 2009).

In addition to the DNA-PK-dependent DDR induced by AAV replication, studies on recombinant AAV (rAAV) vectors (Carter, 2004), have demonstrated the existence of a requirement for DNA-PKcs and Ku70/80 for viral DNA replication (Choi et al., 2010). The inactivation of DNA-PK by a DNA-PK inhibitor or siRNA significantly decreases the replication of rAAV, and any rAAV DNA that is replicated forms head-to-head or tail-to-tail junctions. Moreover, AAV-ITRs interact directly with Ku proteins, suggesting that viral DNA is recognized directly by cellular NHEJ factors (Choi et al., 2010). Furthermore, DNA-PKcs and Artemis have been shown to open the ITR hairpin loops of rAAV *in vivo*, in a tissue-dependent manner. In the absence of either of these factors, double-stranded linear rAAV genomes capped with covalently closed hairpins at their termini accumulate in cells (Inagaki et al., 2007), confirming the importance of host cell NHEJ proteins for viral DNA end processing. By contrast to the "hyperactivation" of DNA-PK observed in response to replicating AAV, the DNA of UV-inactivated AAV particles activates a DDR involving ATM and ATR, leading to the inhibition of cell cycle progression (Jurvansuu et al., 2005). It has been suggested that the UV-treated DNA mimics stalled replication forks (Jurvansuu et al., 2005), whereas DNA-PK activation is consistent with the presence of DSBs as intermediate products during AAV replication.

DNA-PKcs and Ku70/80 as well as other cellular repair or replication factors including Topoisomerases I and II, MSH2-MSH6, RecQL, PARP and scaffold attachment factor A (SAF-A) are involved in Kaposi's sarcoma-associated herpesvirus (KSHV) lytic replication (Wang et al., 2008). KSHV is a large dsDNA virus and the etiologic agent of several AIDS-associated cancers, including Kaposi's sarcoma (Antman & Chang, 2000). The lytic replication of KSHV and the continuous primary infection of fresh cells are responsible for viral tumorigenicity and pathogenesis, by contrast to what has been reported for other oncogenic viruses (Grundhoff & Ganem, 2004). The proteins listed above bind to KSHV DNA fragments and accumulate in viral replication compartments in the nucleus, suggesting a possible role for these host replication and repair proteins in the viral lytic replication process (Wang et al., 2008).

In the case of infection with herpes simplex virus type 1 (HSV-1), which contains a linear dsDNA molecule, a DNA damage signaling is induced which depends principally on ATR (Lilley et al., 2005; Wilkinson & Weller, 2006). Several members of the cellular DNA damage-sensing machinery, including RPA, RAD51 and Nbs1, are activated and redistributed during viral DNA replication, indicating that infection induces the host response to DNA damage. H2AX is phosphorylated but the γ-H2AX signal is marginalized to the periphery of viral replication centers (Wilkinson & Weller, 2006). HSV-1 sequesters hyperphosphorylated RPA away from viral replication compartments, thus preventing a normal ATR-signaling response. The partial and mislocalized activation of the cellular DDR leads ultimately to its disorganization.

ATR is also activated during viral replication of the dsDNA virus human cytomegalovirus (HCMV), leading to an induction of γ-H2AX (Luo et al., 2007). Contrary to what has been observed for HSV-1, γ-H2AX co-localizes with viral replication compartments during late-stage infections with HCMV. Only a subset of proteins in addition to γ-H2AX was specifically sequestered in viral replication centers, with other proteins excluded from these centers, impeding both the efficient repair of viral DNA and checkpoint activation (Luo et al., 2007).

ATM-dependent checkpoint signaling takes place during induction of Epstein Barr virus lytic replication (Kudoh et al., 2005) or polyomavirus replication (Dahl et al., 2005). This is accompanied by the phosphorylation of a number of DNA damage markers including H2AX. The cellular ATM activation in response to both viruses leads to a prolonged S-phase advantageous for viral lytic replication. However, both viruses have developed efficient strategies to block ATM-induced p53 downstream signaling that would eventually lead to apoptosis (Dahl et al., 2005; Kudoh et al., 2005). By contrast, the autonomous minute virus of canines (MVC), a member of the parvovirus family, induces apoptosis and G(2)/M-phase arrest in infected canine cells (Chen et al., 2010). This seems to be the result of the induction of an ATM/p53-mediated DDR (Luo et al., 2011). Infected cells display phosphorylation of H2AX, RPA, ATM and ATR. The inhibition or knockdown of ATM decreased cell death and reduced MVC DNA replication.

In summary, studies of the response of the cell to viral genomic material have demonstrated that the activation of a damage response involving ATM (e.g. in the case of MVC) or ATR (UV-inactivated rAAV) leads to cell cycle arrest or p53-dependent cell death, unless downstream effectors are inactivated or sequestered by viral proteins (HSV-1, HCMV). By contrast, DNA-PK activation (Ad, AAV) leads to pan-nuclear H2AX phosphorylation, which does not seem to be detrimental to the cell. These findings have possible consequences for the choice of viral vectors for gene targeting. It remains to be determined whether the "ectopic" phosphorylation of DNA-PK downstream targets affects the stability of the host cell genome or impairs DNA repair in infected cells. It has also been shown that the specific recruitment of a subset of cellular DNA repair factors is essential for viral DNA replication, suggesting that inhibitors targeting these proteins may have antiviral activity.

3.3.2 DNA damage signals induced by retroviruses

Interaction with the cellular DNA damage sensing machinery is not limited to DNA viruses. Retroviruses, which contain a single-stranded RNA genome, use a viral-encoded reverse transcriptase to generate a cDNA that is then integrated into the host genome. The preintegration complex contains the cDNA and the viral-encoded integrase enzyme. This enzyme then mediates strand transfer to integrate the viral DNA into the host DNA in a non site-specific fashion (Weitzman et al., 2004). The interaction of retroviruses with the cellular DNA repair machinery has been studied in detail (Lilley et al., 2007; Sakurai et al., 2009; Skalka & Katz, 2005). The NHEJ pathway has been implicated in the sensing and processing of the linear cDNA, although the exact step of the viral life-cycle affected by the cellular DNA repair machinery remains unclear Ariumi et al. (2005). It is possible that the viral cDNA acts directly as a substrate for NHEJ, which circularizes the DNA by end ligation (Li et al., 2001). The circularization of unintegrated DNA in this context may protect the viral DNA from degradation and the cell from apoptosis (Kilzer et al., 2003). Consistent with this hypothesis, the infection with retrovirus of cells lacking NHEJ factors results in apoptosis, suggesting that DNA-PKcs and Ku70/80 may protect against the cellular toxicity of high levels of retroviral cDNA (Li et al., 2001).

Another interaction of retroviruses with the DNA repair machinery is constituted by the role of cellular repair and damage signaling factors in the integration of viral DNA into the host genome (Daniel et al., 1999). During retroviral integration, DSBs are created as an intermediate that may be detected as DNA damage by the host cell (Sakurai et al., 2009). Transient phosphorylation of histone H2AX occurs at retroviral integration sites, and it has been suggested that the completion of the integration process is dependent on DNA-PK (Daniel et al., 1999; 2004). DNA-PK-deficient mouse scid cells infected with three different retroviruses display much lower levels of DNA integration than wild-type cells and die by apoptosis. Furthermore, it has been reported that DNA-PKcs is required for efficient transduction by retroviral vectors (Daniel et al., 1999). Other PIKKs have since been shown to be activated after HIV-1 infection and to play a potential role in provirus integration. The use of caffeine or a small-molecule inhibitor to block the ATM activity results in the inhibition of HIV transduction and replication (Daniel et al., 2005; Lau et al., 2005).

DNA-PK and ATM also seem to be important for correct end processing at the junctions between HIV-1 provirus and host DNA (Sakurai et al., 2009). Large numbers of abnormal junctions are observed in Mre11- and DNA-PKcs-deficient cells, and Artemis-deficient cells also display such abnormalities, suggesting a role for NHEJ processing factors in correct viral integration. Another study has reported a role for Ku70/80 in the targeting of retroviral elements to chromatin domains prone to gene silencing. Higher levels of viral DNA expression are observed in the absence of Ku70/80, with no effect on viral transduction (Masson et al., 2007).

The importance of cellular components of the DDR for the replication of some viruses could be exploited for therapeutic purposes. For instance, a small-molecule ATM-inhibitor displayed antiviral activity in a proof-of-concept study with HIV-1, in which ATM deficiency sensitized cells to retrovirus-induced cell death (Lau et al., 2005).

3.4 Tethering of repair factors

Recent studies in yeast and mammals have demonstrated that it is not the DNA lesion that triggers the DDR, leading to the activation of transducer kinases, but the local concentration of signaling factors at repair foci. Soutoglou & Misteli (2008) demonstrated that a DDR can be triggered in the absence of DNA lesions. The artificial localized tethering of repair factors was found to be sufficient to trigger a full DDR response, including cell-cycle arrest, in the absence of DNA breaks. Tethering was achieved by fusing repair proteins to the *Escherichia coli lac* repressor and expressing the resulting constructs in mouse NIH-3T3 cells containing multiple *lacR* binding sites, stably integrated into the genome (Soutoglou & Misteli, 2008). The immobilization of Nbs1, Mre11 or MDC1 alone led to DDR activation. In addition, the tethering of ATM was sufficient to induce ATM kinase activity and autophosphorylation. Consistent with its function downstream from the MRN complex, the induction of ATM activity was not affected by an absence of Mre11 or Nbs1. As similar results were obtained in analogous experiments in *Saccharomyces cerevisiae* (Bonilla et al., 2008), the concentration of key factors on the chromatin may be considered a universal characteristic of DDR initiation and amplification in eukaryotes (Misteli & Soutoglou, 2009). The tethering experiments may be seen as complementary to the experiments with siDNA described below, as the DNA break-mimicking DNA molecules are (i) too short for the formation of repair foci and (ii) not in a chromatin context.

3.5 DDR induction by cofactors, oxidative stress or changes in chromatin state

ATM, and consequently the DDR, can be activated in the absence of DNA breaks, by changes in chromatin structure. Bakkenist & Kastan (2003) showed that ATM is rapidly activated by the exposure of cells to chromatin-active agents, such as mild hypotonic buffers, or treatment with chloroquine. Furthermore, histone deacetylase (HDAC) inhibitors, such as TSA, which induces the global decondensation of chromatin, can also induce ATM activity (Jang et al., 2010; Mazumdar et al., 2006). Consistent with its role as a sensor of chromatin structure, ATM can interact with the chromatin via the nucleosome-binding protein HMGN1 before DNA damage occurs. The loss of this interaction in the absence of HMGN1 compromises ATM activation in response to IR (Kim et al., 2009).

ATM-dependent phosphorylation of H2AX during M-phase has been reported to occur in the absence of DNA damage (Ichijima et al., 2005; Mazumdar et al., 2006). The high degree of compaction of mitotic chromosomes may be the signal responsible for activating DNA damage signaling kinases in the absence of apparent DNA lesions (Ichijima et al., 2005).
Another recent study showed that DNA-damage signaling pathways and ATM could be activated directly by hypoxia, apparently in the absence of lesions (Bencokova et al., 2009). The direct mechanism involved is unknown, but the hypoxia-induced activation of ATM is independent of the MRN complex, and active, autophosphorylated ATM has a pan-nuclear rather than focal distribution. The activation of ATM signaling in response to hypoxia may account for the cessation of replication when oxygen levels are low.
ATM is a also a direct sensor of oxidative stress, in the absence of DNA lesions. Oxidation by ROS results in the formation of an active, disulfide-cross-linked, ATM dimer (Guo et al., 2010). The activation of ATM in response to oxidative stress is independent of the MRN complex and leads to the phosphorylation of DDR effectors including p53 and Chk2, but not the chromatin-associated proteins H2AX or Kap1. This confirms that ATM activation through oxidation may occur without the involvement of the DNA damage recognition machinery.
Consistent with ATM activation, the transducer kinase ATR can also be activated in the absence of DNA damage. Toledo et al. (2008) reported the ectopic activation of ATR following overproduction of a fragment of TopBP1 containing a domain known to stimulate ATR kinase activity (Kumagai et al., 2006). ATR activation was sufficient to drive cell cycle arrest and senescence.

3.6 Systemic response to foreign DNA

DNA fragments trigger a DDR at the cellular level, but the detection of foreign DNA by specific sensors can trigger an innate immune response at the systemic level (for review see Vilaysane & Muruve (2009), Yanai et al. (2009) and Rathinam & Fitzgerald (2011)). The innate immune system is an integral part of the host response to viral and bacterial intrusion. Its activation leads to diverse cellular responses, including the induction of interferon regulatory factors (IRF) 3 and 7, which regulate the production of type I interferon. Furthermore, NFκB is induced, and regulates the expression of pro-inflammatory cytokines (Vilaysane & Muruve, 2009). We provide here a brief overview of the principal sensors of foreign DNA found in humans.
Bacterial DNA differs from mammalian DNA principally in terms of its high CpG dinucleotide content. Furthermore, most of the small number of CpG dinucleotides present in mammalian DNA are methylated, whereas the CpG dinucleotides in bacterial DNA are generally unmethylated (Hemmi et al., 2000). The activation of innate immune responses by nucleic acids is mediated by transmembrane Toll-like receptors (TLRs) and cytosolic receptors. The best understood sensor of microbial DNA is TLR9, which is found principally in plasmacytoid dendritic cells (pDCs) in humans (Hemmi et al., 2000; Wagner, 2004). The endosomal uptake of CpG DNA activates TLR9, which binds MyD88, IRAK4 and IRAK1 that are required for the activation of NFκB and the induction of type I interferons via IRF7 (Akira et al., 2006; Vilaysane & Muruve, 2009). Several studies have also shown that, in addition to responding to bacterial DNA, TLR9 plays an important role in host defense against viruses, including DNA viruses such as herpes simplex virus and murine cytomegalovirus (Delale et al., 2005; Lund et al., 2003).

In addition to the membrane-bound TLR9, cytosolic DNA sensors have recently been identified (Yanai et al., 2009). These sensors include TREX1, DNA-dependent activator of interferon regulatory factors (DAI) and a DNA-sensing inflammasome containing absent in melanoma 2 (AIM2). This protein belongs to the HIN-200 family and is a cytoplasmic sensor mediating caspase 1 activation in response to cytoplasmic dsDNA (Burckstummer et al., 2009; Fernandes-Alnemri et al., 2009; Hornung et al., 2009). Another cytosolic DNA sensor and activator of innate immune responses, DAI (also known as DLM-1 and Z-DNA binding protein 1), has also recently been identified (Takaoka et al., 2007). DAI binds dsDNA, leading to its association with the IRF3 transcription factor and the TBK1 serine/threonine kinase, resulting in a signaling cascade that culminates in NFκB activation. The activation of interferon responses is restricted by the length of the DNA, with little activation observed in response to DNA molecules of less than 100 bp in length, suggesting that DAI activation requires the formation of a multimeric complex over long stretches of DNA (Takaoka & Taniguchi, 2008).

Several studies have identified the 3′→5′ DNA exonuclease DNaseIII/TREX1 as associated with autoimmune and inflammatory diseases in humans (Crow et al., 2006; Lee-Kirsch et al., 2007). TREX1 is a regulator of DNA homeostasis in the cell and has been reported to counteract the activation of ATM by small ssDNA fragments (section 3.1). Indeed, in the absence of TREX1, 60-65 bp ssDNA polynucleotides accumulate, leading to chronic ATM-dependent DNA damage checkpoint signaling (Yang et al., 2007). Thus, TREX1 is not itself a DNA sensor. Instead, it regulates the accumulation of the ssDNA that can trigger an innate immune response. In addition to linking a DDR factor to the immune response, these findings demonstrate that immune responses may be triggered not only by foreign DNA, but also by self-derived DNA.

The most prominent protein involved in both the DDR and the immune response, in addition to TREX1, is DNA-PKcs. In addition to its long known role in V(D)J recombination in developing lymphocytes (Jeggo et al., 1995), DNA-PKcs has also been reported to phosphorylate IFN regulatory factor-3 (IRF-3) directly (Karpova et al., 2002). IRF-3 plays a key role in the host response to viral infection, and its phosphorylation by DNA-PK after viral infection results in its nuclear retention and delayed proteolysis. Another study has suggested that DNA-PKcs mediates Akt activation in response to CpG-DNA in bone marrow-derived macrophages (BMDMs) (Dragoi et al., 2005). In BMDMs, DNA-PKcs associates with Akt upon CpG-DNA stimulation, thereby triggering the nuclear translocation of Akt. It has been suggested that TLR9 is involved in this pathway, but its possible role remains a matter of debate (Dragoi et al., 2005; Sester et al., 2006). The CpG-DNA/DNAPKcs/Akt pathway may account for the induction, by CpG-DNA and synthetic CpG oligonucleotides, of prosurvival signals delivered to the immune system (Dragoi et al., 2005; Park et al., 2002).

4. Signal interfering DNA (siDNA)

As summarized in Figures 1 and 2, difficulties attributing the activation of a specific transducer to a specific type of damage *in vivo* result principally from the multiple type of damage induced by a single treatment, through the mechanism of action of the treatment and metabolism of the initial damage through replication and repair. Moreover, the large DNA molecules sometimes used to induce a damage response (see section 3.1) probably contain sequences recognized by specific proteins that may interfere with DNA damage recognition and repair. We recently tried to overcome these problems by proposing the use of a new class of small molecules (siDNA, for small interfering DNA) each mimicking one particular type of damage and are not degraded, replicated or repaired in the cell.

4.1 SiDNA: principle and properties

We initially designed and tested only a few classes of siDNA molecules, to provide proof-of-concept for this approach. However, this concept can be extended to any specific type of damage. An siDNA is a small nucleic acid molecule carrying a modification recognized as a lesion by the sensor and transducer proteins. In addition to mimicking a specific type of damage, siDNA molecules must (i) be resistant to the action of nucleases, (ii) be as small as possible, to minimize the formation of secondary structures or degradation products, (iii) have no specific sequence likely to be recognized by DNA-binding proteins, such as transcription factors, (iv) mimic one single type of damage, ideally one that cannot be processed and (v) be recognized by at least one molecule involved in the DDR. SiDNAs are oligonucleotides chemically synthesized on solid support, by cycles of nucleotide addition. They are protected from exonuclease degradation by three phosphorothioate groups at the free 3′ and 5′ ends. Most siDNA molecules are double-stranded and have a specific modification characteristic of one type of damage. Dissociation of the short duplex is prevented by a linker tethering the two complementary strands at one or both ends of the molecule. The linker molecule

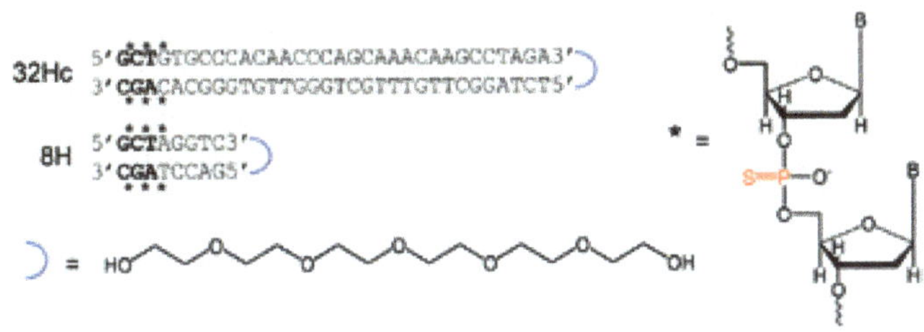

Fig. 4. Structure of the DSB-mimicking Dbait. Dbait 32Hc is a 32 bp DNA molecule tethered to its complementary sequence by a hexaethylene glycol loop (blue half circle) at one end and protected against exonuclease by phosphorothioate nucleotides (asterisks, phosphorothioate bond highlighted in red) at the other end. In the name 32Hc, H stands for hexaethylene glycol and c refers to the sequence. The sequence is not important for recognition as a DSB. The corresponding negative control, 8H, has the same basic structural features as 32Hc, but is too short to bind the central NHEJ components. B, base.

consists of a polyethylene glycol chain that is inert and stable in living systems. The resulting molecules are very stable, with melting temperatures of about 85 to 90°C, despite their small size (between 16 and 64 bp). They are resistant to incubation for six hours with serum or cell extract (unpublished data). Like most nucleic acid-based molecules, siDNAs penetrate cells poorly and complexing with transfection agents (Patil et al., 2005) or lipophilic molecules (Rossi, 2004) is required for efficient entry. Three classes of molecules have already been tested: molecules mimicking double-strand breaks (Dbait), molecules mimicking single-strand breaks (Pbait) and molecules mimicking single-strand DNA stretches (Sbait). An example of the structure of a Dbait molecule is provided in Figure 4. Every siDNA is recognized by specific sensors and triggers a corresponding partial DDR.

4.2 SiDNAs induce specific, stable and persistent damage responses

PIKKs and PARP enzymes are thought to be the first transducers activated by DNA damage. We threfore monitored the cellular response induced by siDNAs by detecting the modification of the downstream targets of these enzymes in cells. Using mutant cells defective in the various enzymes, we showed that Dbait activated DNA-PK and PARP, Pbait activated only PARP and Sbait activated only ATM ((Quanz et al., 2009b); to be published). These transducer activations resulted in the posttranslational modification of all known targets of these enzymes investigated. For example, Dbait induces the phosphorylation of H2AX, RPA, p53, Nbs1, Chk1, Chk2, DNA-PK, ATM, Hsp90α, and the PARylation of a broad number of proteins. Interestingly, ATM which is also thought to be activated by DSBs, was not activated by Dbait or Pbait, but exclusively by Sbait molecules, which are single-stranded. This is consistent with the model in which DSBs must be partially degraded to activate ATM, as described above. The association of Mre11 with Rad50 and Nbs1 stimulates its endonuclease and exonuclease activities, resulting in the processing of DSB ends, leading to the generation of overhanging ssDNA regions (Paull & Gellert, 1998; 1999). Our results show that DSBs do not directly activate ATM if they remain unprocessed.

The posttranslational modifications induced by the siDNA-mediated activation of transducers persist for more than 24 hours in the cells. Phosphorylated or PARylated effectors have been detected more than one day after treatment and their persistence in cells depends on the turnover rate of the modified protein and the rate of cell division (Quanz et al., 2009b). Phosphorylated histone H2AX, for instance, was detected up to five days after treatment with Dbait, when Dbait molecules were no longer present in the cell. Similar results were obtained for other effectors, suggesting that siDNAs do not induce feedback control mechanisms ensuring the rapid return of cells to an "unactivated" state when repair is completed. At least three phosphatases, protein phosphatase 2A (PP2A), wild-type p53-induced phosphatase (Wip1) and protein phosphatase 5 (PP5), are involved in the DDR. It remains unclear how these phosphatases are activated during DDR, but they are instrumental in ATM activation (Ali et al., 2004; Goodarzi et al., 2004; Shreeram et al., 2006). The results of studies of unrepairable siDNAs suggest that the phosphatases or the proteasome must be activated by a "successful repair" signal instead, rather than simply removing phosphates or the modified proteins as a part of an equilibrium.

4.3 Transducer activation by siDNA is not sufficient to induce complete DDR

Although transducers are fully activated and all their molecular targets seem to be modified, the siDNAs Dbait and Pbait do not trigger the major end-points of the DDR response: cell-cycle arrest and apoptosis. In the absence of genotoxic or other stresses, cells with strong siDNA responses continue to divide at the same rate as untreated cells and do not enter apoptosis (Quanz et al., 2009b). This suggests that the DDR requires a correct spatio-temporal organization and/or more than a single damage signaling input for full execution. This is consistent with the model described above, in which redundant pathways may control the risk of erroneous signaling in cells (Yarosh, 2001). According to this hypothesis, the signal resulting from one siDNA treatment would not be sufficient to trigger a complete DDR response.

SiDNAs also differ from chromosomal DNA damage in their location and the timing of the different activation processes. SiDNAs constitute an artificial form of damage outside the context of chromatin and able to cross the cytoplasm, which contains a subset of effectors and transducers, such as DNA-PK and PARP. These signaling enzymes are therefore activated in the cytoplasm and modify the targets present in this compartment (Quanz et al., submitted, Figure 5). The lack of coordination of target modifications at the site of DNA damage prevents

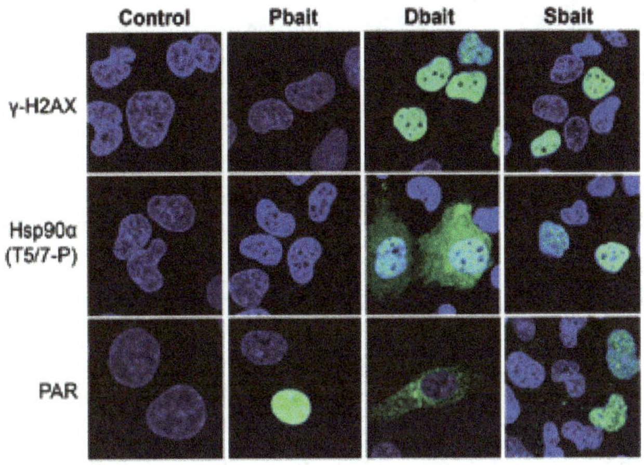

Fig. 5. Differential cytoplasmic and nuclear transducer activation by different siDNAs. Both Dbait and Sbait treatment lead to the phosphorylation of H2AX (green, top) and Hsp90α (green, middle) and induce a PARylation signal (green, bottom). Unlike Sbait, Dbait is already recognized in the cytoplasm, inducing cytoplasmic Hsp90α phosphorylation and a cytoplasmic PARylation signal. Pbait, which activates only PARP, induces PARylation but not the phosphorylation of H2AX or Hsp90α. The negative control is an siDNA molecule that is too short to recruit and activate DNA damage transducers. The cell nuclei are shown in blue.

the further accumulation of DNA repair proteins at repair foci at these sites (Quanz et al., 2009b). For example, in cells treated with Dbait, DNA-PK autophosphorylation is detected in both the cytoplasm and the nucleus and H2AX is phosphorylated along the length of the chromosome. After the irradiation of Dbait-treated cells, repair proteins, such as Nbs1, 53BP1, Rad51, do not relocate to sites of damage or form repair foci. However, despite their incapacity to form repair foci, irradiated siDNA-treated cells display a complete DDR response, with the induction of apoptosis (Quanz et al., 2009b).

4.4 SiDNAs inhibit DNA repair

The disturbance of the spatiotemporal organization of the DDR by siDNA leads to inhibition of the formation of repair foci after irradiation. Cells treated with Dbait or Pbait are therefore sensitive to IR or other DNA damaging agents. Irradiated DNA is repaired with two-component kinetics. Most of the damage is repaired rapidly, with no significant effect of Dbait treatment. By contrast, the repair of the residual damage (15-20%), which takes longer, is strongly affected by Dbait treatment (Quanz et al., Figure 6). The slowly repaired damage is thought to correspond to DSBs with complex ends (Riballo et al., 2004) and/or to be predominantly located at the periphery of genomic heterochromatin, in regions of condensed chromatin (Goodarzi et al., 2010; Mosesso et al., 2010). As a consequence of the inhibition of repair, cells treated with Dbait are highly sensitive to irradiation. This property has been used *in vivo* in the development of new drugs for treating radioresistant tumors. DT01, a clinical product from the Dbait class of siDNAs, increases the survival of nude mice xenografted with radioresistant melanoma (Quanz et al., 2009a). DT01 efficacy is strictly dependent on the dose

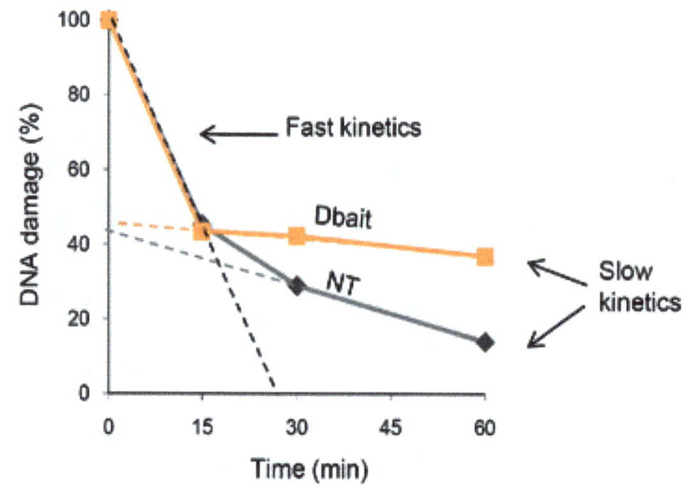

Fig. 6. Dbait inhibits slow DNA repair. MRC5 cells transfected or not transfected with Dbait were irradiated with 8 Gy. DNA damage repair was followed by alkaline comet assays over a period of 60 min.

administered (Figure 7) and is independent of the associated radiotherapy protocol. A phase I/II clinical trial will be initiated in 2011, to assess the efficacy of a treatment combining DT01 and radiotherapy for the treatment of local metastases of melanoma.

5. Conclusion

The study of DNA repair is a complicated task, due to the diversity of damage induced by DNA-damaging agents and the subsequent conversion of the damage by repair pathways or the DNA replication machinery. Furthermore, the damage may be repaired by different repair pathways, depending on the phase of the cell cycle at the time of damage. Finally, if the damage to the chromosome is too extensive, the cell undergoes apoptosis or senescence. The use of different techniques to induce a specific type of damage in the absence of chromosomal DNA damage within the cell has greatly contributed to our understandings of individual repair pathways. The tethering of repair proteins has demonstrated that the local concentration of damage signaling factors is sufficient to trigger a full damage response, independently of the presence of actual cellular damage. Consistent with this, agents modifying chromatin topology can induce DNA damage transducer activity in the absence of DNA lesions. Studies of the recognition of viral genomic material have contributed to our understanding of the cellular DDR. For example, studies of adenovirus interference with damage signaling through degradation of the MRN complex have suggested that MRN plays an upstream role in damage detection. Synthetic ICL constructs, introduced into cells on plasmids, have proved a useful tool for investigating this specific type of DNA damage. This approach made it possible to demonstrate the contribution of the Fanconi anemia pathway to the repair of ICLs. Studies based on the use of DNA fragments have identified ssDNA as the universal signal of the ATM-induced DDR. The introduction into cells of small double-stranded siDNA molecules, which are resistant to exonuclease attack and repair , has made it possible to demonstrate that DSBs alone activate DNA-PK only, leading to the phosphorylation of a multitude of downstream targets. However, unlike

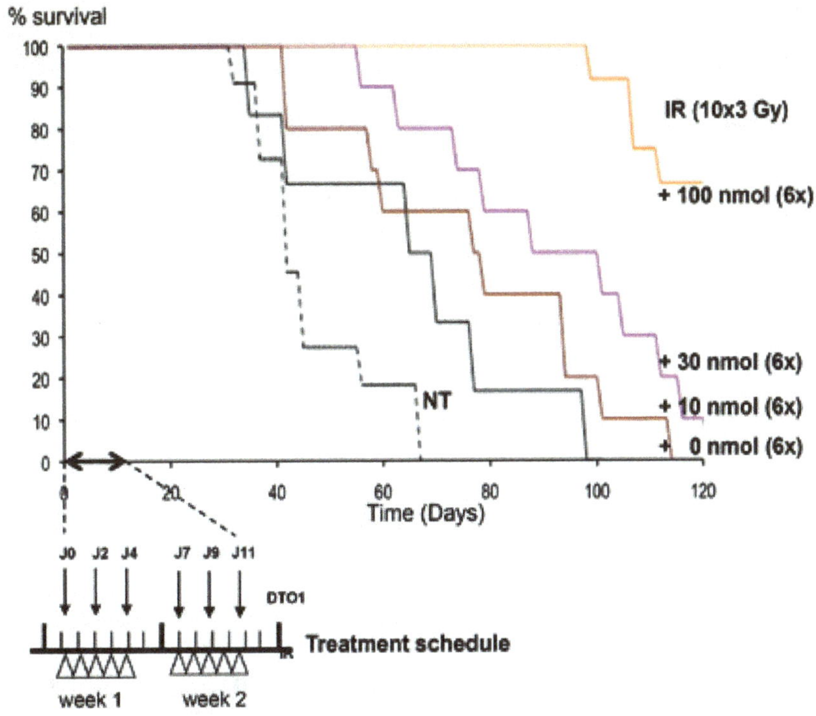

Fig. 7. The survival of xenografted animals is dependent on DT01 dose. Kaplan-Meier representation of the survival of nude mice with xenografted SK28 melanoma tumors. After two weeks of treatment, consisting of six injections of DT01 injections (arrows) at various doses and the administration of 3 Gy in 10 fractions (triangles, tumor volume was assessed. The ethical limit for tumor volume was 2000 mm^3. NT: untreated control group.

ATM activation by ssDNA, DNA-PK activation has a much smaller impact on the cell cycle and apoptosis induction. Thus, siDNA can be used as a tool for the specific activation of individual repair signaling enzymes, making it possible to investigate specific branches of the damage response, which is not possible with conventional DNA damaging agents that induce a plethora of different lesions. A similar approach could now be used for other kinds of DNA damage, to check for activation of the corresponding downstream repair pathways in cells. This should make it possible to answer currently unresolved questions, concerning the impact of PARP-signaling or mismatch-signaling on cell fate, for example. This should not only deepen our understanding of the specific pathways activated in response to a particular type of damage, but should also be useful in cancer treatment. The "jamming" of specific repair signaling pathways may help to overcome resistance to treatment and to enhance the response to cancer treatments targeting DNA.

6. Acknowledgments

We apologize to the many groups whose primary research papers could not be cited owing to space constraints. Work in the authors' laboratory was supported by Institut Curie, CNRS, INSERM, and ANR grant ANR-08-Biot-009-02.

7. References

Ahnesorg, P., Smith, P. & Jackson, S. P. (2006). XLF interacts with the XRCC4-DNA ligase iv complex to promote DNA nonhomologous end-joining, *Cell* 124(2): 301–13.

Akira, S., Uematsu, S. & Takeuchi, O. (2006). Pathogen recognition and innate immunity, *Cell* 124(4): 783–801.

Ali, A., Zhang, J., Bao, S., Liu, I., Otterness, D., Dean, N. M., Abraham, R. T. & Wang, X. F. (2004). Requirement of protein phosphatase 5 in DNA-damage-induced ATM activation, *Genes Dev* 18(3): 249–54.

Antman, K. & Chang, Y. (2000). Kaposi's sarcoma, *N Engl J Med* 342(14): 1027–38.

Ariumi, Y., Turelli, P., Masutani, M. & Trono, D. (2005). DNA damage sensors ATM, ATR, DNA-pkcs, and parp-1 are dispensable for human immunodeficiency virus type 1 integration, *J Virol* 79(5): 2973–8.

Audebert, M., Salles, B. & Calsou, P. (2004). Involvement of poly(adp-ribose) polymerase-1 and xrcc1/DNA ligase iii in an alternative route for DNA double-strand breaks rejoining, *J Biol Chem* 279(53): 55117–26.

Bailone, A., Brandenburger, A., Levine, A., Pierre, M., Dutreix, M. & Devoret, R. (1984). Indirect sos induction is promoted by ultraviolet light-damaged minif and requires the minif lyna locus, *J Mol Biol* 179(3): 367–90.

Bakkenist, C. J. & Kastan, M. B. (2003). DNA damage activates ATM through intermolecular autophosphorylation and dimer dissociation, *Nature* 421(6922): 499–506.

Bandaru, V., Sunkara, S., Wallace, S. S. & Bond, J. P. (2002). A novel human DNA glycosylase that removes oxidative DNA damage and is homologous to escherichia coli endonuclease viii, *DNA Repair (Amst)* 1(7): 517–29.

Bartek, J. & Lukas, J. (2003). Chk1 and chk2 kinases in checkpoint control and cancer, *Cancer Cell* 3(5): 421–9.

Bekker-Jensen, S., Lukas, C., Kitagawa, R., Melander, F., Kastan, M. B., Bartek, J. & Lukas, J. (2006). Spatial organization of the mammalian genome surveillance machinery in response to DNA strand breaks, *J Cell Biol* 173(2): 195–206.

Bencokova, Z., Kaufmann, M. R., Pires, I. M., Lecane, P. S., Giaccia, A. J. & Hammond, E. M. (2009). ATM activation and signaling under hypoxic conditions, *Mol Cell Biol* 29(2): 526–37.

Bianchi, V., Pontis, E. & Reichard, P. (1986). Changes of deoxyribonucleoside triphosphate pools induced by hydroxyurea and their relation to DNA synthesis, *J Biol Chem* 261(34): 16037–42.

Bianco, P. R., Tracy, R. B. & Kowalczykowski, S. C. (1998). DNA strand exchange proteins: a biochemical and physical comparison, *Front Biosci* 3: D570–603.

Boiteux, S. & Radicella, J. P. (2000). The human ogg1 gene: structure, functions, and its implication in the process of carcinogenesis, *Arch Biochem Biophys* 377(1): 1–8.

Bonilla, C. Y., Melo, J. A. & Toczyski, D. P. (2008). Colocalization of sensors is sufficient to activate the DNA damage checkpoint in the absence of damage, *Mol Cell* 30(3): 267–76.

Bonner, W. M., Redon, C. E., Dickey, J. S., Nakamura, A. J., Sedelnikova, O. A., Solier, S. & Pommier, Y. (2008). Gammah2ax and cancer, *Nat Rev Cancer* 8(12): 957–67.

Bouchard, V. J., Rouleau, M. & Poirier, G. G. (2003). Parp-1, a determinant of cell survival in response to DNA damage, *Exp Hematol* 31(6): 446–54.

Brachman, E. E. & Kmiec, E. B. (2002). The 'biased' evolution of targeted gene repair, *Curr Opin Mol Ther* 4(2): 171–6.

Brown, K. E. (2010). The expanding range of parvoviruses which infect humans, *Rev Med Virol* 20(4): 231–44.

Brown, K. L., Roginskaya, M., Zou, Y., Altamirano, A., Basu, A. K. & Stone, M. P. (2010). Binding of the human nucleotide excision repair proteins xpa and xpc/hr23b to the 5r-thymine glycol lesion and structure of the cis-(5r,6s) thymine glycol epimer in the 5′-gtgg-3′ sequence: destabilization of two base pairs at the lesion site, *Nucleic Acids Res* 38(2): 428–40.

Buck, D., Malivert, L., de Chasseval, R., Barraud, A., Fondaneche, M. C., Sanal, O., Plebani, A., Stephan, J. L., Hufnagel, M., le Deist, F., Fischer, A., Durandy, A., de Villartay, J. P. & Revy, P. (2006). Cernunnos, a novel nonhomologous end-joining factor, is mutated in human immunodeficiency with microcephaly, *Cell* 124(2): 287–99.

Burckstummer, T., Baumann, C., Bluml, S., Dixit, E., Durnberger, G., Jahn, H., Planyavsky, M., Bilban, M., Colinge, J., Bennett, K. L. & Superti-Furga, G. (2009). An orthogonal proteomic-genomic screen identifies aim2 as a cytoplasmic DNA sensor for the inflammasome, *Nat Immunol* 10(3): 266–72.

Cadet, J., Berger, M., Douki, T. & Ravanat, J. L. (1997). Oxidative damage to DNA: formation, measurement, and biological significance, *Rev Physiol Biochem Pharmacol* 131: 1–87.

Carson, C. T., Schwartz, R. A., Stracker, T. H., Lilley, C. E., Lee, D. V. & Weitzman, M. D. (2003). The mre11 complex is required for ATM activation and the g2/m checkpoint, *EMBO J* 22(24): 6610–20.

Carter, B. J. (2004). Adeno-associated virus and the development of adeno-associated virus vectors: a historical perspective, *Mol Ther* 10(6): 981–9.

Chan, K. K., Zhang, Q. M. & Dianov, G. L. (2006). Base excision repair fidelity in normal and cancer cells, *Mutagenesis* 21(3): 173–8.

Chapman, J. D., Reuvers, A. P., Borsa, J. & Greenstock, C. L. (1973). Chemical radioprotection and radiosensitization of mammalian cells growing in vitro, *Radiat Res* 56(2): 291–306.

Chappell, C., Hanakahi, L. A., Karimi-Busheri, F., Weinfeld, M. & West, S. C. (2002). Involvement of human polynucleotide kinase in double-strand break repair by non-homologous end joining, *EMBO J* 21(11): 2827–32.

Chaurushiya, M. S. & Weitzman, M. D. (2009). Viral manipulation of DNA repair and cell cycle checkpoints, *DNA Repair (Amst)* 8(9): 1166–76.

Chen, A. Y., Luo, Y., Cheng, F., Sun, Y. & Qiu, J. (2010). Bocavirus infection induces mitochondrion-mediated apoptosis and cell cycle arrest at g2/m phase, *J Virol* 84(11): 5615–26.

Chen, B. P., Uematsu, N., Kobayashi, J., Lerenthal, Y., Krempler, A., Yajima, H., Lobrich, M., Shiloh, Y. & Chen, D. J. (2007). Ataxia telangiectasia mutated (ATM) is essential for DNA-pkcs phosphorylations at the thr-2609 cluster upon DNA double strand break, *J Biol Chem* 282(9): 6582–7.

Chen, J., Silver, D. P., Walpita, D., Cantor, S. B., Gazdar, A. F., Tomlinson, G., Couch, F. J., Weber, B. L., Ashley, T., Livingston, D. M. & Scully, R. (1998). Stable interaction between the products of the BRCA1 and BRCA2 tumor suppressor genes in mitotic and meiotic cells, *Mol Cell* 2(3): 317–28.

Choi, Y. K., Nash, K., Byrne, B. J., Muzyczka, N. & Song, S. (2010). The effect of DNA-dependent protein kinase on adeno-associated virus replication, *PLoS One* 5(12): e15073.

Cleaver, J. E. (2005). Cancer in xeroderma pigmentosum and related disorders of DNA repair, *Nat Rev Cancer* 5(7): 564–73.

Collaco, R. F., Bevington, J. M., Bhrigu, V., Kalman-Maltese, V. & Trempe, J. P. (2009). Adeno-associated virus and adenovirus coinfection induces a cellular DNA damage and repair response via redundant phosphatidylinositol 3-like kinase pathways, *Virology* 392(1): 24–33.

Cornelis, J. J., Su, Z. Z. & Rommelaere, J. (1982). Direct and indirect effects of ultraviolet light on the mutagenesis of parvovirus h-1 in human cells, *EMBO J* 1(6): 693–9.

Costanzo, V., Paull, T., Gottesman, M. & Gautier, J. (2004). Mre11 assembles linear DNA fragments into DNA damage signaling complexes, *PLoS Biol* 2(5): E110.

Craig, N. L. & Roberts, J. W. (1981). Function of nucleoside triphosphate and polynucleotide in escherichia coli reca protein-directed cleavage of phage lambda repressor, *J Biol Chem* 256(15): 8039–44.

Crow, Y. J., Hayward, B. E., Parmar, R., Robins, P., Leitch, A., Ali, M., Black, D. N., van Bokhoven, H., Brunner, H. G., Hamel, B. C., Corry, P. C., Cowan, F. M., Frints, S. G., Klepper, J., Livingston, J. H., Lynch, S. A., Massey, R. F., Meritet, J. F., Michaud, J. L., Ponsot, G., Voit, T., Lebon, P., Bonthron, D. T., Jackson, A. P., Barnes, D. E. & Lindahl, T. (2006). Mutations in the gene encoding the 3′-5′ DNA exonuclease trex1 cause aicardi-goutieres syndrome at the ags1 locus, *Nat Genet* 38(8): 917–20.

Dahl, J., You, J. & Benjamin, T. L. (2005). Induction and utilization of an ATM signaling pathway by polyomavirus, *J Virol* 79(20): 13007–17.

Daniel, R., Katz, R. A. & Skalka, A. M. (1999). A role for DNA-PK in retroviral DNA integration, *Science* 284(5414): 644–7. Daniel, R Katz, R A Skalka, A M AI40721/AI/NIAID NIH HHS/United States AI40835/AI/NIAID NIH HHS/United States CA71515/CA/NCI NIH HHS/United States etc. Research Support, Non-U.S. Gov't Research Support, U.S. Gov't, P.H.S. United states Science (New York, N.Y.) Science. 1999 Apr 23;284(5414):644-7.

Daniel, R., Marusich, E., Argyris, E., Zhao, R. Y., Skalka, A. M. & Pomerantz, R. J. (2005). Caffeine inhibits human immunodeficiency virus type 1 transduction of nondividing cells, *J Virol* 79(4): 2058–65.

Daniel, R., Ramcharan, J., Rogakou, E., Taganov, K. D., Greger, J. G., Bonner, W., Nussenzweig, A., Katz, R. A. & Skalka, A. M. (2004). Histone H2AX is phosphorylated at sites of retroviral DNA integration but is dispensable for postintegration repair, *J Biol Chem* 279(44): 45810–4.

D'Ari, R. & Huisman, O. (1982). DNA replication and indirect induction of the sos response in escherichia coli, *Biochimie* 64(8-9): 623–7.

Davy, C. & Doorbar, J. (2007). G2/m cell cycle arrest in the life cycle of viruses, *Virology* 368(2): 219–26.

De Bont, R. & van Larebeke, N. (2004). Endogenous DNA damage in humans: a review of quantitative data, *Mutagenesis* 19(3): 169–85.

de Jager, M., van Noort, J., van Gent, D. C., Dekker, C., Kanaar, R. & Wyman, C. (2001). Human rad50/mre11 is a flexible complex that can tether DNA ends, *Mol Cell* 8(5): 1129–35.

Delale, T., Paquin, A., Asselin-Paturel, C., Dalod, M., Brizard, G., Bates, E. E., Kastner, P., Chan, S., Akira, S., Vicari, A., Biron, C. A., Trinchieri, G. & Briere, F. (2005). Myd88-dependent and -independent murine cytomegalovirus sensing for ifn-alpha release and initiation of immune responses in vivo, *J Immunol* 175(10): 6723–32.

Doil, C., Mailand, N., Bekker-Jensen, S., Menard, P., Larsen, D. H., Pepperkok, R., Ellenberg, J., Panier, S., Durocher, D., Bartek, J., Lukas, J. & Lukas, C. (2009). Rnf168 binds and amplifies ubiquitin conjugates on damaged chromosomes to allow accumulation of repair proteins, *Cell* 136(3): 435–46.

Dragoi, A. M., Fu, X., Ivanov, S., Zhang, P., Sheng, L., Wu, D., Li, G. C. & Chu, W. M. (2005). DNA-pkcs, but not tlr9, is required for activation of akt by cpg-DNA, *EMBO J* 24(4): 779–89.

D'Silva, I., Pelletier, J. D., Lagueux, J., D'Amours, D., Chaudhry, M. A., Weinfeld, M., Lees-Miller, S. P. & Poirier, G. G. (1999). Relative affinities of poly(adp-ribose) polymerase and DNA-dependent protein kinase for DNA strand interruptions, *Biochim Biophys Acta* 1430(1): 119–26.

Duncan, T., Trewick, S. C., Koivisto, P., Bates, P. A., Lindahl, T. & Sedgwick, B. (2002). Reversal of DNA alkylation damage by two human dioxygenases, *Proc Natl Acad Sci U S A* 99(26): 16660–5.

Durocher, D. & Jackson, S. P. (2001). DNA-PK, ATM and ATR as sensors of DNA damage: variations on a theme?, *Curr Opin Cell Biol* 13(2): 225–31.

Essers, J., Houtsmuller, A. B., van Veelen, L., Paulusma, C., Nigg, A. L., Pastink, A., Vermeulen, W., Hoeijmakers, J. H. & Kanaar, R. (2002). Nuclear dynamics of rad52 group homologous recombination proteins in response to DNA damage, *EMBO J* 21(8): 2030–7.

Fernandes-Alnemri, T., Yu, J. W., Datta, P., Wu, J. & Alnemri, E. S. (2009). Aim2 activates the inflammasome and cell death in response to cytoplasmic DNA, *Nature* 458(7237): 509–13.

Fernandez-Capetillo, O., Celeste, A. & Nussenzweig, A. (2003). Focusing on foci: H2AX and the recruitment of DNA-damage response factors, *Cell Cycle* 2(5): 426–7.

Ferrara, L. & Kmiec, E. B. (2006). Targeted gene repair activates chk1 and chk2 and stalls replication in corrected cells, *DNA Repair (Amst)* 5(4): 422–31.

Fortini, P. & Dogliotti, E. (2007). Base damage and single-strand break repair: mechanisms and functional significance of short- and long-patch repair subpathways, *DNA Repair (Amst)* 6(4): 398–409.

Fragkos, M., Breuleux, M., Clement, N. & Beard, P. (2008). Recombinant adeno-associated viral vectors are deficient in provoking a DNA damage response, *J Virol* 82(15): 7379–87.

Friedberg, E. C. (1995). *DNA repair and mutagenesis*, American Society for Microbiology, Washington, DC.

Friedberg, E. C. (2001). How nucleotide excision repair protects against cancer, *Nat Rev Cancer* 1(1): 22–33.

Fugmann, S. D., Lee, A. I., Shockett, P. E., Villey, I. J. & Schatz, D. G. (2000). The rag proteins and v(d)j recombination: complexes, ends, and transposition, *Annu Rev Immunol* 18: 495–527.

Geoffroy, M. C. & Salvetti, A. (2005). Helper functions required for wild type and recombinant adeno-associated virus growth, *Curr Gene Ther* 5(3): 265–71.

George, J., Devoret, R. & Radman, M. (1974). Indirect ultraviolet-reactivation of phage lambda, *Proc Natl Acad Sci U S A* 71(1): 144–7.

Gerson, S. L. (2004). Mgmt: its role in cancer aetiology and cancer therapeutics, *Nat Rev Cancer* 4(4): 296–307.

Goodarzi, A. A., Jeggo, P. & Lobrich, M. (2010). The influence of heterochromatin on DNA double strand break repair: Getting the strong, silent type to relax, *DNA Repair (Amst)* 9(12): 1273–82.

Goodarzi, A. A., Jonnalagadda, J. C., Douglas, P., Young, D., Ye, R., Moorhead, G. B., Lees-Miller, S. P. & Khanna, K. K. (2004). Autophosphorylation of ataxia-telangiectasia mutated is regulated by protein phosphatase 2a, *EMBO J* 23(22): 4451–61.

Grundhoff, A. & Ganem, D. (2004). Inefficient establishment of kshv latency suggests an additional role for continued lytic replication in kaposi sarcoma pathogenesis, *J Clin Invest* 113(1): 124–36.

Guainazzi, A. & Scharer, O. D. (2010). Using synthetic DNA interstrand crosslinks to elucidate repair pathways and identify new therapeutic targets for cancer chemotherapy, *Cell Mol Life Sci* 67(21): 3683–97.

Guo, Z., Kozlov, S., Lavin, M. F., Person, M. D. & Paull, T. T. (2010). ATM activation by oxidative stress, *Science* 330(6003): 517–21.

Hanawalt, P. C. (2002). Subpathways of nucleotide excision repair and their regulation, *Oncogene* 21(58): 8949–56.

Hartlerode, A. J. & Scully, R. (2009). Mechanisms of double-strand break repair in somatic mammalian cells, *Biochem J* 423(2): 157–68.

Helleday, T., Lo, J., van Gent, D. C. & Engelward, B. P. (2007). DNA double-strand break repair: from mechanistic understanding to cancer treatment, *DNA Repair (Amst)* 6(7): 923–35.

Helleday, T., Petermann, E., Lundin, C., Hodgson, B. & Sharma, R. A. (2008). DNA repair pathways as targets for cancer therapy, *Nat Rev Cancer* 8(3): 193–204.

Hemmi, H., Takeuchi, O., Kawai, T., Kaisho, T., Sato, S., Sanjo, H., Matsumoto, M., Hoshino, K., Wagner, H., Takeda, K. & Akira, S. (2000). A toll-like receptor recognizes bacterial DNA, *Nature* 408(6813): 740–5.

Hornung, V., Ablasser, A., Charrel-Dennis, M., Bauernfeind, F., Horvath, G., Caffrey, D. R., Latz, E. & Fitzgerald, K. A. (2009). Aim2 recognizes cytosolic dsdna and forms a caspase-1-activating inflammasome with asc, *Nature* 458(7237): 514–8. Hornung, Veit Ablasser, Andrea Charrel-Dennis, Marie Bauernfeind, Franz Horvath, Gabor Caffrey, Daniel R Latz, Eicke Fitzgerald, Katherine A AI-065483/AI/NIAID NIH HHS/United States AI-067497/AI/NIAID NIH HHS/United States R01 AI067497-03/AI/NIAID NIH HHS/United States R01 AI067497-04/AI/NIAID NIH HHS/United States Research Support, N.I.H., Extramural Research Support, Non-U.S. Gov't England Nature Nature. 2009 Mar 26;458(7237):514-8. Epub 2009 Jan 21.

Hsiang, Y. H., Lihou, M. G. & Liu, L. F. (1989). Arrest of replication forks by drug-stabilized topoisomerase i-DNA cleavable complexes as a mechanism of cell killing by camptothecin, *Cancer Res* 49(18): 5077–82.

Huang, L. C., Clarkin, K. C. & Wahl, G. M. (1996). Sensitivity and selectivity of the DNA damage sensor responsible for activating p53-dependent g1 arrest, *Proc Natl Acad Sci U S A* 93(10): 4827–32.

Huen, M. S., Grant, R., Manke, I., Minn, K., Yu, X., Yaffe, M. B. & Chen, J. (2007). Rnf8 transduces the DNA-damage signal via histone ubiquitylation and checkpoint protein assembly, *Cell* 131(5): 901–14.

Ichijima, Y., Sakasai, R., Okita, N., Asahina, K., Mizutani, S. & Teraoka, H. (2005). Phosphorylation of histone H2AX at m phase in human cells without DNA damage response, *Biochem Biophys Res Commun* 336(3): 807–12.

Igoucheva, O., Alexeev, V. & Yoon, K. (2004). Oligonucleotide-directed mutagenesis and targeted gene correction: a mechanistic point of view, *Curr Mol Med* 4(5): 445–63.

Ikegami, S., Taguchi, T., Ohashi, M., Oguro, M., Nagano, H. & Mano, Y. (1978). Aphidicolin prevents mitotic cell division by interfering with the activity of DNA polymerase-alpha, *Nature* 275(5679): 458–60.

Iliakis, G. (2009). Backup pathways of nhej in cells of higher eukaryotes: cell cycle dependence, *Radiother Oncol* 92(3): 310–5.

Inagaki, A., Schoenmakers, S. & Baarends, W. M. (2010). DNA double strand break repair, chromosome synapsis and transcriptional silencing in meiosis, *Epigenetics* 5(4).

Inagaki, K., Ma, C., Storm, T. A., Kay, M. A. & Nakai, H. (2007). The role of DNA-pkcs and artemis in opening viral DNA hairpin termini in various tissues in mice, *J Virol* 81(20): 11304–21.

Jang, E. R., Choi, J. D., Park, M. A., Jeong, G., Cho, H. & Lee, J. S. (2010). ATM modulates transcription in response to histone deacetylase inhibition as part of its DNA damage response, *Exp Mol Med* 42(3): 195–204.

Jazayeri, A., Balestrini, A., Garner, E., Haber, J. E. & Costanzo, V. (2008). Mre11-rad50-nbs1-dependent processing of DNA breaks generates oligonucleotides that stimulate ATM activity, *Embo J* 27(14): 1953–62.

Jeggo, P. A., Taccioli, G. E. & Jackson, S. P. (1995). Menage a trois: double strand break repair, v(d)j recombination and DNA-PK, *Bioessays* 17(11): 949–57. Bioessays. 1995 Nov;17(11):949-57.

Jeggo, P. & Lavin, M. F. (2009). Cellular radiosensitivity: how much better do we understand it?, *Int J Radiat Biol* 85(12): 1061–81.

Johnson, R. D. & Jasin, M. (2000). Sister chromatid gene conversion is a prominent double-strand break repair pathway in mammalian cells, *EMBO J* 19(13): 3398–407.

Jungmichel, S. & Stucki, M. (2010). Mdc1: The art of keeping things in focus, *Chromosoma* .

Jurvansuu, J., Raj, K., Stasiak, A. & Beard, P. (2005). Viral transport of DNA damage that mimics a stalled replication fork, *J Virol* 79(1): 569–80.

Karpova, A. Y., Trost, M., Murray, J. M., Cantley, L. C. & Howley, P. M. (2002). Interferon regulatory factor-3 is an in vivo target of DNA-PK, *Proc Natl Acad Sci U S A* 99(5): 2818–23.

Kastan, M. B. & Bartek, J. (2004). Cell-cycle checkpoints and cancer, *Nature* 432(7015): 316–23.

Kilzer, J. M., Stracker, T., Beitzel, B., Meek, K., Weitzman, M. & Bushman, F. D. (2003). Roles of host cell factors in circularization of retroviral DNA, *Virology* 314(1): 460–7.

Kim, W. J., Rajasekaran, B. & Brown, K. D. (2007). Mlh1- and ATM-dependent mapk signaling is activated through c-abl in response to the alkylator n-methyl-n′-nitro-n′-nitrosoguanidine, *J Biol Chem* 282(44): 32021–31.

Kim, Y. C., Gerlitz, G., Furusawa, T., Catez, F., Nussenzweig, A., Oh, K. S., Kraemer, K. H., Shiloh, Y. & Bustin, M. (2009). Activation of ATM depends on chromatin interactions occurring before induction of DNA damage, *Nat Cell Biol* 11(1): 92–6.

Knipscheer, P., Raschle, M., Smogorzewska, A., Enoiu, M., Ho, T. V., Scharer, O. D., Elledge, S. J. & Walter, J. C. (2009). The fanconi anemia pathway promotes replication-dependent DNA interstrand cross-link repair, *Science* 326(5960): 1698–701.

Koch, C. A., Agyei, R., Galicia, S., Metalnikov, P., O'Donnell, P., Starostine, A., Weinfeld, M. & Durocher, D. (2004). XRCC4 physically links DNA end processing by polynucleotide kinase to DNA ligation by DNA ligase iv, *EMBO J* 23(19): 3874–85.

Kohn, K. W. (1999). Molecular interaction map of the mammalian cell cycle control and DNA repair systems, *Mol Biol Cell* 10(8): 2703–34.

Kohn, K. W., Pommier, Y., Kerrigan, D., Markovits, J. & Covey, J. M. (1987). Topoisomerase ii as a target of anticancer drug action in mammalian cells, *NCI Monogr* (4): 61–71.

Kolas, N. K., Chapman, J. R., Nakada, S., Ylanko, J., Chahwan, R., Sweeney, F. D., Panier, S., Mendez, M., Wildenhain, J., Thomson, T. M., Pelletier, L., Jackson, S. P. & Durocher, D. (2007). Orchestration of the DNA-damage response by the rnf8 ubiquitin ligase, *Science* 318(5856): 1637–40.

Kudoh, A., Fujita, M., Zhang, L., Shirata, N., Daikoku, T., Sugaya, Y., Isomura, H., Nishiyama, Y. & Tsurumi, T. (2005). Epstein-barr virus lytic replication elicits ATM checkpoint signal transduction while providing an s-phase-like cellular environment, *J Biol Chem* 280(9): 8156–63.

Kumagai, A., Lee, J., Yoo, H. Y. & Dunphy, W. G. (2006). Topbp1 activates the ATR-atrip complex, *Cell* 124(5): 943–55.

Kunkel, T. A. & Erie, D. A. (2005). DNA mismatch repair, *Annu Rev Biochem* 74: 681–710.

Lau, A., Swinbank, K. M., Ahmed, P. S., Taylor, D. L., Jackson, S. P., Smith, G. C. & O'Connor, M. J. (2005). Suppression of hiv-1 infection by a small molecule inhibitor of the ATM kinase, *Nat Cell Biol* 7(5): 493–500.

Lee, J. H. & Paull, T. T. (2004). Direct activation of the ATM protein kinase by the mre11/rad50/nbs1 complex, *Science* 304(5667): 93–6.

Lee, J. H. & Paull, T. T. (2005). ATM activation by DNA double-strand breaks through the mre11-rad50-nbs1 complex, *Science* 308(5721): 551–4.

Lee-Kirsch, M. A., Gong, M., Chowdhury, D., Senenko, L., Engel, K., Lee, Y. A., de Silva, U., Bailey, S. L., Witte, T., Vyse, T. J., Kere, J., Pfeiffer, C., Harvey, S., Wong, A., Koskenmies, S., Hummel, O., Rohde, K., Schmidt, R. E., Dominiczak, A. F., Gahr, M., Hollis, T., Perrino, F. W., Lieberman, J. & Hubner, N. (2007). Mutations in the gene encoding the 3'-5' DNA exonuclease trex1 are associated with systemic lupus erythematosus, *Nat Genet* 39(9): 1065–7.

Li, G. M. (1999). The role of mismatch repair in DNA damage-induced apoptosis, *Oncol Res* 11(9): 393–400.

Li, G. M. (2008). Mechanisms and functions of DNA mismatch repair, *Cell Res* 18(1): 85–98.

Li, J. J. & Deshaies, R. J. (1993). Exercising self-restraint: discouraging illicit acts of s and m in eukaryotes, *Cell* 74(2): 223–6.

Li, L., Olvera, J. M., Yoder, K. E., Mitchell, R. S., Butler, S. L., Lieber, M., Martin, S. L. & Bushman, F. D. (2001). Role of the non-homologous DNA end joining pathway in the early steps of retroviral infection, *EMBO J* 20(12): 3272–81.

Li, L. & Zou, L. (2005). Sensing, signaling, and responding to DNA damage: organization of the checkpoint pathways in mammalian cells, *J Cell Biochem* 94(2): 298–306.

Lilley, C. E., Carson, C. T., Muotri, A. R., Gage, F. H. & Weitzman, M. D. (2005). DNA repair proteins affect the lifecycle of herpes simplex virus 1, *Proc Natl Acad Sci U S A* 102(16): 5844–9.

Lilley, C. E., Schwartz, R. A. & Weitzman, M. D. (2007). Using or abusing: viruses and the cellular DNA damage response, *Trends Microbiol* 15(3): 119–26.

Liu, Y. & Maizels, N. (2000). Coordinated response of mammalian rad51 and rad52 to DNA damage, *EMBO Rep* 1(1): 85–90.

Liu, Y. & West, S. C. (2004). Happy hollidays: 40th anniversary of the holliday junction, *Nat Rev Mol Cell Biol* 5(11): 937–44.

Lobrich, M. & Jeggo, P. A. (2007). The impact of a negligent g2/m checkpoint on genomic instability and cancer induction, *Nat Rev Cancer* 7(11): 861–9.

Lopez-Contreras, A. J. & Fernandez-Capetillo, O. (2010). The ATR barrier to replication-born DNA damage, *DNA Repair (Amst)* 9(12): 1249–55.

Lukas, C., Falck, J., Bartkova, J., Bartek, J. & Lukas, J. (2003). Distinct spatiotemporal dynamics of mammalian checkpoint regulators induced by DNA damage, *Nat Cell Biol* 5(3): 255–60.

Lukas, J., Lukas, C. & Bartek, J. (2004). Mammalian cell cycle checkpoints: signalling pathways and their organization in space and time, *DNA Repair (Amst)* 3(8-9): 997–1007.

Lund, J., Sato, A., Akira, S., Medzhitov, R. & Iwasaki, A. (2003). Toll-like receptor 9-mediated recognition of herpes simplex virus-2 by plasmacytoid dendritic cells, *J Exp Med* 198(3): 513–20.

Lundin, C., Erixon, K., Arnaudeau, C., Schultz, N., Jenssen, D., Meuth, M. & Helleday, T. (2002). Different roles for nonhomologous end joining and homologous recombination following replication arrest in mammalian cells, *Mol Cell Biol* 22(16): 5869–78.

Luo, M. H., Rosenke, K., Czornak, K. & Fortunato, E. A. (2007). Human cytomegalovirus disrupts both ataxia telangiectasia mutated protein (ATM)- and ATM-rad3-related kinase-mediated DNA damage responses during lytic infection, *J Virol* 81(4): 1934–50.

Luo, Y., Chen, A. Y. & Qiu, J. (2011). Bocavirus infection induces a DNA damage response that facilitates viral DNA replication and mediates cell death, *J Virol* 85(1): 133–45.

Ma, Y., Pannicke, U., Schwarz, K. & Lieber, M. R. (2002). Hairpin opening and overhang processing by an artemis/DNA-dependent protein kinase complex in nonhomologous end joining and v(d)j recombination, *Cell* 108(6): 781–94.

Malanga, M. & Althaus, F. R. (2005). The role of poly(adp-ribose) in the DNA damage signaling network, *Biochem Cell Biol* 83(3): 354–64.

Malanga, M., Pleschke, J. M., Kleczkowska, H. E. & Althaus, F. R. (1998). Poly(adp-ribose) binds to specific domains of p53 and alters its DNA binding functions, *J Biol Chem* 273(19): 11839–43.

Masson, C., Bury-Mone, S., Guiot, E., Saez-Cirion, A., Schoevaert-Brossault, D., Brachet-Ducos, C., Delelis, O., Subra, F., Jeanson-Leh, L. & Mouscadet, J. F. (2007). Ku80 participates in the targeting of retroviral transgenes to the chromatin of cho cells, *J Virol* 81(15): 7924–32.

Matsuoka, S., Ballif, B. A., Smogorzewska, A., McDonald, E. R., r., Hurov, K. E., Luo, J., Bakalarski, C. E., Zhao, Z., Solimini, N., Lerenthal, Y., Shiloh, Y., Gygi, S. P. & Elledge, S. J. (2007). ATM and ATR substrate analysis reveals extensive protein networks responsive to DNA damage, *Science* 316(5828): 1160–6.

Mazumdar, M., Lee, J. H., Sengupta, K., Ried, T., Rane, S. & Misteli, T. (2006). Tumor formation via loss of a molecular motor protein, *Curr Biol* 16(15): 1559–64.

McAdams, H. H. & Arkin, A. (1999). It's a noisy business! genetic regulation at the nanomolar scale, *Trends Genet* 15(2): 65–9.

Misteli, T. & Soutoglou, E. (2009). The emerging role of nuclear architecture in DNA repair and genome maintenance, *Nat Rev Mol Cell Biol* 10(4): 243–54.

Moreno-Herrero, F., de Jager, M., Dekker, N. H., Kanaar, R., Wyman, C. & Dekker, C. (2005). Mesoscale conformational changes in the DNA-repair complex rad50/mre11/nbs1 upon binding DNA, *Nature* 437(7057): 440–3.

Mosesso, P., Palitti, F., Pepe, G., Pinero, J., Bellacima, R., Ahnstrom, G. & Natarajan, A. T. (2010). Relationship between chromatin structure, DNA damage and repair following x-irradiation of human lymphocytes, *Mutat Res* 701(1): 86–91.

Moshous, D., Callebaut, I., de Chasseval, R., Corneo, B., Cavazzana-Calvo, M., Le Deist, F., Tezcan, I., Sanal, O., Bertrand, Y., Philippe, N., Fischer, A. & de Villartay, J. P. (2001). Artemis, a novel DNA double-strand break repair/v(d)j recombination protein, is mutated in human severe combined immune deficiency, *Cell* 105(2): 177–86.

Nash, K., Chen, W., Salganik, M. & Muzyczka, N. (2009). Identification of cellular proteins that interact with the adeno-associated virus rep protein, *J Virol* 83(1): 454–69.

Nichols, G. J., Schaack, J. & Ornelles, D. A. (2009). Widespread phosphorylation of histone H2AX by species c adenovirus infection requires viral DNA replication, *J Virol* 83(12): 5987–98.

Nick McElhinny, S. A., Havener, J. M., Garcia-Diaz, M., Juarez, R., Bebenek, K., Kee, B. L., Blanco, L., Kunkel, T. A. & Ramsden, D. A. (2005). A gradient of template dependence defines distinct biological roles for family x polymerases in nonhomologous end joining, *Mol Cell* 19(3): 357–66.

Nur, E. K. A., Li, T. K., Zhang, A., Qi, H., Hars, E. S. & Liu, L. F. (2003). Single-stranded DNA induces ataxia telangiectasia mutant (ATM)/p53-dependent DNA damage and apoptotic signals, *J Biol Chem* 278(14): 12475–81.

Orelli, B., McClendon, T. B., Tsodikov, O. V., Ellenberger, T., Niedernhofer, L. J. & Scharer, O. D. (2010). The xpa-binding domain of ercc1 is required for nucleotide excision repair but not other DNA repair pathways, *J Biol Chem* 285(6): 3705–12.

Park, Y., Lee, S. W. & Sung, Y. C. (2002). Cutting edge: Cpg DNA inhibits dendritic cell apoptosis by up-regulating cellular inhibitor of apoptosis proteins through the phosphatidylinositide-3'-oh kinase pathway, *J Immunol* 168(1): 5–8.

Patil, S. D., Rhodes, D. G. & Burgess, D. J. (2005). DNA-based therapeutics and DNA delivery systems: a comprehensive review, *Aaps J* 7(1): E61–77.

Paull, T. T. & Gellert, M. (1998). The 3' to 5' exonuclease activity of mre 11 facilitates repair of DNA double-strand breaks, *Mol Cell* 1(7): 969–79.

Paull, T. T. & Gellert, M. (1999). Nbs1 potentiates atp-driven DNA unwinding and endonuclease cleavage by the mre11/rad50 complex, *Genes Dev* 13(10): 1276–88.

Pellegrini, L., Yu, D. S., Lo, T., Anand, S., Lee, M., Blundell, T. L. & Venkitaraman, A. R. (2002). Insights into DNA recombination from the structure of a rad51-BRCA2 complex, *Nature* 420(6913): 287–93.

Peng, Y., Woods, R. G., Beamish, H., Ye, R., Lees-Miller, S. P., Lavin, M. F. & Bedford, J. S. (2005). Deficiency in the catalytic subunit of DNA-dependent protein kinase causes down-regulation of ATM, *Cancer Res* 65(5): 1670–7.

Perry, J. J., Yannone, S. M., Holden, L. G., Hitomi, C., Asaithamby, A., Han, S., Cooper, P. K., Chen, D. J. & Tainer, J. A. (2006). Wrn exonuclease structure and molecular mechanism imply an editing role in DNA end processing, *Nat Struct Mol Biol* 13(5): 414–22.

Polo, S. E. & Jackson, S. P. (2011). Dynamics of DNA damage response proteins at DNA breaks: a focus on protein modifications, *Genes Dev* 25(5): 409–33.

Quanz, M., Berthault, N., Roulin, C., Roy, M., Herbette, A., Agrario, C., Alberti, C., Josserand, V., Coll, J. L., Sastre-Garau, X., Cosset, J. M., Larue, L., Sun, J. S. & Dutreix, M. (2009). Small-molecule drugs mimicking DNA damage: a new strategy for sensitizing tumors to radiotherapy, *Clin Cancer Res* 15(4): 1308–16.

Quanz, M., Chassoux, D., Berthault, N., Agrario, C., Sun, J. S. & Dutreix, M. (2009). Hyperactivation of DNA-PK by double-strand break mimicking molecules disorganizes DNA damage response, *PLoS One* 4(7): e6298.

Raderschall, E., Golub, E. I. & Haaf, T. (1999). Nuclear foci of mammalian recombination proteins are located at single-stranded DNA regions formed after DNA damage, *Proc Natl Acad Sci U S A* 96(5): 1921–6.

Radford, I. R. (1985). The level of induced DNA double-strand breakage correlates with cell killing after x-irradiation, *Int J Radiat Biol Relat Stud Phys Chem Med* 48(1): 45–54.

Raschle, M., Knipscheer, P., Enoiu, M., Angelov, T., Sun, J., Griffith, J. D., Ellenberger, T. E., Scharer, O. D. & Walter, J. C. (2008). Mechanism of replication-coupled DNA interstrand crosslink repair, *Cell* 134(6): 969–80.

Rathinam, V. A. & Fitzgerald, K. A. (2011). Innate immune sensing of DNA viruses, *Virology* 411(2): 153–62.

Reardon, J. T. & Sancar, A. (2005). Nucleotide excision repair, *Prog Nucleic Acid Res Mol Biol* 79: 183–235.

Riballo, E., Kuhne, M., Rief, N., Doherty, A., Smith, G. C., Recio, M. J., Reis, C., Dahm, K., Fricke, A., Krempler, A., Parker, A. R., Jackson, S. P., Gennery, A., Jeggo, P. A. & Lobrich, M. (2004). A pathway of double-strand break rejoining dependent upon ATM, artemis, and proteins locating to gamma-H2AX foci, *Mol Cell* 16(5): 715–24.

Rosidi, B., Wang, M., Wu, W., Sharma, A., Wang, H. & Iliakis, G. (2008). Histone h1 functions as a stimulatory factor in backup pathways of nhej, *Nucleic Acids Res* 36(5): 1610–23.

Rossi, J. J. (2004). Medicine: a cholesterol connection in rnai, *Nature* 432(7014): 155–6.

Rouleau, M., Patel, A., Hendzel, M. J., Kaufmann, S. H. & Poirier, G. G. (2010). Parp inhibition: Parp1 and beyond, *Nat Rev Cancer* 10(4): 293–301.

Rupnik, A., Grenon, M. & Lowndes, N. (2008). The mrn complex, *Curr Biol* 18(11): R455–7.

Sakurai, Y., Komatsu, K., Agematsu, K. & Matsuoka, M. (2009). DNA double strand break repair enzymes function at multiple steps in retroviral infection, *Retrovirology* 6: 114.

Sartori, A. A., Lukas, C., Coates, J., Mistrik, M., Fu, S., Bartek, J., Baer, R., Lukas, J. & Jackson, S. P. (2007). Human ctip promotes DNA end resection, *Nature* 450(7169): 509–14.

Schiavone, N., Papucci, L., Luciani, P., Lapucci, A., Donnini, M. & Capaccioli, S. (2000). Induction of apoptosis and mitosis inhibition by degraded DNA lipotransfection mimicking genotoxic drug effects, *Biochem Biophys Res Commun* 270(2): 406–14.

Schlacher, K. & Goodman, M. F. (2007). Lessons from 50 years of sos DNA-damage-induced mutagenesis, *Nat Rev Mol Cell Biol* 8(7): 587–94.

Schwartz, R. A., Carson, C. T., Schuberth, C. & Weitzman, M. D. (2009). Adeno-associated virus replication induces a DNA damage response coordinated by DNA-dependent protein kinase, *J Virol* 83(12): 6269–78.

Scully, R., Chen, J., Ochs, R. L., Keegan, K., Hoekstra, M., Feunteun, J. & Livingston, D. M. (1997). Dynamic changes of BRCA1 subnuclear location and phosphorylation state are initiated by DNA damage, *Cell* 90(3): 425–35.

Sester, D. P., Brion, K., Trieu, A., Goodridge, H. S., Roberts, T. L., Dunn, J., Hume, D. A., Stacey, K. J. & Sweet, M. J. (2006). Cpg DNA activates survival in murine macrophages through tlr9 and the phosphatidylinositol 3-kinase-akt pathway, *J Immunol* 177(7): 4473–80.

Shell, S. M., Li, Z., Shkriabai, N., Kvaratskhelia, M., Brosey, C., Serrano, M. A., Chazin, W. J., Musich, P. R. & Zou, Y. (2009). Checkpoint kinase ATR promotes nucleotide excision repair of uv-induced DNA damage via physical interaction with xeroderma pigmentosum group a, *J Biol Chem* 284(36): 24213–22.

Shimodaira, H., Yoshioka-Yamashita, A., Kolodner, R. D. & Wang, J. Y. (2003). Interaction of mismatch repair protein pms2 and the p53-related transcription factor p73 in apoptosis response to cisplatin, *Proc Natl Acad Sci U S A* 100(5): 2420–5.

Shreeram, S., Hee, W. K., Demidov, O. N., Kek, C., Yamaguchi, H., Fornace, A. J., J., Anderson, C. W., Appella, E. & Bulavin, D. V. (2006). Regulation of ATM/p53-dependent suppression of myc-induced lymphomas by wip1 phosphatase, *J Exp Med* 203(13): 2793–9.

Skalka, A. M. & Katz, R. A. (2005). Retroviral DNA integration and the DNA damage response, *Cell Death Differ* 12 Suppl 1: 971–8.

Smith, J., Tho, L. M., Xu, N. & Gillespie, D. A. (2010). The ATM-chk2 and ATR-chk1 pathways in DNA damage signaling and cancer, *Adv Cancer Res* 108: 73–112.

Soutoglou, E. & Misteli, T. (2008). Activation of the cellular DNA damage response in the absence of DNA lesions, *Science* 320(5882): 1507–10.

Stewart, G. S., Panier, S., Townsend, K., Al-Hakim, A. K., Kolas, N. K., Miller, E. S., Nakada, S., Ylanko, J., Olivarius, S., Mendez, M., Oldreive, C., Wildenhain, J., Tagliaferro, A., Pelletier, L., Taubenheim, N., Durandy, A., Byrd, P. J., Stankovic, T., Taylor, A. M. & Durocher, D. (2009). The riddle syndrome protein mediates a ubiquitin-dependent signaling cascade at sites of DNA damage, *Cell* 136(3): 420–34.

Stiff, T., O'Driscoll, M., Rief, N., Iwabuchi, K., Lobrich, M. & Jeggo, P. A. (2004). ATM and DNA-PK function redundantly to phosphorylate H2AX after exposure to ionizing radiation, *Cancer Res* 64(7): 2390–6.

Stracker, T. H., Carson, C. T. & Weitzman, M. D. (2002). Adenovirus oncoproteins inactivate the mre11-rad50-nbs1 DNA repair complex, *Nature* 418(6895): 348–52.

Stracker, T. H., Cassell, G. D., Ward, P., Loo, Y. M., van Breukelen, B., Carrington-Lawrence, S. D., Hamatake, R. K., van der Vliet, P. C., Weller, S. K., Melendy, T. & Weitzman, M. D. (2004). The rep protein of adeno-associated virus type 2 interacts with single-stranded DNA-binding proteins that enhance viral replication, *J Virol* 78(1): 441–53.

Strumberg, D., Pilon, A. A., Smith, M., Hickey, R., Malkas, L. & Pommier, Y. (2000). Conversion of topoisomerase i cleavage complexes on the leading strand of ribosomal DNA into 5′-phosphorylated DNA double-strand breaks by replication runoff, *Mol Cell Biol* 20(11): 3977–87.

Sy, S. M., Huen, M. S. & Chen, J. (2009). Palb2 is an integral component of the BRCA complex required for homologous recombination repair, *Proc Natl Acad Sci U S A* 106(17): 7155–60.

Takaoka, A. & Taniguchi, T. (2008). Cytosolic DNA recognition for triggering innate immune responses, *Adv Drug Deliv Rev* 60(7): 847–57.

Takaoka, A., Wang, Z., Choi, M. K., Yanai, H., Negishi, H., Ban, T., Lu, Y., Miyagishi, M., Kodama, T., Honda, K., Ohba, Y. & Taniguchi, T. (2007). Dai (dlm-1/zbp1) is a cytosolic DNA sensor and an activator of innate immune response, *Nature* 448(7152): 501–5.

Toledo, L. I., Murga, M., Gutierrez-Martinez, P., Soria, R. & Fernandez-Capetillo, O. (2008). ATR signaling can drive cells into senescence in the absence of DNA breaks, *Genes Dev* 22(3): 297–302.

Van Dyck, E., Stasiak, A. Z., Stasiak, A. & West, S. C. (2001). Visualization of recombination intermediates produced by rad52-mediated single-strand annealing, *EMBO Rep* 2(10): 905–9.

van Heemst, D., Brugmans, L., Verkaik, N. S. & van Gent, D. C. (2004). End-joining of blunt DNA double-strand breaks in mammalian fibroblasts is precise and requires DNA-PK and XRCC4, *DNA Repair (Amst)* 3(1): 43–50.

Vilaysane, A. & Muruve, D. A. (2009). The innate immune response to DNA, *Semin Immunol* 21(4): 208–14.

Wagner, H. (2004). The immunobiology of the tlr9 subfamily, *Trends Immunol* 25(7): 381–6.

Wang, S., Guo, M., Ouyang, H., Li, X., Cordon-Cardo, C., Kurimasa, A., Chen, D. J., Fuks, Z., Ling, C. C. & Li, G. C. (2000). The catalytic subunit of DNA-dependent protein kinase selectively regulates p53-dependent apoptosis but not cell-cycle arrest, *Proc Natl Acad Sci U S A* 97(4): 1584–8.

Wang, X., Ohnishi, K., Takahashi, A. & Ohnishi, T. (1998). Poly(adp-ribosyl)ation is required for p53-dependent signal transduction induced by radiation, *Oncogene* 17(22): 2819–25.

Wang, X., Peterson, C. A., Zheng, H., Nairn, R. S., Legerski, R. J. & Li, L. (2001). Involvement of nucleotide excision repair in a recombination-independent and error-prone pathway of DNA interstrand cross-link repair, *Mol Cell Biol* 21(3): 713–20.

Wang, Y., Li, H., Tang, Q., Maul, G. G. & Yuan, Y. (2008). Kaposi's sarcoma-associated herpesvirus ori-lyt-dependent DNA replication: involvement of host cellular factors, *J Virol* 82(6): 2867–82.

Ward, I. & Chen, J. (2004). Early events in the DNA damage response, *Curr Top Dev Biol* 63: 1–35.

Ward, I. M. & Chen, J. (2001). Histone H2AX is phosphorylated in an ATR-dependent manner in response to replicational stress, *J Biol Chem* 276(51): 47759–62.

Ward, J. F. (1975). Radiation-induced strand breakage in DNA, *Basic Life Sci* 5B: 471–2.

Weitzman, M. D., Carson, C. T., Schwartz, R. A. & Lilley, C. E. (2004). Interactions of viruses with the cellular DNA repair machinery, *DNA Repair (Amst)* 3(8-9): 1165–73.

Weitzman, M. D. & Ornelles, D. A. (2005). Inactivating intracellular antiviral responses during adenovirus infection, *Oncogene* 24(52): 7686–96.

Weterings, E. & Chen, D. J. (2007). DNA-dependent protein kinase in nonhomologous end joining: a lock with multiple keys?, *J Cell Biol* 179(2): 183–6.

Weterings, E. & van Gent, D. C. (2004). The mechanism of non-homologous end-joining: a synopsis of synapsis, *DNA Repair (Amst)* 3(11): 1425–35.

Wieler, S., Gagne, J. P., Vaziri, H., Poirier, G. G. & Benchimol, S. (2003). Poly(adp-ribose) polymerase-1 is a positive regulator of the p53-mediated g1 arrest response following ionizing radiation, *J Biol Chem* 278(21): 18914–21.

Wilkinson, D. E. & Weller, S. K. (2006). Herpes simplex virus type i disrupts the ATR-dependent DNA-damage response during lytic infection, *J Cell Sci* 119(Pt 13): 2695–703.

Wyman, C. & Kanaar, R. (2006). DNA double-strand break repair: all's well that ends well, *Annu Rev Genet* 40: 363–83.

Yanai, H., Savitsky, D., Tamura, T. & Taniguchi, T. (2009). Regulation of the cytosolic DNA-sensing system in innate immunity: a current view, *Curr Opin Immunol* 21(1): 17–22.

Yang, J., Yu, Y., Hamrick, H. E. & Duerksen-Hughes, P. J. (2003). ATM, ATR and DNA-PK: initiators of the cellular genotoxic stress responses, *Carcinogenesis* 24(10): 1571–80.

Yang, Y. G., Lindahl, T. & Barnes, D. E. (2007). Trex1 exonuclease degrades ssdna to prevent chronic checkpoint activation and autoimmune disease, *Cell* 131(5): 873–86.

Yarosh, D. B. (2001). Why is DNA damage signaling so complicated? chaos and molecular signaling, *Environ Mol Mutagen* 38(2-3): 132–4.

Yoshioka, K., Yoshioka, Y. & Hsieh, P. (2006). ATR kinase activation mediated by mutsalpha and mutlalpha in response to cytotoxic o6-methylguanine adducts, *Mol Cell* 22(4): 501–10.

Yun, M. H. & Hiom, K. (2009). Ctip-BRCA1 modulates the choice of DNA double-strand-break repair pathway throughout the cell cycle, *Nature* 459(7245): 460–3.

Zhu, Y., Hu, J., Hu, Y. & Liu, W. (2009). Targeting DNA repair pathways: a novel approach to reduce cancer therapeutic resistance, *Cancer Treat Rev* 35(7): 590–6.

10

Mechanisms of Mutagenic DNA Nucleobase Damages and their Chemical and Enzymatic Repairs Investigated by Quantum Chemical Methods

Eric A. C. Bushnell[1], Jorge Llano[2], Leif A. Eriksson[3] and James W. Gauld[1]
[1]*University of Windsor, Department of Chemistry and Biochemistry, Windsor, Ontario*
[2]*Grant MacEwan University, Department of Physical Sciences, Edmonton, Alberta*
[3]*School of Chemistry, National University of Ireland, Galway*
[1,2]*Canada*
[3]*Ireland*

1. Introduction

A cells genetic information, its 'blueprint of life', is contained within its DNA. This biologically important molecule, however, can be attacked by high-energy ionizing radiation and oxidizing agents resulting in a range of possible damage. For instance, nucleobases can undergo chemical modifications or degradation such as oxidation, deamination, alkylation or be cleaved from the sugar-phosphate backbone. (De Bont & van Larebeke 2004; Friedberg et al. 2004; Hecht 1999; Kamiya et al. 1998; Labet et al. 2008a; Lindahl 1993; Lysetska et al. 2002; Neeley & Essigmann 2006; Rydberg & Lindahl 1982; Taylor 1994; Wang 2008) Similarly, the deoxyribose sugar moieties may also undergo various chemical modifications. These events can lead further to the formation of DNA-DNA or DNA-protein cross-links or DNA-strand breaks. (Kumar & Sevilla 2010; Lipfert et al. 2004) Importantly, damage to DNA can significantly affect its replication and transcription. This can ultimately result in cell apoptosis or protein mutations and pathological diseases such as cancer. (Pages & Fuchs 2002)

Experimentally, there have been numerous detailed *in vivo* and *in vitro* investigations into the processes and pathways involved in the damage of DNA. (See, for instance, Kumar & Sevilla 2010; Mishina et al. 2006, Wetmore et al. 2001) Radiolysis experiments with photometric, electrochemical and electron paramagnetic resonance detection, enzymatic inhibition and mutagenesis studies have identified a large number of reaction intermediates and rate constants for many damage and repair processes. For more in-depth reviews of experimental investigations on DNA damage processes the reader is also directed to relevant chapters in this present book. Unfortunately, however, many uncertainties and questions still remain about DNA damage and repair.

Computational chemistry provides an alternate and also complementary approach for obtaining a deeper understanding of chemical processes. This is in part because it can not only be applied to systems that are amenable to experimental investigation but also to those systems or reactions that may be too challenging or even impossible to study using such experimental techniques. Furthermore, it is nowadays possible to apply highly accurate and reliable computational methods to larger, more complete biochemical models. Thus, using such approaches one can not only reconcile theory with experiment but, for example, compare the feasibility of differing proposed reaction mechanisms or identify new pathways.

There have been numerous computational investigations on or related to DNA damage and repair. In this chapter the application of Computational Chemistry to the study of DNA damage and repair is illustrated through a review of a number of relevant computational investigations that we have performed. More specifically, we have applied high accuracy density functional theory (DFT)-based methods to the study of several important primary and secondary nucleobase damage pathways and repair mechanisms. The chapter is divided into sections, each of which focuses on select results concerning a damage and/or repair process involving either the nucleobase or phosphate components of DNA:

2. **Nucleobase oxidation via ionizing radiation**: describes primary redox damage in nucleobases. In particular, the Gibbs Free Energies of solution-phase electron (ET), proton (PT) and proton-coupled electron (PTET) transfers for all DNA bases are examined. In addition, the potential of alkylthiols to act as repair agents of such damage is considered.
3. **8-Oxopurine formation in purine, adenine and guanine**: focuses on secondary damage of purine nucleobases. Specifically, the mechanisms of •OH attack leading to formation of 8-oxopurine derivatives are discussed as well as the Gibbs Free Energy changes of possible associated ET, PT and PTET processes.
4. **Deamination of oxidized cytosine**: examines the thermochemistry of several possible mechanisms by which oxidized cytosine, a pyrimidine nucleobase, may undergo deamination.
5. **Oxidation of serine phosphate: Implications for DNA**: investigates radicals formed from radiation-induced damage of serine phosphate.
6. **Oxidative repair of alkylated nucleobases: The catalytic mechanism of AlkB**: describes key results of our studies on the enzymatic mechanism of AlkB, a member of the family of α-ketoglutarate-Fe(II)-dependent dioxygenase enzymes that catalyse the oxidative repair of alkylated nucleobases.

1.1 Methods

For the detailed study of electronic properties of biochemical systems the current computational chemistry methods of choice for investigators are those of density functional theory (DFT). The principle reasons for this is that they inherently include electron correlation effects via their basis upon the electron density of the chemical system. Such effects are often important, for example, in accurately describing bond making and breaking processes, or weakly bound systems such as reaction transition structures. Furthermore, regardless of the number of electrons in the chemical system, the electron density is only ever a function of the three Cartesian coordinates. Thus, with such methods one can use larger and more complete chemical models consisting of 150 or more atoms. In addition, they are usually highly reliable and accurate.(See, for example, Llano 2010) For biochemical systems, the currently most widely used DFT functional is B3LYP,(Becke 1993a; Becke 1993b; Lee et al. 1988) and it has been used throughout this chapter.

Many biochemical processes occur within a polar environment, in particular an enzyme active site or aqueous medium. This can influence the properties and reactions of a biomolecule. Hence, it can be important to include such effects in the computational model. Each study described in this chapter has used a polarizable continuum (PCM)-based approach(Cammi & Tomasi 1995; Miertus et al. 1981) in the integral equation formulism (IEF).(Cances & Mennucci 1998; Cances et al. 1997; Mennucci et al. 1997) In this method the chemical system is effectively 'wrapped' in a density-fitting polar dielectric medium. Within this chapter a dielectric constant (ε) value of 4.0 has been used when modeling reactions within a protein active site, while the standard value for water at 298 K has been used for reactions modeled in aqueous environments. The specific computational details of each investigation are outlined in their respective section and in the appropriate article.
In order to determine relative free energies of reactions in which protons and electrons act as independent ions, it can be necessary to use 'fundamental values' such as the chemical potential of an electron or proton in a vacuum or aqueous solution under standard conditions. The values used in this chapter are given in **Table 1.** These have been obtained by means of a first principles quantum and statistical mechanics approach, the details of which are provided in a recent paper by Llano and Eriksson.(Llano & Eriksson 2002)

Quantity	eV	kcal mol^{-1}
$\mu_{0K}^{vac}(e^-)$	0.0	0.0
$\mu_{298K,1atm}^{\Theta,SHE}(e^-)$	-4.34 ± 0.02	-100.03 ± 0.5
$\mu_{298K,1atm}^{\Theta,aq}(e^-)$	-1.6638 ± 0.04	-38.37 ± 0.5
$\mu_{298K,1atm}^{\Theta,aq}(H^+)$	-11.6511 ± 0.02	-268.68 ± 0.5

Table 1. Chemical potentials of an electron in vacuum and an electron and proton in aqueous reference states.(Llano & Eriksson 2002).

2. Nucleobase oxidation via ionizing radiation

Ionizing radiation can potentially be absorbed by any of the three nucleotide components of DNA (i.e., phosphate, sugar or nucleobase) or its surrounding waters; also an essential part of DNA structure.(Kumar & Sevilla 2010) Primary damage of, for example, nucleobases, is caused by their direct absorption of radiation. Secondary damage (such as that described later in this chapter) can also occur, for instance, when the radiation is absorbed by the solvent, thus generating radicals or solvated electrons which then attack the nucleobase.(von Sonntag 1987; von Sonntag 1996)
Direct absorption (primary damage) can cause the formation of a radical-cationic base via the loss of an electron, i.e., generation of an electron hole. Due to the stacking of nucleobases within DNA charge transfer (transfer of the hole) can then occur along the strand. Consequently, this enables 'primary damage related' reactions to occur distant from the site of initial damage. The potential for charge transfer due to the π-orbital interactions between bases was proposed as early as 1962. (Eley & Spivey 1962) Alternatively, however, it may enable charge recombination to occur further along the chain. This is because radical-anionic bases can be formed by the capture of the free electrons, where the resulting damage to the nucleobase also constitutes primary damage. Guanine has the lowest ionization potential of

the four DNA nucleobases, followed by adenine.(Hush & Cheung 1975; Kumar & Sevilla 2010; Steenken & Jovanovic 1997; Yang et al. 2004) Consequently, they are in general oxidized to give their radical-cations while thymine and cytosine act as electron sinks and form their radical-anions. However, vice versa, in the transfer of electron holes guanine typically acts as a sink for DNA radiative oxidation.(Cadet et al. 2008; Kumar & Sevilla 2010) Reduction/oxidation of a nucleobase can significantly affect its properties. In particular, it has been shown that their oxidation greatly increases their acidity (lowers their pK_a).(Kumar & Sevilla 2010) Indeed, the formation of a radical base is often associated with proton transfer reactions that can lead to further nucleobase damage. However, as has also been noted, these same proton transfers can result in nucleobase repair.(Llano & Eriksson 2004b)

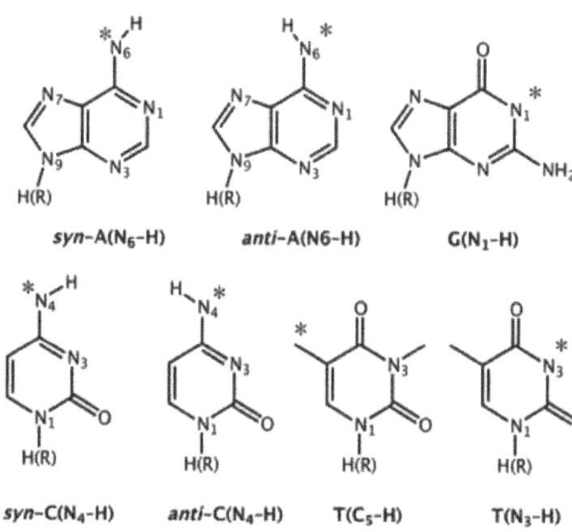

Fig. 1. Structures of the dehydrogenated nucleobases for both the cations and anions. The position of the missing hydrogen is marked by the asterisk.

Unfortunately, our understanding of these important electron- (ET) and proton-transfer (PT) reactions is incomplete.(Llano & Eriksson 2004a) This is not only due to the highly transient and reactive nature of key species involved, but also because experimental measurements of free energies for such processes can only be obtained indirectly.(Llano & Eriksson 2004a) Moreover, at times, the available experimental techniques (photoelectron spectroscopy, mass spectroscopy, pulse radiolysis and electrochemical techniques) appear to give contradictory results.(Seidel et al. 1996) Using computational methods we have investigated the processes involved in the oxidation and reduction of DNA nucleobases.(Llano & Eriksson 2004a) In particular, the nature of the ET process, the effect of PT on such processes, and vice versa, was examined using the chemical models shown in **Figure 1**.

All optimizations were performed at the B3LYP/6-31(+)G(d,p) level of theory; diffuse functions only being included for anionic species'. Harmonic vibrational frequencies and zero-point vibrational energies (ZPVE) were calculated at this same level of theory. Relative energies and absolute chemical potentials were then obtained via single point calculations at the IEF-PCM/B3LYP/6-311+G(2df,p) level of theory, in aqueous solvent, based on the above optimized structures with inclusion of the appropriate Gibbs corrections. In combination with the values listed in **Table 1**, the free energies for oxidation of the four neutral DNA bases and the corresponding anions was determined. Specifically, the free energies were calculated for the three different reference states used to define the absolute chemical potential of the electron: in vacuum, aqueous or the SHE reference state.

$B^{\bullet -}_{(aq)}$	→			$B_{(aq)}$	→			$B^{\bullet +}_{(aq)}$
	$-e^-_{(vac)}$	$-e^-_{(aq)}$	$-e^-_{(SHE)}$		$-e^-_{(vac)}$	$-e^-_{(aq)}$	$-e^-_{(SHE)}$	
$A^{\bullet -}$	40.7	2.3	-59.3 (-56.0)[a]	A	136.7	98.3	36.7 (32.7)[c]	$A^{\bullet +}$
$G^{\bullet -}$	37.9	-0.5	-62.1 (-63.2)[a]	G	125.9	87.5	25.9 (29.7)[c]	$G^{\bullet +}$
$T^{\bullet -}$	51.9	13.5	-48.1 (-25.6)[b]	T	145.2	106.8	45.2 (39.2)[c]	$T^{\bullet +}$
$C^{\bullet -}$	43.3	9.9	-51.7 (-25.8)[b]	C	147.6	109.2	47.6 (36.9)[c]	$C^{\bullet +}$

Table 2. Calculated (see text) standard free energies (in kcal mol^{-1}) of primary ionizations of the four nucleobases in aqueous solution. Experimental values are in parenthesis and taken from references: [a] (Seidel et al. 1996), [b] (Steenken et al. 1992), [c] (Steenken & Jovanovic 1997).

ET is a common process that occurs upon absorption of radiation by nucleobases. Using a first principles approach the free energy changes involved with such a process for all four DNA nucleobases were calculated and are shown in **Table 2**.(Llano & Eriksson 2002) It can be seen that the ionization of each of the anionic bases ($B^{\bullet -}_{(aq)}$) can be either endothermic or exothermic depending on the reference state of the electron. For example, in the vacuum or aqueous state the oxidation of the anionic bases is generally an endothermic process. The only exception occurs for guanine in the aqueous state in which the process is marginally exothermic (-0.5 kcal mol^{-1}). In contrast, in the case of the SHE reference state, oxidation of each base is markedly exothermic. For $A^{\bullet -}$ and $G^{\bullet -}$ the values calculated are in close agreement to those obtained experimentally.(Seidel et al. 1996; Steenken & Jovanovic 1997; Steenken et al. 1992) In contrast, those calculated for $C^{\bullet -}$ and $T^{\bullet -}$ are not in as good agreement, being almost twice the corresponding experimental values. However, the overall trends are consistent; the oxidation of $C^{\bullet -}$ or $T^{\bullet -}$ is thermodynamically less favorable than that of $A^{\bullet -}$ or $G^{\bullet -}$. Conversely, the reverse process, capture of a solvated electron by C or T (i.e., $C/T_{(aq)} + e^-_{(aq)} \rightarrow C/T^{\bullet -}_{(aq)}$) is thermodynamically preferred (-9.9 kcal mol^{-1} and -13.5 kcal mol^{-1}, respectively) compared to that involving A or G (-2.3 kcal mol^{-1} and 0.5 kcal mol^{-1}, respectively).

Oxidation of the neutral bases is calculated to be endothermic for each reference state of the electron (**Table 2**). The degree of endothermicity, however, depends on the reference state being most endothermic in vacuum and least for the SHE reference state. Unlike that observed for the radical anion bases, the SHE calculated values for the neutral bases are all in good agreement with experiment. The largest difference occurs for C and is now only 10.7 kcal mol^{-1} compared to the 25.9 kcal mol^{-1} difference for $C^{\bullet -}$, while the smallest difference (-3.8 kcal mol^{-1}) is observed for guanine. In addition, neutral G is calculated to have the lowest free energy of oxidation and is thus the easiest of the four DNA nucleobases to be ionized, in agreement with experimental observations.

The free energies associated with the loss of a proton from the resulting radical-cationic bases to solution were calculated and are given in **Table 3**. For $A/G^{\bullet +}$ the energy changes associated with deprotonations to form *syn*-A(N_6-H), *anti*-A(N_6-H), and G(N_1-H) were determined to be quite small at just -0.6, -0.7 and -0.3 kcal mol^{-1} respectively.(Llano & Eriksson 2004a) In contrast, the energy changes associated with deprotonation of $C/T^{\bullet +}$ to give *syn*-C(N_4-H) or *anti*-C(N4-H) and T(C_5-H) are larger at -5.2, -4.5 and -22.3 kcal mol^{-1}, respectively.(Llano & Eriksson 2004a) It is noted that T(C_5-H) has only been observed in the solid state and not in solution,(Steenken 1989) and thus will not be discussed herein. Unlike the other deprotonation processes, formation of T(N_3-H) was found to be endothermic and

Cationic Radical Base	ΔG (kcal mol^{-1})	Deprotonated Radical Base
$A^{•+}$	-0.7 (≤ 1.4)[a]	*syn*-A(N_6-H),
$A^{•+}$	-0.6 (≤ 1.4)[a]	*anti*-A(N_6-H)
$G^{•+}$	-0.3 (5.3)[a]	G(N_1-H)
$T^{•+}$	-22.3	T(C_5-H)
$T^{•+}$	9.9 (4.9)[a]	T(N_3-H)
$C^{•+}$	-5.2 (~5.4)[a]	*syn*-C(N_4-H),
$C^{•+}$	-4.5 (~5.4)[a]	*anti*-C(N_4-H)

Table 3. Calculated (see text) standard Gibbs energies (in kcal mol^{-1}) of the decay of the radical cations. Experimental values included in parenthesis taken from references: [a] (Steenken 1989; Steenken 1992).

had the largest absolute free energy change (9.9 kcal mol^{-1}).(Llano & Eriksson 2004a) Thus, the loss of a proton in aqueous conditions is thermodynamically favorable for the radical-cationic bases except for proton loss from N_3—H in thymine. The unfavourable decay of $T^{•+}$ via deprotonation of N_3-H suggests that the ion may have a long enough lifetime such that it may instead obtain an electron, a thermodynamically favourable process (**Table 2**). Thus, $T^{•+}$ may instead preferably react to regenerate the neutral base T rather than decay.(Llano & Eriksson 2004a)

Having established an understanding of the energies associated with oxidation of the anionic and neutral bases, energy changes associated with possible repair mechanisms of this damage were then investigated. For the deprotonated neutral radical bases ($B(-H)^{•}_{(aq)}$) regeneration can occur via three possible pathways: (i) ET followed by PT (**Table 4**); (ii) a proton-coupled electron transfer (PTET) (**Table 5**) or (iii) direct transfer of a hydrogen atom. From **Table 4** it can be seen that reduction of the deprotonated bases is exothermic under all reference states with the exception of T(N_3-H)$^{•}$ in the SHE reference state. However, the energy change for protonating all of the reduced bases ($B(-H)^{-}_{(aq)}$) is favorable. Protonation of G(N_1-H)$^{-}$ has the smallest free energy change suggesting that the conjugate acid is relatively stronger than the other neutral bases. Importantly, the more acidic a molecule, the more powerful it is as a reducing agent. Thus, as G has the smallest energy cost of deprotonation of any of the DNA bases it is more likely to reduce the other bases and thereby act as an electron hole sink, as observed experimentally.

$B(-H)^{•}_{(aq)}$	→			$B(-H)^{-}_{(aq)}$	→	$B_{(aq)}$
	$+e^{-}_{(vac)}$	$+e^{-}_{(aq)}$	$+e^{-}_{(SHE)}$		$+H^{+}_{(aq)}$	
syn-A(N_6-H)$^{•}$	-113.2	-74.9	-13.2	*syn*-A(N_6-H)$^{-}$	-22.7 (≥ -19.1)[a]	A
anti-A(N_6-H)$^{•}$	-113.9	-75.6	-13.9	*anti*-A(N_6-H)$^{-}$	-22.2 (≥ -19.1)[a]	A
G(N_1-H)$^{•}$	-111.5	-73.2	-11.5	G(N_1-H)$^{-}$	-14.4 (-13.0)[a]	G
T(N_3-H)$^{•}$	-72.3	-34.0	27.7	T(N_3-H)$^{-}$	-50.6	T
syn-C(N_4-H)$^{•}$	-123.0	-84.6	-23.0	*syn*-C(N_4-H)$^{-}$	-19.4 (-17.7)[a]	C
anti-C(N_4-H)$^{•}$	-123.4	-85.0	-23.4	*anti*-C(N_4-H)$^{-}$	-19.6 (-17.7)[a]	C

Table 4. Calculated (see text) standard Gibbs energies (in kcal mol^{-1}) of the regeneration of the nucleobases via a ET then PT process. Experimental values included in parenthesis taken from references: [a] (Steenken 1989; Steenken 1992).

Under alkaline conditions it is expected that ET would occur prior to PT, as seen in **Table 4**. However, under acidic conditions a PTET process may occur. The associated calculated energy values are given in **Table 5**. As can be seen, the free energy changes for ET are exothermic for all reference states when it occurs simultaneously with a PT. Importantly, the free energies associated with electron addition are decidedly more favorable in the case of a PTET process compared to that observed in the previous ET process (cf. **Table 4**).

$B(-H)^{\bullet}_{(aq)}$	→			$B_{(aq)}$
	$+e^-_{(vac)}$	$+e^-_{(aq)}$	$+e^-_{(SHE)}$	
syn-A(N$_6$-H)$^\bullet$	-136.0	-97.6	-36.0 (-46.8)[a]	A
anti-A(N$_6$-H)$^\bullet$	-136.1	-97.7	-36.1 (-46.8)[a]	A
G(N$_1$-H)$^\bullet$	-125.6	-87.3	-26.5 (-19.7)[a]	G
T(N$_3$-H)$^\bullet$	-155.1	-116.7	-55.1	T
syn-C(N$_4$-H)$^\bullet$	-142.4	-104.0	-42.4	C
anti-C(N$_4$-H)$^\bullet$	-143.0	-104.6	-43.0	C

Table 5. Calculated (see text) standard Gibbs energies of the regeneration of the nucleobases via a PTET process. Experimental values included in parenthesis taken from references: [a] (Steenken & Jovanovic 1997).

The aqueous state reduction of the neutral radical bases ($B(-H)^{\bullet}_{(aq)}$) by addition of $H^{\bullet}_{(aq)}$ was calculated to be exothermic for all DNA bases. More specifically, the free energy changes for reduction of *syn / anti*-A(N$_6$-H)$^\bullet$ and -C(N$_4$-H)$^\bullet$ are -85.0, -85.1, -91.4 and -92.0 kcal mol^{-1}, respectively while for G(N$_1$-H)$^\bullet$ and T(N$_3$-H)$^\bullet$ they are -74.6 and -104.1 kcal mol^{-1}, respectively. It is likely that this process is important under low pH conditions where the free protons would scavenge the hydrated electrons to yield H$^\bullet$. These free energy changes are less exothermic than those seen in the PTET process (cf. **Table 5**; $e^-_{(aq)}$ results). However, under acidic conditions the PTET and H$^\bullet$ processes would likely compete as they both react at diffusion-limited rates. Of all possible three reduction mechanisms for B(-H)$^\bullet$, PTET processes show the greatest change in free energy.

Deprotonated Radical Base	$\Delta_{ET}G^{\ominus}$	$\Delta_{PTET}G^{\ominus}$
syn-A(N$_6$-H)$^\bullet$	-5.1	-13.5
anti-A(N$_6$-H)$^\bullet$	-5.8	-13.6
G(N$_1$-H)$^\bullet$	-3.4	-3.1
T(N$_3$-H)$^\bullet$	-32.6	-32.6
syn-C(N$_4$-H)$^\bullet$	-14.9	-19.9
anti-C(N$_4$-H)$^\bullet$	-15.3	-20.5

Table 6. Calculated (see text) standard Gibbs energies (in kcal mol^{-1}) of the regeneration of the nucleobases by methylthiol. $\Delta_{ET}G^{\ominus}$ is the free energy change for $B(-H)^{\bullet}_{(aq)} + MeS^-_{(aq)} = B(-H)^-_{(aq)} + MeS^{\bullet}_{(aq)}$ while $\Delta_{PTET}G^{\ominus}$ is the free energy change for $B(-H)^{\bullet}_{(aq)} + MeSH_{(aq)} = B_{(aq)} + MeS^{\bullet}_{(aq)}$.

Clearly, the possible processes by which the neutral bases may be regenerated are inherently favorable regardless of whether the electrons originate from vacuum, dilute aqueous

solutions or SHE reference states. However, they still require that there be a suitable reductant. It has been noted that in solution a free thiol could be a likely reductant for transfer of a H• to a radical-cationic DNA base, thereby repairing the lesion.(von Sonntag 1987; von Sonntag 1996). Hence, the applicability of thiols to act as such a reductant was also investigated. It should be noted that although the process of repairing the nucleobase can occur via enzymatic or other chemical processes, only the latter involving methylthiol is discussed here. The calculated free energy costs associated with regeneration of the deprotonated radical bases by methylthiol (CH_3SH) are given in **Table 6**.
Two possible reduction pathways exist:

i. $B(-H)^{\bullet}_{(aq)} + MeS^{-}_{(aq)} \rightarrow B(-H)^{-}_{(aq)} + MeS^{\bullet}_{(aq)}$
ii. $B(-H)^{\bullet}_{(aq)} + MeSH_{(aq)} \rightarrow B_{(aq)} + MeS^{\bullet}_{(aq)}$

Pathway i most likely only occurs under basic conditions. However, as can be seen from **Table 6**, for *syn*- / *anti*-A(N_6-H)• and -C(N_4-H)• an initial loss of the -SH proton markedly lowers the reductive ability of the thiol. That is, the overall free energy change associated with regeneration of the nucleobases is reduced, i.e., $\Delta_{ET}G^{\ominus}$ is less exothermic than $\Delta_{PTET}G^{\ominus}$. However, for G(N_1-H)• and T(N_3-H)• the free energy changes are quite close for both possible regeneration pathways. The markedly larger values of $\Delta_{PTET}G^{\ominus}$ compared to $\Delta_{ET}G^{\ominus}$ for all adenine and cytosine species considered suggests that PTET is the favoured process at any pH for these nucleobases. However, the negligible difference observed for guanine and thymine suggest that the preferred path will depend on the reaction conditions, e.g., pH. Importantly, regardless of the preferred pathway the calculated free energies indicate they are both favorable, exothermic processes.

3. 8-Oxopurine formation in purine, adenine and guanine

A major type of secondary DNA damage is that caused by the attack of hydroxyl radicals.(Llano & Eriksson 2004a; von Sonntag 1987; von Sonntag 1996) Such radicals can be formed when metals or hydrogen peroxide are present.(Burrows & Muller 1998) In addition, however, the absorption of radiation by water can lead to not only the formation of solvated electrons but also of reactive oxygen species such as •OH. Furthermore, related modifications of nucleobases can occur via the reaction of their radical cation with water. For instance, reaction of $G^{\bullet+}$ with H_2O has been suggested to be an important alternative pathway in DNA modification.(Candeias & Steenken 2000) Unfortunately, due to the high reactivity of these radicals where the rates of reaction are typically diffusion controlled,(Llano & Eriksson 2004a) it is impossible for radical scavengers to prevent them from damaging DNA. It has been suggested that approximately half of the damage done by •OH occurs at the nucleobases. In the purine bases the hydroxyl has been observed to attack at their double bonds to form the C_4, C_5 and C_8 adducts with the latter (i.e., **B8OH•**$_{(aq)}$) being the major product of oxidation and radiolysis.(Hagen 1986; Hatahet 1998; Kasai et al. 1986; Llano & Eriksson 2004b; Teoule 1987)
The subsequent oxidation of **B8OH•**$_{(aq)}$ to give **8-OHB**$_{(aq)}$ may occur via either of the two pathways shown in **Figure 2**: (i) a PT followed by an ET(Cullis et al. 1996) or (ii) a PTET mechanism(Candeias & Steenken 2000). The resulting common **8-OHB**$_{(aq)}$ product of both pathways can then undergo tautomerization to yield the corresponding 8-oxo derivative (**8-oxoB**$_{(aq)}$). It is noted that the barrier for tautomerization of 8-hydroxy-purine (**8-OHPu**$_{(aq)}$) has been calculated to be quite low at only 7.0 kcal mol^{-1} with the keto form (**8-oxoPu**$_{(aq)}$) being favoured over the enol form by 10.6 kcal mol^{-1}. (Llano & Eriksson 2004b)

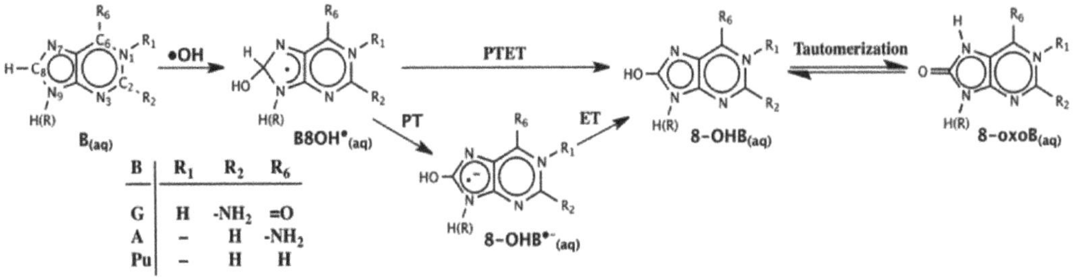

Fig. 2. Two proposed pathways for •OH attack at the C8 position of a purine base and subsequent oxidation to generate the 8-oxo purine derivative.

The **8-oxoG/A** products are in fact major stable DNA purine oxidation products produced via the radiolysis of water.(Hagen 1986; Hatahet 1998; Kasai et al. 1986; Teoule 1987) However, it is been observed that the adenine derivative (**8-oxoA**) is formed only about one-third of the time compared to the guanine derivative (**8-oxoG**).(Burrows & Muller 1998; Llano & Eriksson 2004b) Importantly, however, the formation of either **8-oxoB** species promotes the formation of mutagenic lesions that can cause mispairings resulting in G:C and T:A transversions.(Cheng et al. 1992; Cullis et al. 1996; Llano & Eriksson 2004b; Newcomb 1998; Pavlov et al. 1994) Such lesions are in fact caused by the further oxidation of **8-oxoB** to their corresponding **8-oxoB•(-H7)** derivatives. Moreover, it has been shown that depending on the reaction conditions both spiroiminodi- and guanidino-hydantoin are also major products formed by further oxidation of **8-oxoG**.(Munk et al. 2008) It has been suggested that these further reactions occur because the **8-oxoB** species' have lower ionization potentials than any other native base.(Cadet & Vigny 1990; Chatgilialoglu et al. 2000) Hence, they could act as a trap for a migrating electron hole.(Sponer et al. 2004; Yao et al. 2005) Unfortunately, however, despite detailed experimental study, the exact route by which such species' (**8-oxoB** and **8-oxoB•(-H7)**) may be formed remains unclear.(Llano & Eriksson 2004b)

We performed a computational investigation on the processes by which **$8-OHB_{(aq)}$** may be formed for purine, adenine and guanine.(Llano & Eriksson 2004b) In addition, the subsequent oxidations by which **8-oxoB** and **8-oxoB•(-H7)** may be formed were also examined using a first principles approach.(Llano & Eriksson 2002) Optimized structures, harmonic vibrational frequencies and ZPVEs were calculated at the B3LYP/6-31(+)G(d,p) level theory; diffuse functions only being included for anionic species'. Relative Gibbs Free energies were obtained by performing single point calculations at the IEF-PCM/B3LYP/6-311+G(2df,p) level of theory, in aqueous solvent, based on the above structures with inclusion of the appropriate Gibbs corrections.

Attack of •OH at the C_8 position in purine, adenine or guanine results in formation of the corresponding radical hydroxylated intermediates **B8OH•** (**Figure 3**). Notably, they are stabilized relative to the isolated reactants by -13.4, -14.9 and -15.8 kcal mol^{-1} for purine, adenine and guanine respectively.

The oxidation of **$B8OH^{\bullet}{}_{(aq)}$** may then be initiated via PT from its $-C_8-H$ moiety (**Figure 3**). This step, resulting in formation of the corresponding radical-anionic derivatives **$8-OHB^{\bullet -}{}_{(aq)}$** was calculated to be significantly endothermic for all three purine bases considered with a minimum free energy cost of ~28 kcal mol^{-1}. Notably, the largest costs of 35.4 and 47.4 kcal mol^{-1} are observed for adenine and guanine, respectively. This suggests that a strong base is

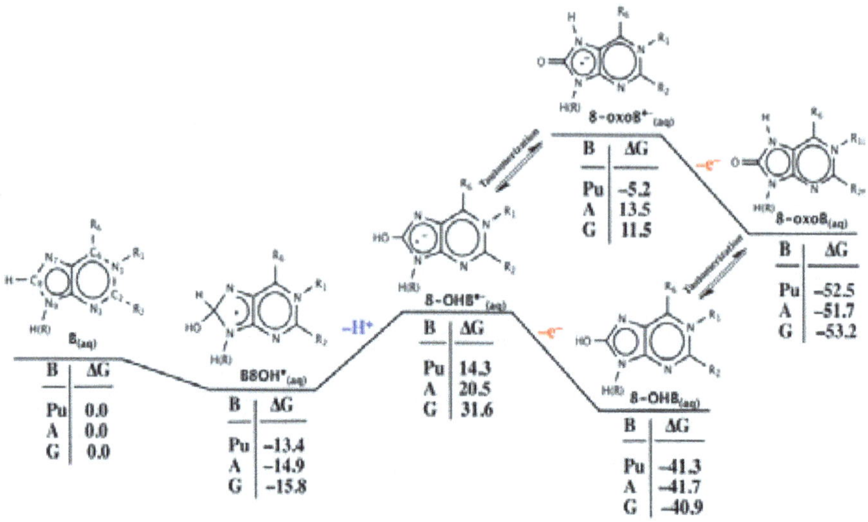

Fig. 3. Calculated (see text) standard Gibbs energies (kcal mol-1) for PT initiated oxidation of **B8OH•**.

required for deprotonation of C_8 in **B8OH•$_{(aq)}$** and is unlikely to occur under neutral or acidic conditions. The resulting **8-OHB•-$_{(aq)}$** ions can then either oxidize further via loss of an electron to give **8-OHB$_{(aq)}$** or tautomerize to give **8-oxoB•-$_{(aq)}$**. As can be seen in **Figure 3**, both possible processes are thermodynamically preferred. Importantly, however, these latter two species can subsequently undergo tautomerization and electron loss, respectively to give the same **8-oxoB$_{(aq)}$** product species. The barriers for tautomerization of the radical-anionic (**8-OHPu•-$_{(aq)}$**) and neutral purine (**8-OHPu$_{(aq)}$**) are both low at just 5.2 and 7.1 kcal mol-1, respectively. (Llano & Eriksson 2004b) Thus, the choice of pathway from **8-OHB•-$_{(aq)}$** to **8-oxoB$_{(aq)}$** may in fact be controlled by the thermodynamics of the loss of an electron. From **Figure 3** it can be seen that for purine and guanine the largest decreases in free energy observed for electron loss along either of these two paths occurs for the oxidation of the enol radical anion **8-OHB•-$_{(aq)}$** to give **8-OHB$_{(aq)}$** with decreases of 55.6 and 72.5 kcal mol-1 respectively. In contrast, for adenine the largest decrease (65.2 kcal mol-1) is observed for loss of an electron from the keto radical anion **8-oxoB•-$_{(aq)}$** to give **8-oxoB$_{(aq)}$**. Thus for purine and guanine it is likely that formation of **8-oxoB$_{(aq)}$** occurs via tautomerization of **8-OHB$_{(aq)}$**, while for adenine it involves oxidation of **8-oxoB•-$_{(aq)}$**.

As shown in **Figure 4**, oxidation of **B8OH•$_{(aq)}$** may alternatively be initiated by ET, giving rise to **B8OH+$_{(aq)}$** ions. Similar to that observed for an initial PT from **B8OH•$_{(aq)}$** (cf. **Figure 3**), this process is also found to be endothermic for all three purine nucleobases. However, with the exception of purine, the energy costs incurred are now significantly less. Indeed, for **A/G8OH•$_{(aq)}$** ET is thermodynamically preferred to PT by 24.1 and 47.2 kcal mol-1 respectively. It is further noted that for guanine, the reactant **G8OH•$_{(aq)}$** is essentially thermoneutral with the **G8OH+$_{(aq)}$** intermediate. Furthermore, the subsequent PT from **B8OH+$_{(aq)}$** to give **8-OHB$_{(aq)}$** is highly exothermic for all bases by 57.1, 45.3 and 25.3 kcal mol-1 for purine, adenine and guanine, respectively. This is in contrast to the highly endothermic initial PT observed in **B8OH•$_{(aq)}$** (cf. **Figure 3**). For the ET initiated oxidation pathway tautomerization can only happen once PT has occurred, that is, once **8-OHB$_{(aq)}$** has been formed. This rearrangement, which results directly in formation of **8-oxoB$_{(aq)}$**, is exothermic for all bases considered by 10.0 - 12.3 kcal mol-1. It should be noted that in addition to the possible ET and PT initiated processes, a PTET (i.e., the concerted loss of electron and proton) process may also occur. However, the overall free energy change for formation of **8-OHB** via this alternate path is -27.9, -26.8 and -25.1 kcal mol-1 relative to **B8OH**$^{\bullet}$$_{(aq)}$ for purine, adenine and guanine, respectively.

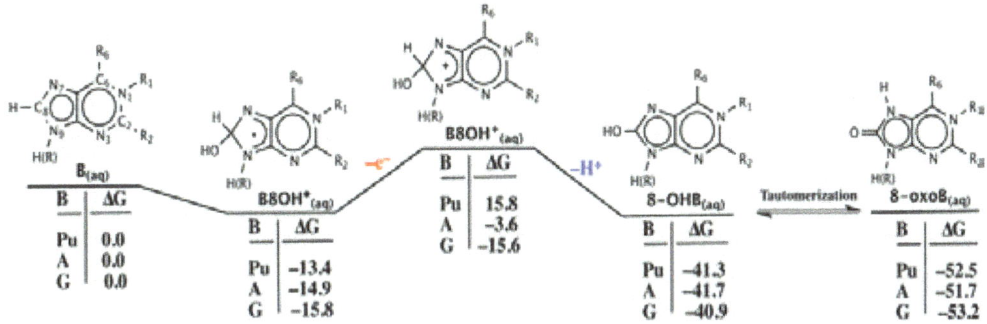

Fig. 4. Calculated (see text) standard Gibbs energies (kcal mol-1) for the ET initiated oxidation pathway in **B8OH**$^{\bullet}$.

The formation of **8-oxoB**$^{\bullet}$**(-H7)**$_{(aq)}$ can potentially be achieved by further oxidation of the neutral tautomers **8-oxoB**$_{(aq)}$ and **8-OHB**$_{(aq)}$, initiated by loss of an electron (**Figure 5**). For both species', however, this ET process is endothermic. For purine and adenine the lowest associated energy costs (46.1 and 30.5 kcal mol-1 respectively) are incurred for ET from **8-oxoB**$_{(aq)}$ while for guanine it is incurred from **8-OHB**$_{(aq)}$ with a cost of 20.1 kcal mol-1. Notably, for both **8-oxoB**$_{(aq)}$ and **8-OHB**$_{(aq)}$ the loss of an electron from the guanine-derivative (**8-oxoG**$_{(aq)}$ and **8-OHG**$_{(aq)}$) is preferred to that from the corresponding adenine or purine-derivatives. Regardless, however, a suitable oxidant is required in order to oxidize either **8-oxoB**$_{(aq)}$ or **8-OHB**$_{(aq)}$. The barriers for tautomerization for both the neutral **8-oxoB**$_{(aq)}$/**8-OHB**$_{(aq)}$ and radical-cationic **8-OHB**$^{\bullet+}$$_{(aq)}$/**8-oxoB**$^{\bullet+}$$_{(aq)}$ species' are quite low at

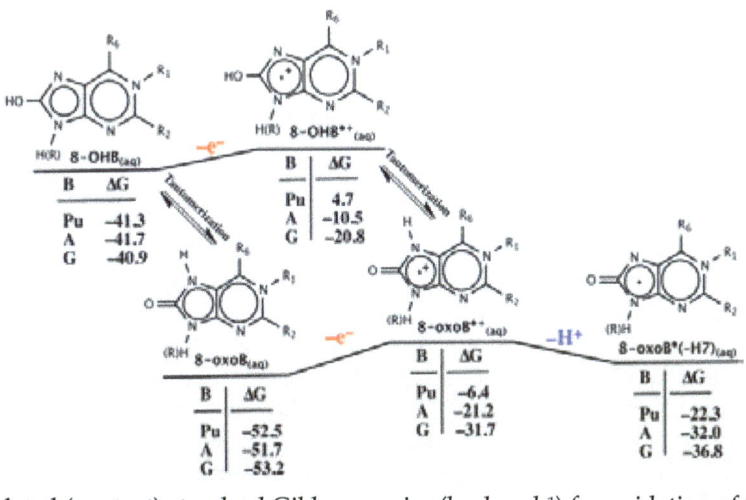

Fig. 5. Calculated (see text) standard Gibbs energies (kcal mol-1) for oxidation of **8-OHB** and **8-oxoB**.

just 7.0 and 9.2 kcal mol^{-1}, respectively.(Llano & Eriksson 2004b) Thus, once formed, such species are expected to be able to easily interconvert between their enol and keto forms with equilibrium favouring the latter. However, once the **8-oxoB**$^{\bullet+}_{(aq)}$ species is formed, loss of a proton (H^+) from N7 to give **8-oxoB**$^{\bullet}$**(-H7)**$_{(aq)}$ is exothermic for all bases (**Figure 5**). Notably, **8-oxoG**$^{\bullet}$**(-H7)**$_{(aq)}$ is calculated to lie 4.8 kcal mol^{-1} lower in energy than the corresponding adenine derivative **8-oxoA**$^{\bullet}$**(-H7)**$_{(aq)}$ and may thus help explain the preference of its formation over that of **8-oxoA**.

4. Deamination of oxidized cytosine

In addition to damage by ionizing radiation it has been found that nucleobases are susceptible to oxidation by one-electron oxidants, e.g., nitrosoperoxycarbonate present during inflammatory processes.(Cadet et al. 2006; Lee et al. 2007) The purine base guanine, despite having the lowest ionization potential, is not the sole target for oxidants. In particular it has been observed that the pyrimidine bases are also susceptible to oxidation.(Decarroz et al. 1986; Douki & Cadet 1999; Wagner et al. 1990) Importantly, this oxidation leads to degradation via two possible competing pathways that are initiated by deprotonation of: (i) the methylene carbon of the sugar moiety (C_1') attached to the pyrimidine nitrogen (N_1) or (ii) the exocyclic amine attached to C_4 of the ring. Notably, the latter path has been suggested to lead to hydrolytic deamination of the pyrimidine ring.(Decarroz et al. 1987)

Previous computational investigations have investigated the deamination of non-oxidized cytosine, in particular via the attack of water or an hydroxyl anion (^-OH) at its C_4 centre and via $NO^{\bullet}$ attack at N_4.(Almatarneh et al. 2006; Labet et al. 2009) While the lowest barrier was obtained for the nucleophilic attack of OH^- at C_4, the calculated value was 9.6 kcal mol^{-1} higher than that obtained experimentally. However, the susceptibility of cytosine to one-electron oxidation suggests that possible mechanisms for deamination of $C^{\bullet+}$ should also be taken into consideration. The importance of considering such reactions is further underlined by the fact that the product of oxidation and deamination of cytosine is the highly mutagenic uracil residue.

We used computational chemistry methods to investigate the deamination of cytosine via the oxidized cytosine intermediate $C^{\bullet+}$ and via a deprotonated cytosine. Optimized structures and their corresponding harmonic vibrational frequencies were obtained at the IEF-PCM/B3LYP/6-311G(d,p) level of theory in aqueous solvent. Relative free energies were obtained at the same level of theory with inclusion of the appropriate Gibbs energy corrections.

In **section 2** it was shown that the one-electron oxidation of cytosine with the loss of the electron and proton in aqueous solution (i.e. $C \rightarrow e^-_{(aq)} + H^+_{(aq)} + C(-N_4)^{\bullet}_{(aq)}$) occurs with a sizeable free energy cost of approximately 104 kcal mol^{-1} (**Table 4**). The optimized structure of the oxidized $C(-N_4)^{\bullet}_{(aq)}$ ring (not shown) is similar to that of neutral cytosine being planar with similar bond lengths, in agreement with other theoretical studies.(Cauet et al. 2006; Wetmore et al. 2000; Wetmore et al. 1998) The calculated spin densities and Mulliken charges showed that the positive charge is delocalized over the ring with the greatest change in partial charges occurring at C_5 (+0.24e) while for spin densities they occur at C_5 (0.64) and N_1 (0.30).

The loss of a proton from N_4 in $C^{\bullet+}$ can result in the formation of either *syn*- or *anti*-$C(N_4$-$H)^{\bullet}$ with the former being slightly more stable (**Table 4**). However, in the resulting *anti*-form it was found that when H_2O is added, analogous to spontaneous deamination of the neutral base,(Labet et al. 2008a) it forms a hydrogen-bond bridge between N_3 and N_4 (**RC**: **Figure 6**). Thus, only the *anti*- form is discussed herein. It is noted that the addition of H_2O has negligible effect on the Mulliken charges and spin densities of *anti*-C(N_4-H)$^\bullet$ and with no delocalization onto the water itself.

Deamination is then initiated by transfer of a H$^\bullet$ from the water onto the N_3 ring centre (**Figure 6**). This process proceeds via **TS1** with a barrier of 16.8 kcal mol^{-1} to give intermediate **I1**, lying 11.5 kcal mol^{-1} higher in free energy than **RC** and is thus endergonic. Intermediate **I1** resembles a complex between a cytosine tautomer and a hydroxyl radical. Interestingly, upon H$^\bullet$ transfer the partial charge on C_4 has increased by +0.29e to 0.38e close to that observed on C_4 (0.37e) in neutral cytosine. Thus, in **I1** C_4 has the same electrophilicity as in the neutral base. Indeed, the next step is nucleophilic attack of the $^\bullet$OH moiety at the C_4 centre. This occurs via **TS2** with a barrier of 8.6 kcal mol^{-1} relative to **I1**; 20.1 kcal mol^{-1} with respect to **RC**. It should be noted that for spontaneous deamination of cytosine in water the analogous hydroxylation also occurs via attack of water at the C_4 position with simultaneous transfer of a proton from the H_2O moiety onto the amino N_4 centre with concomitant cleavage of the C_4-N_4 bond. However, it proceeds with a barrier four to five times larger than that observed above for reaction via **TS2**.(Labet et al. 2008b) In the resulting intermediate **I2**, lying just 4.2 kcal mol^{-1} higher in energy than the initial complex **RC**, the C_4 centre is now tetrahedral with a C_4-OH bond length of 1.432 Å. There are then five possible pathways by which deamination of **I2** may occur, hereafter referred to as **Path A, B, C, D,** and **E**. The free energy changes associated with each are summarized in **Table 7**.

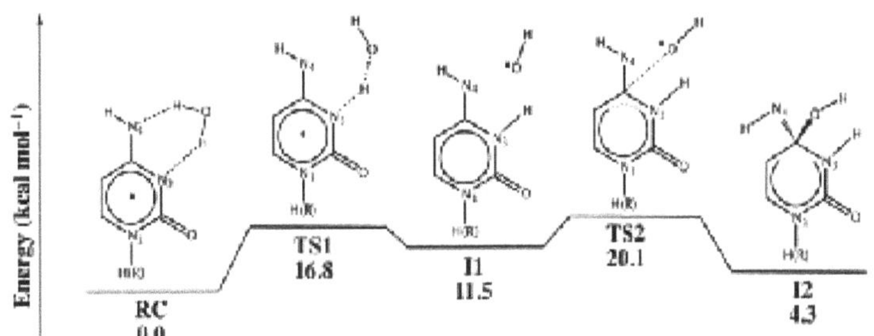

Fig. 6. Calculated (see text) relative free energies for initial abstraction of H$^\bullet$ from H_2O by *anti*-C(N_4-H)$^\bullet$ with subsequent attack of $^\bullet$OH at the C_4 centre.

Path A	ΔG	Path B	ΔG	Path C	ΔG	Path D	ΔG	Path E	ΔG
I2	4.3	**I2**	4.3	**I2**	4.3	**I2**	4.3	**I2**	4.3
^{A}**I3**	-9.0	^{B}**TS3**	38.3	^{A}**I3**	-9.0	^{D}**TS3**	31.1	^{A}**I3**	-9.0
^{A}**I4**	-0.2	^{B}**I3**	13.1	^{C}**TS3**	30.4	^{D}**I3**	6.5	^{E}**TS3**	24.9
^{A}**TS3**	7.1	^{B}**I4**	7.5	^{B}**I4**	7.5	^{D}**I4**	0.1	^{D}**I4**	0.1
^{A}**P**	-7.5	^{B}**TS4**	9.4	^{B}**TS4**	9.4	^{D}**TS4**	2.2	^{D}**TS4**	2.2
		^{B}**P**	11.4	^{B}**P**	11.4	^{D}**P**	-22.0	^{D}**P**	-22.0

Table 7. Calculated (see text) relative free energies for stationary points along **Path A, B, C, D** and **E** for deamination of **I2** in aqueous solution.

Path A begins with protonation of the N_4 centre in **I2** where the proton originates from the surrounding dilute aqueous solvent. The resulting intermediate ^{A}**I3** lies 13.3 kcal mol^{-1} lower in energy than **I2**. This is followed by a second protonation of N_4 with the proton again originating from the surrounding dilute aqueous solvent. In contrast to the first, this second protonation is endergonic by 8.8 kcal mol^{-1}. However, the resulting intermediate ^{A}**I4** still lies lower in energy than **I2** by 4.5 kcal mol^{-1}. In ^{A}**I4** the initial $-N_4H$ group in **I2** has now formally become an $-N_4H_3^+$ group. Consequently, the next step is the loss of NH_3 by simple cleavage of the C−N bond. This occurs with a barrier of 7.3 kcal mol^{-1} relative to ^{A}**I4** (**Table 7**). It should be noted that the resulting product complex of ^{A}**P** lies 11.8 kcal mol^{-1} lower in energy than **I2** and resembles a complex between $NH_3^{\bullet+}$ and protonated uracil.(Labet et al. 2008b)

In contrast, in **Path B** the initial 'protonation' of N_4 is achieved via an intramolecular rearrangement from the N_3-H group and does not originate from solution. This reaction proceeds via the four-membered ring TS ^{B}**TS3** at a significant cost of 34.0 kcal mol^{-1} to give intermediate ^{B}**I3**, lying 8.8 kcal mol^{-1} higher in energy than **I2** (**Table 7**). However, similar to **Path A** the second step is protonation of N_4 with the proton originating from solution. This process is exergonic with the resulting intermediate ^{B}**I4** lying 5.6 kcal mol^{-1} lower in free energy than ^{B}**I3**. The subsequent cleavage of the $C_4-N_4H_3^+$ bond occurs via ^{B}**TS4** to give the product complex ^{B}**P**. However, unlike for **Path A**, ^{B}**P** is higher in energy than **I2** by 7.1 kcal mol^{-1} and instead resembles a complex between NH_3 and the oxidized enol form of Uracil.

Like **Path A**, the alternate **Path C** begins with the exothermic protonation of N_4 by a proton originating from solution to give ^{A}**I3** (**Table 7**). Now, however, the second proton is obtained via the intramolecular proton transfer that initiated **Path B**, i.e., by transfer from the N_3-H group. This reaction proceeds via ^{C}**TS3** with a considerable barrier of 39.4 kcal mol^{-1}, even higher than that observed in **Path B**, to give intermediate ^{B}**I4**. The remaining step, cleavage of the C_4-N_4 bond, is then identical to that of **Path B** as is the product formed.

Path D, unlike the previous paths, involves an initial intramolecular proton transfer from the C_4-OH hydroxyl onto the N_4 centre (**Table 7**). This reaction proceeds via ^{D}**TS3** at a cost of 26.8 kcal mol^{-1}. While this barrier is still quite high, it is 7.2 and 12.6 kcal mol^{-1} lower than the analogous intramolecular rearrangements in **Paths B** and **C** and is thus kinetically favoured. The resulting intermediate formed ^{D}**I3** lies only 2.2 kcal mol^{-1} higher in energy than **I2**. This is then followed by protonation of the N_4 centre by a proton originating from solution, similar to **Paths A** and **B**. This step is exothermic with the intermediate formed, ^{D}**I4**, lying 6.4 kcal mol^{-1} lower in energy than ^{D}**I3**. The next and final step is the loss of NH_3 and occurs via ^{D}**TS4** with a quite small barrier of just 2.1 kcal mol^{-1}. The resulting product ^{D}**P**, resembling a complex between NH_3 and oxidized uracil, is markedly lower in energy than **I2** by 26.3 kcal mol^{-1}. Importantly, it is in fact the lowest energy product complex obtained of all those considered herein.

The final path considered, **Path E**, begins with the same exothermic intermolecular protonation of N_4 as in **Paths A** and **C** and again leads to formation of ^{A}**I3**. The next step, however, is intramolecular proton transfer from the C_4-OH group to N_4 as occurs in **Path D**. Importantly, it proceeds via ^{E}**TS3** with a higher barrier (33.9 kcal mol^{-1}) than observed in **Path D** (26.8 kcal mol^{-1}) to give ^{D}**I4**. The final step is then cleavage of the C_4-N_4 bond as in **Path D** to give ^{D}**P**.

Thus, while deamination via donation of both protons from the aqueous solution (**Path A**) may have the lowest associated barriers, the resulting product is not the most thermodynamically favoured. In contrast, in those cases in which only one proton originates from solution (**Paths B - E**), only those involving intramolecular rearrangement of a proton from C_4−OH (**Paths D** and **E**) are exothermic and lead to formation of the most thermodynamically preferred product (**^{D}P**). Furthermore, the barrier for this rearrangement is lowest when it occurs prior to proton donation from the solvent. Lastly in the case where both protonations occur via intermolecular processes, $NH_3^{\bullet+}$ is formed (**^{A}P**) while NH_3 is formed when only a single proton originates from exogenous sources (**^{B}P** and **^{D}P**).

5. Oxidation of serine phosphate: Implications for DNA

As mentioned in **section 2**, the exposure of DNA to high-energy radiation can also cause damage at its phosphate backbone. In particular, it can cause strand breaks via cleavage of the phosphoester bonds.(Lipfert et al. 2004) When the absorption of radiation causes the ionization of the phosphate it has been shown that it then abstracts a H• from the deoxyribose ring at either its $C_{4'}$ or $C_{5'}$ position. This is then followed by heterolytic cleavage of the phosphoester bond.(Lipfert et al. 2004; Steenken & Goldbergerova 1998) Alternatively, the strand break may be preceded by chemical modification of the nucleobase or deoxyribose ring or the phosphoester bond may simply undergo a direct cleavage.(Lipfert et al. 2004)

Experimentally it can be difficult to clearly observe and characterize damage within DNA due to its size. Thus, it is common to either use short fragments or model compounds that can reproduce or mimic the damage and associated processes that may occur. For example, serine phosphate contains a phosphate bond as well as a carboxylate that can act as an electron scavenger much like the bases within DNA itself. Thus, it is often used in experimental studies on the processes of DNA damage at its phosphate and subsequent bond cleavage reactions and in fact has led to a deeper understanding of those processes involved.

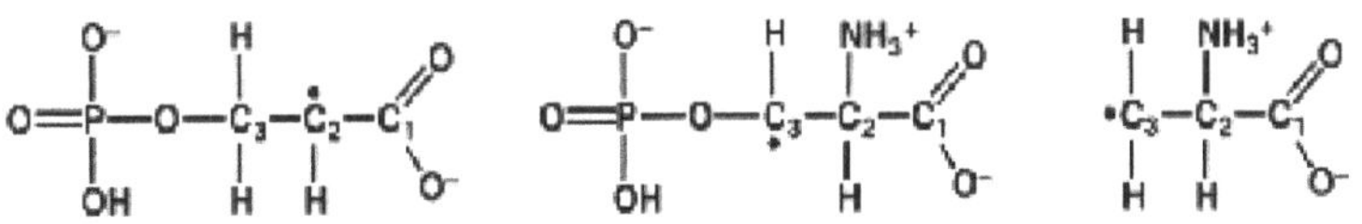

(I) (II) (III)

Fig. 7. The C_2-centered radical **I** and C_3-centered radicals **II** and **III** proposed to be formed upon the irradiation of non- and partially-deuterated single crystals of L-*O*-serine phosphate. (Sanderud & Sagstuen 1996)

In particular, evidence has been obtained suggesting the formation of several different radical species. Specifically, the irradiation of non- and partially-deuterated single crystals of L-*O*-serine phosphate has been suggested to produce the three radicals **I, II** and **III** shown in **Figure 7**.(Sanderud & Sagstuen 1996) In particular, it is thought that upon irradiation serine phosphate can take up a now free electron to form a C_1-centered radical anion. This may then undergo deamination to form the C_2-centered radical anion **I**. Alternatively, a serine phosphate may lose an electron to form a neutral C_1-centered radical which then undergoes decarboxylation to give a C_2-centered radical. This latter radical may then abstract a H• from the C_3 position of another serine phosphate to generate the C_3-centered radical anion **II**. In contrast, the neutral C_3-centered radical **III** is proposed to be formed via the uptake of a free electron by serine phosphate to give a P-centered radical anion which then simply undergoes loss of the phosphate group.

We investigated the nature of radicals **I**, **II** and **III** by obtaining optimized structures at the B3LYP/6-31G(d) level of theory. Hyperfine coupling constants (HFCCs) were then calculated via single point calculations at the B3LYP/6-311+G(2df,p) level of theory on the above structures and are listed for all three radicals in **Table 8**.(Lipfert et al. 2004)

In the optimized structure of radical **I** the largest spin density is located on C_2 (0.71) while the carbonylic oxygen of the carboxylate group also has significant spin density (0.18). This delocalization of spin density is due to conjugation between the singly occupied molecular orbital (SOMO) on C_2 and the C_1=O π-bond. In addition, it is noted that near planarity was observed for C_1 and C_2 and their substituents, in agreement with experiment.(Sanderud & Sagstuen 1996) With respect to its calculated HFCCs, as can be seen in **Table 8** the values calculated for the α-hydrogen are in good agreement with experiment. The slight deviation in A_{iso} from experiment is possibly due to the fact that the calculations are performed in the gas-phase on an isolated molecule and hence effects due to crystal packing are ignored. The calculated HFCCs for the two β-hydrogens are also in good agreement with the experiment. However, a rotational scan was performed in order to obtain the dihedral angle between the β-hydrogens and SOMO that gave HFCCs in best agreement between theory and experiment. It was found that this occurred for dihedral angles of -1.7° and 117.2°.

Radical	Atom	A_{iso}	T_{xx}	T_{yy}	T_{zz}
I	α-$H_{(calcd)}$	-43.1	28.2	-1.2	-29.5
	α-$H_{(exp)}$	-54.2	32.3	3.3	-29.0
	β-$H_{1(calcd)}$	105.6	8.7	-2.4	-6.3
	β-$H_{1(exp)}$	104.3	7.2	-2.0	-5.3
	β-$H_{2(calcd)}$	57.8	8.3	-3.6	-4.7
	β-$H_{2(exp)}$	57.4	8.1	-3.9	-4.2
II	α-$H_{(calcd)}$	-53.3	-36.1	-1.4	37.5
	α-$H_{(exp)}$	-51.0	-34.5	3.8	30.7
	β-$H_{(calcd)}$	15.4	10.8	-4.0	-6.8
	β-$H_{(exp)}$	25.0	14.0	-7.0	-8.0
	β-$N_{(calcd)}$	12.7	2.1	-0.9	-1.2
	β-$N_{(exp)}$	15.9	2.1	-0.3	-1.8
	γ-$H_{(calcd)}$	1.9	4.3	-1.5	-2.8
	γ-$H_{(exp)}$	5.9	10.1	-4.1	-5.8
III	α-$H_{1(calcd)}$	-48.8	-37.3	-1.7	39.0
	α-$H_{1(exp)}$	-47.1	-22.0	-1.5	23.6
	α-$H_{2(calcd)}$	-59.3	-37.4	-1.5	38.8
	α-$H_{2(exp)}$	-50.8	-24.6	0.5	24.2
	β-$H_{(calcd)}$	73.0	8.9	-2.2	-6.7
	β-$H_{(exp)}$	73.0	(13.3)	(-6.6)	(-6.6)

Table 8. Comparison of calculated (see text) and experimental (Sanderud & Sagstuen 1996) isotropic and anisotropic components (MHz) of the hyperfine coupling tensor of radicals **I**, **II**, and **III**.

In contrast to radical **I**, the best agreement between computational and experimental HFCCs for radicals **II** and **III** was not obtained for their proposed structures shown in **Figure 7**. Rather, the structures that gave best agreement were found to be the radical-cationic forms of **II** and **III**; that is, structures in which their phosphate and carboxylic acid groups are neutral while the amino group is protonated. Hence, these latter structures were used in all HFCC studies on radicals **II** and **III**.

For radical-cationic **II** the calculated HFCCs for the α-hydrogen are generally in good agreement with the experimental values with A_{iso} differing by just 2.3 MHz (**Table 8**). However, for both β-hydrogens, less satisfactory agreement between theory and experiment is observed. Specifically, the calculated A_{iso} values of 15.4 and 12.7 MHz differ from their corresponding experimental values by 9.6 and 3.2 MHz, respectively. As noted for the α-hydrogen in **I**, these differences are likely due to bulk crystal effects not being modeled in the calculations. Similarly, for the γ-hydrogens on the amino group, a difference of 4.0 MHz is seen between the calculated and experimental values. However, it has been stated that the given experimental value is associated with a degree of uncertainty.(Sanderud & Sagstuen 1996) In the optimized structure of **II** the C_3 centre is not completely planar where an angle between the hydrogen on C_3 and the plane defined by C_3-C_2-O was found to be 22.0°.(Lipfert et al. 2004) This is in good agreement with the corresponding experimentally determined value of 19.5°.(Sanderud & Sagstuen 1996) It is noted that the C_3 centre and adjacent oxygen have spin densities of 0.84 and 0.11 respectively, suggesting slight delocalization of the SOMO. Dobbs et al.(Dobbs et al. 1971; Dobbs et al. 1972) have suggested that this is due to incomplete rehybridization of the carbon-centered radical and is common when the carbon is bonded to an oxygen.

Indeed, in radical-cationic **III** in which the phosphate group on C_3 has been lost, i.e., there is no C_3—O bond, the radical is now fully localized on C_3. Furthermore, from **Table 8** it can be seen that quite good agreement is obtained for α-H_1 and the β-hydrogen with differences of 1.7 and 0.0 MHz respectively, while α-H_2 differs slightly more by 8.5 MHz. It should be noted that in order to obtain the best agreement for the HFCCs of the α-hydrogens they had to be tilted out of the plane by 5°. That is, the planarity of the C_3 centre had to be reduced. This is similar to that observed need in related studies on the methyl radical ($^{\bullet}CH_3$) to slightly pyramidalize the carbon centre in order to obtain best agreement between the calculated and experimentally measured HFCCs.(Eriksson et al. 1994)

6. Oxidative repair of alkylated nucleobases: the catalytic mechanism of AlkB

A common type of DNA damage is the alkylation of nucleobases at one or more of their oxygen and nitrogen centres.(Liu et al. 2009) This can be caused by endo- or exogenous agents such as S-adenosylmethionine or tobacco smoke, respectively.(Hecht 1999; Rydberg & Lindahl 1982) Consequently, cells have developed several methods by which to mediate or repair such damage. One approach is to use enzymes known as DNA glycolsylases to simply excise the damaged nucleobase via an acid-base cleavage of its N-glycosidic bond.(Mishina et al. 2006; Sedgwick et al. 2007) Alternatively, repair enzymes may use a non-redox mechanism to remove only the alkyl group. For example, O^6-methylguanine-DNA methyltransferase transfers the methyl of O^6-methylguanine onto an active site cysteinyl residue.(Lindahl et al. 1988) However, a third approach is alkyl group removal using a redox mechanism catalysed by the AlkB family of enzymes.

Although included in the α-ketoglutarate-Fe(II)-dependant dioxygenase superfamily, the AlkB family is the only one known to oxidatively dealkylate nucleobases.(Falnes et al. 2002; Trewick et al. 2002) Specifically, under physiological conditions they oxidatively repair the methylated nucleobases 1-meA, 1-meG, 3-meC and 3-meT (**Figure 8**).(Yang et al. 2008) It is noted, however, that they have been demonstrated to also be able to remove longer alkyl chains.(Delaney et al. 2005; Duncan et al. 2002; Koivisto et al. 2003; Mishina et al. 2005)

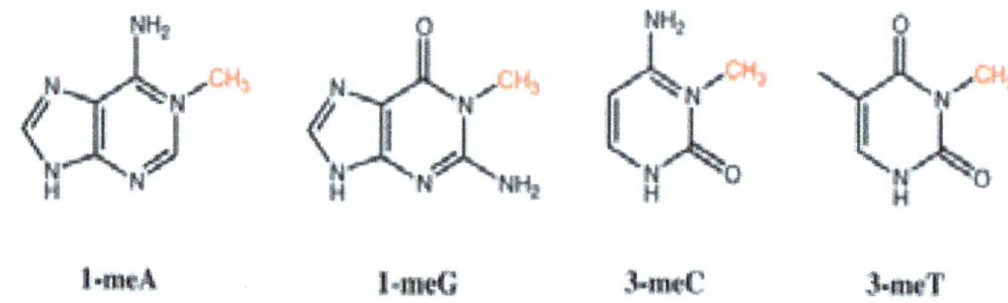

Fig. 8. Examples of methylated substrates that are dealkylated by the AlkB family of enzymes. The methyl groups to be removed have been colored in red.

Several X-ray crystal structures have been obtained of AlkB complexed with, for instance, cosubstrate or coproducts.(Yang et al. 2008; Yu et al. 2006) From these structures it was concluded that the active site of AlkB contains an Fe(II) ion ligated via two histidyl (His_{131}, His_{187}) and an aspartyl (Asp_{133}) residue. Furthermore, the α-ketoglutarate (α–KG) co-substrate bidentately ligates to the Fe(II) centre via carboxyl and ketone oxygens,(Falnes et al. 2002; Mishina et al. 2005; Trewick et al. 2002) while the methylated nucleobase sits adjacent to the Fe(II) centre. Based on these structures it was proposed that the mechanism of AlkB begins with activation of O_2: on binding to the Fe(II) centre the O_2 moiety is reduced to $O_2^{\bullet -}$ while the Fe centre is oxidized to Fe(III).(Berglund et al. 2002; Nakajima & Yamazaki 1987) The $O_2^{\bullet -}$ moiety formed then attacks the α–KG cosubstrate converting it to succinate with concomitant formation of an oxo-ferryl Fe(IV)=O species, a strong oxidizing agent.(Clifton et al. 2006; Kovaleva & Lipscomb 2008; Liu et al. 2009) However, the =O group of the oxo-ferryl sits in the apical position and thus is not ideally situated to react with the methylated nucleobase. Hence, it reorients to an equatorial position.(Yu et al. 2006)
An X-ray crystal structure (PDB: 2FD8) has been obtained under anaerobic conditions of AlkB with the single-strand trinucleotide dT-(1-me-dA)-dT bound within its active site.(Yu et al. 2006) Based on this experimental structure we obtained an appropriate chemical model for our computational studies. In particular, key active site residues, the Fe(II) centre, and α–KG modeled by pyruvate were included. A crystal structure water observed to be ligated to the Fe(II) centre in the apical position was replaced by O_2 while the substrate 1-methyladenine was modeled as 3-methyl-4-amino pyrimidinyl cation (3me4amPym$^+$). Calculations were then performed at the IEF-PCM(ε=4.0)-B3LYP/LACV3P+(d,p)//B3LYP/LACVP(d) level of theory. For complete details on the model and methods used please refer to Liu et al. 2009.(Liu et al. 2009)
In this chapter we focus on key findings of the oxidative demethylation stage of the mechanism, shown schematically in **Figure 9**. However, it should be noted that the initial O_2 activation process preferentially occurs in the quintet spin state with a rate-limiting barrier of just 9.1 kcal mol^{-1}. The lowest energy pathway for the subsequent reorientation of the Fe(IV)=O species was also found to occur for the quintet spin state. Furthermore, it was found to proceed via a concerted mechanism with a barrier of 11.3 kcal mol^{-1}. For the oxidative demethylation itself, the lowest energy pathway also occurred on the quintet

surface; the next lowest spin state, the triplet, at all times being higher in energy. Thus, herein, only the results for the quintet spin state are discussed. However, the energies for the triplet surface have been included in **Figure 9** for purposes of comparison.

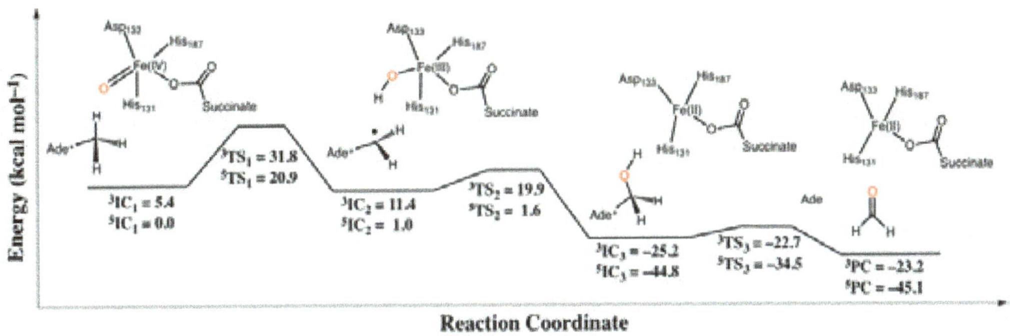

Fig. 9. Potential energy surface for the dealkylation of the methylated adenine nucleobase model 3me4amPym+ in the triplet and quintet spin states.

In the apical position, the Fe(IV)=O oxygen is approximately 4.12 Å from the nearest target methyl hydrogen of the 3me4amPym+ substrate. However, in **^{5}IC$_1$**, where it now lies in the equatorial position trans to His$_{187}$, this distance has been reduced dramatically to 2.68 Å. Demethylation is initiated by abstraction of a hydrogen (H•) from the target methyl group of the substrate by the Fe(IV)=O oxygen. This step proceeds via the transition structure **^{5}TS$_1$** at a cost of 20.9 kcal mol^{-1} to give intermediate **^{5}IC$_2$** lying just 1.0 kcal mol^{-1} higher in energy than **^{5}IC$_1$**. In **^{5}TS$_1$** the cleaving -CH$_2$—H bond has lengthened to 1.30 Å while the corresponding FeO···H• distance is quite short at 1.22 Å.(Liu et al. 2009)
This step is not only the rate limiting step in the actual demethylation of 3me4amPym+, but is also the highest reaction barrier obtained in the overall mechanism of AlkB.(Liu et al. 2009) In the related α-KG-Fe(II) non-heme enzyme TauD, which catalyses hydroxylation of propene, abstraction of a methyl hydrogen by the Fe(IV)=O species was also calculated to be the rate limiting step.(de Visser 2006) The barrier in AlkB, however, is significantly higher. It has been observed that in C—H activating heme enzymes the barrier for such an abstraction is linearly related to the BDE of the substrates C—H bond being cleaved.(de Visser et al. 2004; Kaizer et al. 2004) Thus, the significantly higher barrier observed in AlkB compared to TauD is likely due to the 14.3 kcal mol^{-1} greater -CH$_2$—H bond energy in its substrate, 3me4amPym+. It should be noted that experimentally k_{cat} for AlkB has been measured to be 4.5 min^{-1},(Koivisto et al. 2003; Yu et al. 2006) corresponding to a rate-limiting barrier of 19.8 kcal mol^{-1}; in good agreement with the present calculated barrier height for **^{5}TS$_1$**.
In **^{5}IC$_2$** the Fe(IV)=O has been reduced to Fe(III)—OH while the substrate now contains a methylene-carbon centered radical (see **Figure 9**). The next step is a 'rebound', transfer, of the hydroxyl group from the Fe-OH moiety to the substrate's radical centre. This reaction is almost barrierless proceeding via **^{5}TS$_2$** with a cost of only 0.6 kcal mol^{-1}. Significantly, the resulting intermediate **^{5}IC$_3$** lies markedly lower in energy than **^{5}IC$_1$** by -44.8 kcal mol^{-1}. Thus, effectively, the result of the first two steps in demethylation are exothermic insertion of an oxygen into a C—H bond of the substrates methyl group with reduction of the Fe(IV) centre to Fe(II). The much lower relative energy of **^{5}IC$_3$** may also reflect the structural rearrangement that occurs at the Fe centre which has gone from penta- to tetra-coordinate.

The final step in the demethylation of 3me4amPym$^+$ is decomposition of the hydroxylated intermediate to give 4-amino pyrimidine, the model for the demethylated nucleobase, and formaldehyde (**Figure 9**). In this step an active site Glu_{136} residue acts as a general base and deprotonates the Ade-CH_2OH hydroxyl with concomitant cleavage of the $_{Ade}N-CH_2OH$ bond.(Liu et al. 2009) This reaction proceeds via ^{5}**TS$_3$** at the modest cost of 10.3 kcal mol^{-1}. It is noted that in ^{5}**TS$_3$** the $_{Ade}N\cdots CH_2OH$ and Ade-CH_2O-H bonds have lengthened to 1.58 and 1.22 Å, respectively, highlighting their concomitant cleavage. The product-bound complex ^{5}**PC** lies 45.1 kcal mol^{-1} lower in relative energy than the initial reactant complex ^{5}**IC$_1$**. Thus, demethylation of 1-methyladenine is calculated to be a quite exothermic process.

7. Conclusion

In this chapter the application of density functional theory (DFT)-based methods to the study of DNA damage and repair mechanisms has been illustrated.

In particular, it was shown how they may be used to provide accurate detailed insights into the thermochemistry of fundamental chemical processes such as electron and proton transfers and thus, help to explain a number of experimental observations. Furthermore, through such studies they were able to show differences in the preferred oxidation pathways for the various DNA nucleobases. Similarly, by the careful examination of calculated hyperfine coupling constants, the nature *and* structure of radicals that may be formed upon exposure of DNA to radiation were deduced. Such an understanding also aids in determining the mechanism by which they may be formed. Finally, their versatility for the investigation of damage and repair mechanisms was highlighted. Indeed, by examining several pathways using seemingly quite simple chemical models, we have been able to deduce the preferred mechanism by which the deamination of cytosine radical may occur including (i) the preferred proton source(s), (ii) the order in which they are added to the leaving nitrogen centre, and (iii) the thermodynamically preferred products. Finally, similar methods in combination with much larger chemical models were used to also elucidate the oxidative dealkylation repair mechanism of AlkB. Together, these studies highlight the versatility and accuracy of DFT methods when used in combination with well-chosen chemical models for the study of DNA damage and repair.

8. Acknowledgements

JWG, JL and EACB acknowledge the Natural Sciences and Engineering Research Council (NSERC, Canada) for funding and CGS & PGSD scholarships (EACB) and JL and LAE thank the Swedish Science Research Council (VR) for funding. LAE also acknowledges the National University of Ireland (Galway) for financial support. SHARCNET (Canada) and the National Supercomputing Centre (Linköping, Sweden) are acknowledged for additional computational resources.

9. References

Almatarneh, M. H., Flinn, C. G., Poirier, R. A., & Sokalski, W. A. (2006). "Computational study of the deamination reaction of cytosine with H_2O and OH." *J. Phys. Chem. A*, 110(26), 8227-8234.

Becke, A. D. (1993a). "A Mixing of Hartree-Fock and Local Density-Functional Theories." *J. Chem. Phys.*, 98, 1372.

Becke, A. D. (1993b). "Density-Functional Thermochemistry .3. The Role of Exact Exchange." *J. Chem. Phys.*, 98(7), 5648-5652.

Berglund, G. I., Carlsson, G. H., Smith, A. T., Szoke, H., Henriksen, A., & Hajdu, J. (2002). "The catalytic pathway of horseradish peroxidase at high resolution." *Nature*, 417(6887), 463-468.

Burrows, C. J., & Muller, J. G. (1998). "Oxidative nucleobase modifications leading to strand scission." *Chem. Rev.*, 98(3), 1109-1151.

Cadet, J., Douki, T., & Ravanat, J. L. (2006). "One-electron oxidation of DNA and inflammation processes." *Nat. Chem. Biol.*, 2(7), 348-349.

Cadet, J., Douki, T., & Ravanat, J. L. (2008). "Oxidatively generated damage to the guanine moiety of DNA: Mechanistic aspects and formation in cells." *Accounts Chem. Res.*, 41(8), 1075-1083.

Cadet, J., & Vigny, P. (1990). Bioorganic Photochemistry. Photochemistry and the Nucleic Acids, H. Morrison, ed., Wiley, New York, 1-272.

Cammi, R., & Tomasi, J. (1995). "Remarks on the use of the apparent surface-charges (ASC) methods in solvation problems - Iterative versus matrix-inversion procedures and the renormalization of the apparent charges." *J. Comput. Chem.*, 16(12), 1449-1458.

Cances, E., & Mennucci, B. (1998). "New applications of integral equations methods for solvation continuum models: ionic solutions and liquid crystals." *J. Math. Chem.*, 23(3-4), 309-326.

Cances, E., Mennucci, B., & Tomasi, J. (1997). "A new integral equation formalism for the polarizable continuum model: Theoretical background and applications to isotropic and anisotropic dielectrics." *J. Chem. Phys.*, 107(8), 3032-3041.

Candeias, L. P., & Steenken, S. (2000). "Reaction of HO center dot with guanine derivatives in aqueous solution: Formation of two different redox-active OH-Adduct radicals and their unimolecular transformation reactions. Properties of G(-H)(center dot)." *Chem.-Eur. J.*, 6(3), 475-484.

Cauet, E., Dehareng, D., & Lievin, J. (2006). "Ab initio study of the ionization of the DNA bases: Ionization potentials and excited states of the cations." *J. Phys. Chem. A*, 110(29), 9200-9211.

Chatgilialoglu, C., Ferreri, C., Bazzanini, R., Guerra, M., Choi, S. Y., Emanuel, C. J., Horner, J. H., & Newcomb, M. (2000). "Models of DNA C1 ' radicals. Structural, spectral, and chemical properties of the thyminylmethyl radical and the 2 '-deoxyuridin-1 '-yl radical." *J. Am. Chem. Soc.*, 122(39), 9525-9533.

Cheng, K. C., Cahill, D. S., Kasai, H., Nishimura, S., & Loeb, L. A. (1992). "8-hydroxyguanine, an abundant form of oxidative dna damage, causes g -> t and a -> c substitutions." *J. Biol. Chem.*, 267(1), 166-172.

Clifton, I. J., McDonough, M. A., Ehrismann, D., Kershaw, N. J., Granatino, N., & Schofield, C. J. (2006). "Structural studies on 2-oxoglutarate oxygenases and related double-stranded beta-helix fold proteins." *J. Inorg. Biochem.*, 100(4), 644-669.

Cullis, P. M., Malone, M. E., & MersonDavies, L. A. (1996). "Guanine radical cations are precursors of 7,8-dihydro-8-oxo-2'-deoxyguanosine but are not precursors of immediate strand breaks in DNA." *J. Am. Chem. Soc.*, 118(12), 2775-2781.

De Bont, R., & van Larebeke, N. (2004). "Endogenous DNA damage in humans: a review of quantitative data." *Mutagenesis*, 19(3), 169-185.

de Visser, S. P. (2006). "Propene activation by the oxo-iron active species of taurine/alpha-ketoglutarate dioxygenase (TauD) enzyme. How does the catalysis compare to heme-enzymes?" *J. Am. Chem. Soc.*, 128(30), 9813-9824.

de Visser, S. P., Kumar, D., Cohen, S., Shacham, R., & Shaik, S. (2004). "A predictive pattern of computed barriers for C-H hydroxylation by compound I of cytochrome P450." *J. Am. Chem. Soc.*, 126(27), 8362-8363.

Decarroz, C., Wagner, J. R., & Cadet, J. (1987). *Free Radical Res. Commun.*(2), 295-301.

Decarroz, C., Wagner, J. R., Vanlier, J. E., Krishna, C. M., Riesz, P., & Cadet, J. (1986). "Sensitized photooxidation of thymidine by 2-methyl-1-1,4-naphthoquinone - characterization of the stable photoproducts." *Int. J. Radiat. Biol.*, 50(3), 491-505.

Delaney, J. C., Smeester, L., Wong, C. Y., Frick, L. E., Taghizadeh, K., Wishnok, J. S., Drennan, C. L., Samson, L. D., & Essigmann, J. M. (2005). "AlkB reverses etheno DNA lesions caused by lipid oxidation in vitro and in vivo." *Nat. Struct. Mol. Biol.*, 12(10), 855-860.

Dobbs, A. J., Gilbert, B. C., & Norman, R. O. C. (1971). "Electron spin resonance studies .27. geometry of oxygen-substituted alkyl radicals." *J. Chem. Soc. A*(1), 124-&.

Dobbs, A. J., Gilbert, B. C., & Norman, R. O. C. (1972). "Electron-spin resonance studies .32. information from hyperfine splittings for aliphatic radicals about shape and conformation." *J. Chem. Soc.-Perkin Trans. 2*(6), 786-&.

Douki, T., & Cadet, J. (1999). "Modification of DNA bases by photosensitized one-electron oxidation." *Int. J. Radiat. Biol.*, 75(5), 571-581.

Duncan, T., Trewick, S. C., Koivisto, P., Bates, P. A., Lindahl, T., & Sedgwick, B. (2002). "Reversal of DNA alkylation damage by two human dioxygenases." *Proc. Natl. Acad. Sci. U. S. A.*, 99(26), 16660-16665.

Eley, D. D., & Spivey, D. I. (1962). "Semiconductivity of organic substances .9. Nucleic acid in dry state." *Trans. Faraday Soc.*, 58, 411.

Eriksson, L. A., Malkin, V. G., Malkina, O. L., & Salahub, D. R. (1994). "The effects of nonlocal gradient corrections in density-functional calculations of hydrocarbon radical hyperfine structures." *Int. J. Quantum Chem.*, 52(4), 879-901.

Falnes, P. O., Johansen, R. F., & Seeberg, E. (2002). "AlkB-mediated oxidative demethylation reverses DNA damage in Escherichia coli." *Nature*, 419(6903), 178-182.

Friedberg, E. C., McDaniel, L. D., & Schultz, R. A. (2004). "The role of endogenous and exogenous DNA damage and mutagenesis." *Curr. Opin. Genet. Dev.*, 14(1), 5-10.

Hagen, U. (1986). "Current aspects on the radiation-induced base damage in dna." *Radiat. Environ. Biophys.*, 25(4), 261-271.

Hatahet, A., & Wallace, Z.Z. (1998). DNA Damage and Repair, DNA Repair in Prokaryotes and Lower Eukaryotes, J. A. Nickoloff, Hoekstra, M.F., ed., Humana Press, New Jersey.

Hecht, S. S. (1999). "DNA adduct formation from tobacco-specific N-nitrosamines." *Mutat. Res.-Fundam. Mol. Mech. Mutagen.*, 424(1-2), 127-142.

Hush, N. S., & Cheung, A. S. (1975). "Ionization-potentials and donor properties of nucleic-acid bases and related compounds." *Chem. Phys. Lett.*, 34(1), 11-13.

Kaizer, J., Klinker, E. J., Oh, N. Y., Rohde, J. U., Song, W. J., Stubna, A., Kim, J., Munck, E., Nam, W., & Que, L. (2004). "Nonheme (FeO)-O-IV complexes that can oxidize the C-H bonds of cyclohexane at room temperature." *J. Am. Chem. Soc.*, 126(2), 472-473.

Kamiya, H., Iwai, S., & Kasai, H. (1998). "The (6-4) photoproduct of thymine-thymine induces targeted substitution mutations in mammalian cells." *Nucleic Acids Res.*, 26(11), 2611-2617.

Kasai, H., Crain, P. F., Kuchino, Y., Nishimura, S., Ootsuyama, A., & Tanooka, H. (1986). "Formation of 8-hydroxyguanine moiety in cellular dna by agents producing oxygen radicals and evidence for its repair." *Carcinogenesis*, 7(11), 1849-1851.

Koivisto, P., Duncan, T., Lindahl, T., & Sedgwick, B. (2003). "Minimal methylated substrate and extended substrate range of Escherichia coli AlkB protein, a 1-methyladenine-DNA dioxygenase." *J. Biol. Chem.*, 278(45), 44348-44354.

Kovaleva, E. G., & Lipscomb, J. D. (2008). "Versatility of biological non-heme Fe(II) centers in oxygen activation reactions." *Nat. Chem. Biol.*, 4(3), 186-193.

Kumar, A., & Sevilla, M. D. (2010). "Proton-Coupled Electron Transfer in DNA on Formation of Radiation-Produced Ion Radicals." *Chem. Rev.*, 110(12), 7002-7023.

Labet, V., Grand, A., Cadet, J., & Eriksson, L. A. (2008a). "Deamination of the radical cation of the base moiety of 2 '-deoxycytidine: A theoretical study." *ChemPhysChem*, 9(8), 1195-1203.

Labet, V., Grand, A., Morell, C., Cadet, J., & Eriksson, L. A. (2008b). "Proton catalyzed hydrolytic deamination of cytosine: a computational study." *Theor. Chem. Acc.*, 120(4-6), 429-435.

Labet, V., Grand, A., Morell, C., Cadet, J., & Eriksson, L. A. (2009). "Mechanism of nitric oxide induced deamination of cytosine." *Phys. Chem. Chem. Phys.*, 11, 2379-2386.

Lee, C. T., Yang, W. T., & Parr, R. G. (1988). "Development of the colle-salvetti correlation-energy formula into a functional of the electron-density." *Phys. Rev. B*, 37(2), 785-789.

Lee, Y. A., Yun, B. H., Kim, S. K., Margolin, Y., Dedon, P. C., Geacintov, N. E., & Shafirovich, V. (2007). "Mechanisms of oxidation of guanine in DNA by carbonate radical anion, a decomposition product of nitrosoperoxycarbonate." *Chem.-Eur. J.*, 13(16), 4571-4581.

Lindahl, T. (1993). "Instability and decay of the primary structure of dna." *Nature*, 362(6422), 709-715.

Lindahl, T., Sedgwick, B., Sekiguchi, M., & Nakabeppu, Y. (1988). "Regulation and expression of the adaptive response to alkylating-agents." *Annu. Rev. Biochem.*, 57, 133-157.

Lipfert, J., Llano, J., & Eriksson, L. A. (2004). "Radiation-induced damage in serine phosphate-insights into a mechanism for direct DNA strand breakage." *J. Phys. Chem. B*, 108(23), 8036-8042.

Liu, H. N., Llano, J., & Gauld, J. W. (2009). "A DFT Study of Nucleobase Dealkylation by the DNA Repair Enzyme AlkB." *J. Phys. Chem. B*, 113(14), 4887-4898.

Llano, J., & Eriksson, L. A. (2002). "First principles electrochemistry: Electrons and protons reacting as independent ions." *J. Chem. Phys.*, 117(22), 10193-10206.

Llano, J., & Eriksson, L. A. (2004a). "First principles electrochemical study of redox events in DNA bases and chemical repair in aqueous solution." *Phys. Chem. Chem. Phys.*, 6(9), 2426-2433.

Llano, J., & Eriksson, L. A. (2004b). "Oxidation pathways of adenine and guanine in aqueous solution from first principles electrochemistry." *Phys. Chem. Chem. Phys.*, 6(19), 4707-4713.

Llano, J., & Gauld, J.W. (2010). Mechanistics of Enzyme Catalysis: From Small to Large Active-Site Models, In: *Quantum Biochemistry: Electronic Structure and Biological Activity*, Matta, C. F., 643-666, Wiley-VCH, Weinheim.

Lysetska, M., Knoll, A., Boehringer, D., Hey, T., Krauss, G., & Krausch, G. (2002). "UV light-damaged DNA and its interaction with human replication protein A: an atomic force microscopy study." *Nucleic Acids Res.*, 30(12), 2686-2691.

Mennucci, B., Cances, E., & Tomasi, J. (1997). "Evaluation of solvent effects in isotropic and anisotropic dielectrics and in ionic solutions with a unified integral equation method: Theoretical bases, computational implementation, and numerical applications." *J. Phys. Chem. B*, 101(49), 10506-10517.

Miertus, S., Scrocco, E., & Tomasi, J. (1981). "Electrostatic interaction of a solute with a continuum - a direct utilization of abinitio molecular potentials for the prevision of solvent effects." *Chem. Phys.*, 55(1), 117-129.

Mishina, Y., Duguid, E. M., & He, C. (2006). "Direct reversal of DNA alkylation damage." *Chem. Rev.*, 106(2), 215-232.

Mishina, Y., Yang, C. G., & He, C. (2005). "Direct repair of the exocyclic DNA adduct 1,N-6-ethenoadenine by the DNA repair AlkB proteins." *J. Am. Chem. Soc.*, 127(42), 14594-14595.

Munk, B. H., Burrows, C. J., Schlegel, H. B. (2008). "An Exploration of Mechanisms for the Transformation of 8-Oxoguanine to Guanidinohydantoin and Spiroiminodihydantoin by Density Functional Theory." *J. Am. Chem. Soc.*, 130, 5245-5256

Nakajima, R., & Yamazaki, I. (1987). "The mechanism of oxyperoxidase formation from ferryl peroxidase and hydrogen-peroxide." *J. Biol. Chem.*, 262(6), 2576-2581.

Neeley, W. L., & Essigmann, J. M. (2006). "Mechanisms of formation, genotoxicity, and mutation of guanine oxidation products." *Chem. Res. Toxicol.*, 19(4), 491-505.

Newcomb, T. G., & Loeb, L.A. (1998). DNA Damage and Repair, DNA Repair in Prokaryotes and Lower Eukaryotes, J. A. Nickoloff, Hoekstra, M.F., ed., Humana Press, New Jersey.

Pages, V., & Fuchs, R. P. P. (2002). "How DNA lesions are turned into mutations within cells?" *Oncogene*, 21(58), 8957-8966.

Pavlov, Y. I., Minnick, D. T., Izuta, S., & Kunkel, T. A. (1994). "DNA-replication fidelity with 8-oxodeoxyguanosine triphosphate." *Biochemistry*, 33(15), 4695-4701.

Rydberg, B., & Lindahl, T. (1982). "Non-enzymatic methylation of DNA by the intracellular methyl-group donor s-adenosyl-l-methionine is a potentially mutagenic reaction." *Embo J.*, 1(2), 211-216.

Sanderud, A., & Sagstuen, E. (1996). "EPR and ENDOR studies of H-1 and N-14 hyperfine and quadrupolar couplings in crystals of L-O-serine phosphate after X-irradiation at 295 K." *J. Phys. Chem.*, 100(22), 9545-9555.

Sedgwick, B., Bates, P. A., Paik, J., Jacobs, S. C., & Lindahl, T. (2007). "Repair of alkylated DNA: Recent advances." *DNA Repair*, 6(4), 429-442.

Seidel, C. A. M., Schulz, A., & Sauer, M. H. M. (1996). "Nucleobase-specific quenching of fluorescent dyes .1. Nucleobase one-electron redox potentials and their correlation with static and dynamic quenching efficiencies." *J. Phys. Chem.*, 100(13), 5541-5553.

Sponer, J. E., Miguel, P. J. S., Rodriguez-Santiago, L., Erxleben, A., Krumm, M., Sodupe, M., Sponer, J., & Lippert, B. (2004). "Metal-mediated deamination of cytosine: Experiment and DFT calculations." *Angew. Chem.-Int. Edit.*, 43(40), 5396-5399.

Steenken, S. (1989). "Purine-bases, nucleosides, and nucleotides - aqueous-solution redox chemistry and transformation reactions of their radical cations and e- and OH adducts." *Chem. Rev.*, 89(3), 503-520.

Steenken, S. (1992). "Electron-transfer-induced acidity basicity and reactivity changes of purine and pyrimidine-bases - consequences of redox processes for DNA-base pairs." *Free Radic. Res. Commun.*, 16(6), 349-379.

Steenken, S., & Goldbergerova, L. (1998). "Photoionization of organic phosphates by 193 nm laser light in aqueous solution: Rapid intramolecular H-transfer to the primarily formed phosphate radical. A model for ionization-induced chain-breakage in DNA?" *J. Am. Chem. Soc.*, 120(16), 3928-3934.

Steenken, S., & Jovanovic, S. V. (1997). "How easily oxidizable is DNA? One-electron reduction potentials of adenosine and guanosine radicals in aqueous solution." *J. Am. Chem. Soc.*, 119(3), 617-618.

Steenken, S., Telo, J. P., Novais, H. M., & Candeias, L. P. (1992). "One-electron-reduction potentials of pyrimidine-bases, nucleosides, and nucleotides in aqueous-solution - consequences for DNA redox chemistry." *J. Am. Chem. Soc.*, 114(12), 4701-4709.

Taylor, J. S. (1994). "Unraveling the molecular pathway from sunlight to skin-cancer." *Accounts Chem. Res.*, 27(3), 76-82.

Teoule, R. (1987). "Radiation-induced DNA damage and its repair." *Int. J. Radiat. Biol.*, 51(4), 573-589.

Trewick, S. C., Henshaw, T. F., Hausinger, R. P., Lindahl, T., & Sedgwick, B. (2002). "Oxidative demethylation by Escherichia coli AlkB directly reverts DNA base damage." *Nature*, 419(6903), 174-178.

von Sonntag, C. (1987). *The Chemical Basis of Radiation Biology*, Taylor & Francis, London.

von Sonntag, C., Schuchmann, H.P. (1996). Encyclopedia of Molecular Biology and Molecular Medicine, R. A. Meyers, ed., VCH, Weinheim.

Wagner, J. R., Vanlier, J. E., Decarroz, C., Berger, M., & Cadet, J. (1990). "Photodynamic methods for oxy radical-induced dna-damage." *Method Enzymol.*, 186, 502-511.

Wang, Y. S. (2008). "Bulky DNA lesions induced by reactive oxygen species." *Chem. Res. Toxicol.*, 21(2), 276-281.

Wetmore, S. D., Boyd, R. J., & Eriksson, L. A. (2000). "Electron affinities and ionization potentials of nucleotide bases." *Chem. Phys. Lett.*, 322(1-2), 129-135.

Wetmore, S. D., Eriksson, L. A. & Boyd, R. J., (2001). A Multi-Component Model for Radiation Damage to DNA from its Constituents in Theoretical Biochemistry Processes and Properties of Biological Systems, In: *Theoretical and Computational Chemistry*, Eriksson, L. A., 409-466, Elsevier, Amsterdam.

Wetmore, S. D., Himo, F., Boyd, R. J., & Eriksson, L. A. (1998). "Effects of ionizing radiation on crystalline cytosine monohydrate." *J. Phys. Chem. B*, 102(38), 7484-7491.

Yang, C. G., Yi, C. Q., Duguid, E. M., Sullivan, C. T., Jian, X., Rice, P. A., & He, C. (2008). "Crystal structures of DNA/RNA repair enzymes AlkB and ABH2 bound to dsDNA." *Nature*, 452(7190), 961-U4.

Yang, X., Wang, X. B., Vorpagel, E. R., & Wang, L. S. (2004). "Direct experimental observation of the low ionization potentials of guanine in free oligonucleotides by using photoelectron spectroscopy." *Proc. Natl. Acad. Sci. U. S. A.*, 101(51), 17588-17592.

Yao, L. S., Li, Y., Wu, Y., Liu, A. Z., & Yan, H. G. (2005). "Product release is rate-limiting in the activation of the prodrug 5-fluorocytosine by yeast cytosine deaminase." *Biochemistry*, 44(15), 5940-5947.

Yu, B., Edstrom, W. C., Benach, J., Hamuro, Y., Weber, P. C., Gibney, B. R., & Hunt, J. F. (2006). "Crystal structures of catalytic complexes of the oxidative DNA/RNA repair enzyme AlkB." *Nature*, 439(7078), 879-884.

Permissions

All chapters in this book were first published in STDNAR, by InTech Open; hereby published with permission under the Creative Commons Attribution License or equivalent. Every chapter published in this book has been scrutinized by our experts. Their significance has been extensively debated. The topics covered herein carry significant findings which will fuel the growth of the discipline. They may even be implemented as practical applications or may be referred to as a beginning point for another development.

The contributors of this book come from diverse backgrounds, making this book a truly international effort. This book will bring forth new frontiers with its revolutionizing research information and detailed analysis of the nascent developments around the world.

We would like to thank all the contributing authors for lending their expertise to make the book truly unique. They have played a crucial role in the development of this book. Without their invaluable contributions this book wouldn't have been possible. They have made vital efforts to compile up to date information on the varied aspects of this subject to make this book a valuable addition to the collection of many professionals and students.

This book was conceptualized with the vision of imparting up-to-date information and advanced data in this field. To ensure the same, a matchless editorial board was set up. Every individual on the board went through rigorous rounds of assessment to prove their worth. After which they invested a large part of their time researching and compiling the most relevant data for our readers.

The editorial board has been involved in producing this book since its inception. They have spent rigorous hours researching and exploring the diverse topics which have resulted in the successful publishing of this book. They have passed on their knowledge of decades through this book. To expedite this challenging task, the publisher supported the team at every step. A small team of assistant editors was also appointed to further simplify the editing procedure and attain best results for the readers.

Apart from the editorial board, the designing team has also invested a significant amount of their time in understanding the subject and creating the most relevant covers. They scrutinized every image to scout for the most suitable representation of the subject and create an appropriate cover for the book.

The publishing team has been an ardent support to the editorial, designing and production team. Their endless efforts to recruit the best for this project, has resulted in the accomplishment of this book. They are a veteran in the field of academics and their pool of knowledge is as vast as their experience in printing. Their expertise and guidance has proved useful at every step. Their uncompromising quality standards have made this book an exceptional effort. Their encouragement from time to time has been an inspiration for everyone.

The publisher and the editorial board hope that this book will prove to be a valuable piece of knowledge for researchers, students, practitioners and scholars across the globe.

List of Contributors

Yi-Shan Tsai
Center of Excellence for Environmental Medicine, Kaohsiung Medical University, Kaohsiung

Jau-Ling Huang
Department of Bioscience Technology, Chang Jung Christian University, Tainan

Chang-Shen Lin
Graduate Institute of Medicine, Kaohsiung Medical University, Kaohsiung Taiwan

Jelena Markovic, Nancy Mora, Amparo Gimeno, Consuelo Burguete, José Luis García-Gimenez and Federico V. Pallardó
University of Valencia School of Medicine, Spain

Laurence A. Marchat
Escuela Nacional de Medicina y Homeopatía-IPN, Programa Institucional de Biomedicina Molecular
Programa de Doctorado en Biotecnología en Red-IPN

Mavil López-Casamichana, Esther Orozco and César López-Camarillo
Universidad Autónoma de la Ciudad de México, Posgrado en Ciencias Genómicas México

Kiyotsugu Yoshida
Medical Research Institute, Tokyo Medical and Dental University, Tokyo, Japan

Mirta Milić, Ružica Rozgaj and Vilena Kašuba
Institute for Medical Research and Occupational Health, Mutagenesis Unit, Zagreb, Croatia

Ana Marija Jazbec
Faculty of Forestry, University of Zagreb, Zagreb, Croatia

Patrizia Hrelia and Sabrina Angelini
Department of Pharmacology, University of Bologna, Bologna, Italy

Svetlana Khodyreva and Olga Lavrik
Institute of Chemical Biology and Fundamental Medicine, Siberian Branch of the Russian Academy of Sciences, Russia

Marie-Eve Dextraze and Darel J. Hunting
Department of Nuclear Medicine & Radiobiology, Faculté de medicine, Université de Sherbrooke, Sherbrooke, Québec, Canada

Tsvetan G. Gantchev
Department of Nuclear Medicine & Radiobiology, Faculté de medicine, Université de Sherbrooke, Sherbrooke, Québec, Canada
Department of Gene Regulations, Institute of Molecular Biology, Bulgarian Academy of Sciences, Sofia, Bulgaria

Alice A. Ramos and Cristina Pereira-Wilson
CBMA - Molecular and Environmental Biology Centre

Cristóvão F. Lima
CITAB - Centre for the Research and Technology of Agro-Environmental and Biological Sciences Department of Biology, School of Sciences, University of Minho, Campus de Gualtar, Braga, Portugal

Marie Dutreix
Institut Curie, Centre National de Recherche Scientifique (CNRS) UMR3347, Institut National de la Santé et de Recherche Médicale (INSERM) U1021, Université Paris-Sud 11, Centre Universitaire, 91405 Orsay

Jorge Llano
Grant MacEwan University, Department of Physical Sciences, Edmonton, Alberta, Canada

Maria Quanz and Amélie Croset
Institut Curie, Centre National de Recherche Scientifique (CNRS) UMR3347, Institut National de la Santé et de Recherche Médicale (INSERM) U1021, Université Paris-Sud 11, Centre Universitaire, 91405 Orsay
DNA Therapeutics SA, 91058 Evry France

Eric A. C. Bushnell and James W. Gauld
University of Windsor, Department of Chemistry and Biochemistry, Windsor, Ontario, Canada

Leif A. Eriksson
School of Chemistry, National University of Ireland, Galway, Ireland

Index

A

Aliquots, 7, 9, 107

Anticancer Drugs, 1-2, 4, 6-8, 10-14, 16, 66-67, 100

Antiparasitic drugs, 41, 54-55, 216

Apoptosis, 1-3, 19-21, 24-25, 34-35, 40, 60-71, 98-100, 147-155, 164-167, 174-181, 184-185, 188-191, 194-195, 200-205, 210-215, 217

Areca nut extracts, 10-13

Arecoline, 4-9, 16-18

Ataxia telangiectasia mutated, 2-3, 16-17, 62-63, 182-183, 204-205, 210-211

B

Biosynthesis, 20-23, 38-39, 166-167

C

Carcinogenesis, 14-15, 18-19, 40-41, 61, 74-75, 90-99, 142-143, 152-153, 162-171, 174-180, 204-205, 216, 238-239

Carcinogenicity, 1, 4-5, 16-17, 100, 174-175

Centrosome duplication, 2-3, 14-15

Chemotherapy, 2-7, 12-18, 24-25, 76-77, 124-125, 166-169, 174-175, 181, 208-209

Cisplatin resistance, 2-5, 14-15

D

Deoxyribonucleotides, 22-23, 132-133

Dithiothreitol, 22-25

Dual-luciferase assay, 6-7, 10-11

E

Electrophoresis, 10-11, 74-75, 78-81, 86-87, 90-95, 98-99, 104-105, 110-111, 116-117, 130-131, 142-143, 147, 154-157, 170-173, 176-177

Electrophoretic mobility, 104-107, 112-113, 116-117, 130-131

Enzymatic activity, 20-21, 102-103, 108-109, 118-121

Ethylenediaminetetraacetic acid, 74-75, 78-79

F

Fluorochrome, 32-33

G

Gene polymorphisms, 76-77, 86-89, 94-95

Genome integrity, 1-3, 12-13, 54-55, 72, 100-101, 148-149

Genomic instability, 1, 14-15, 94-95, 100

Genotoxic stress, 40-41, 61-67, 216

Global genome repair, 41, 184-185, 216

Glutathione, 19-40, 61, 96-97, 158-163, 174-175, 180

H

Head and neck squamous cell carcinoma, 2-3, 14-18

Helix-loop-helix proteins, 26-27, 38-39

Hepatocyte, 26-27, 38-39

Heteroduplex, 52-53, 132-133

Homologous recombination, 1-3, 10-17, 41, 44-45, 48-49, 54-59, 73, 100, 112-113, 127, 146, 150-153, 182-185, 206-207, 214-216

Host Cell Reactivation, 1-4, 6-10, 12, 14, 16, 100

Human malignancies, 4-5, 12-13

Hydroxyurea, 114-115, 124-125, 186-187, 204-205

I

Ionising radiation, 28-29, 73-77, 84-91, 94-99, 146

Ionizing radiation, 1, 18, 24-25, 41, 60, 62-63, 66-67, 72-74, 76, 78, 80, 82, 84, 86, 88, 90-103, 106-107, 114-115, 120-121, 124-133, 136-137, 144-146, 181, 216-219, 228-229, 240-241

K

Kinase activity, 62-63, 126, 184-185, 196-197

L

Luciferase activity, 6-13

Lymphocytes, 1, 22-23, 40, 61, 78-79, 86-100, 154-155, 158-179, 198-199, 212-213

M

Malabsorption syndrome, 42-43

Malignancies, 2-5, 12-13, 18, 174-175

Mammalian genome, 6-27, 204-205

Meiotic recombination machinery, 43
Mouse embryonic fibroblast, 112-113
Mutagenesis, 16-17, 34-35, 40, 48-49, 60-61, 73, 90-99, 122-123, 142-143, 146, 148-149, 154-155, 170-175, 178-179, 204-209, 212-213, 217, 238-239

N
Neutral denaturation, 74-75
Nuclear matrix, 26-29, 34-35, 156-157
Nucleophilic attack, 72, 101, 228-229
Nucleoprotein filament, 52-53, 186-187

O
Oligonucleotide, 104-107, 110-111, 116-119, 132-133, 184-185, 208-209
Oxidative damage, 19-21, 24-25, 34-35, 38-39, 44-45, 73, 86-87, 122-123, 146, 148-149, 156-157, 160-165, 170-171, 174-177, 180, 204-205
Oxidative stimuli, 19, 180
Oxidative stress, 19-25, 30-39, 62-67, 70-71, 148-149, 160-161, 168-171, 174-177, 180, 196-197, 208-209
Oxidized pyrimidines, 112-113, 147, 156-157

P
Peptide nucleic acids, 132-133, 142-145
Phosphatidylinositol, 40, 61, 206-207, 214-215
Phosphoesterase motifs, 52-53
Plasmodium falciparum, 42-43, 54-59
Posttranslational modification, 22-23, 28-29, 62-63, 188-189, 200-201
Prognostic marker, 4-5
Prokaryotic cells, 20-21, 32-33
Proliferation, 19-33, 36-37, 62-63, 66-67, 147-149, 154-155, 176-180

R
RAD51 recombinase, 52-53, 186-187
Radiosensitizers, 73, 132-133, 146
Radiotherapy, 2-7, 12-13, 76-79, 90-93, 96-97, 127, 144-145, 181, 202-203, 212-213
Redox buffer, 20-21, 28-29
Redox state, 19-21, 28-29, 34-39, 180
Renilla luciferase gene, 8-13
Ribonucleotide reductase, 22-23, 38-40, 61

S
Schiff base formation, 102-105, 110-111
Somatic, 2-3, 147, 208-209
Sporadic, 2-3, 152-153
Synergistic effect, 4-5, 154-155

T
Telomerase regulation, 22-25
Telomere length, 22-25, 34-37
Thioredoxin, 22-23, 32-33, 38-39
Transcription-coupled repair, 41, 176-177, 184-185, 216
Tumorigenesis, 2-3, 6-7, 12-13, 16-17, 38-39, 168-169

U
Ubiquitin proteasome-mediated pathway, 62-65

V
Venous blood, 78-79

X
Xeroderma pigmentosum, 2-3, 13, 15, 49, 79, 150 182, 206, 214

www.ingramcontent.com/pod-product-compliance
Lightning Source LLC
LaVergne TN
LVHW080637210926
848485LV00003B/278